Rebuilding after Disasters

Rebuilding after Disasters
From emergency to sustainability

Edited by Gonzalo Lizarralde, Cassidy Johnson and Colin Davidson

Preface by Hernando de Soto

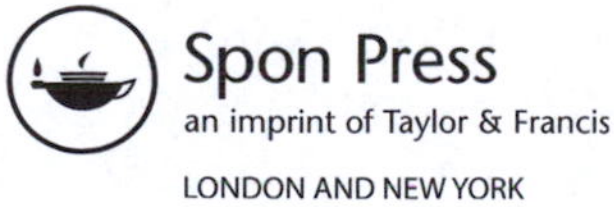

LONDON AND NEW YORK

First published 2010
by Spon Press
2 Park Square, Milton Park, Abingdon, Oxon OX14 4RN

Simultaneously published in the USA and Canada
by Spon Press
270 Madison Avenue, New York, NY 10016, USA

Spon Press is an imprint of the Taylor & Francis Group, an informa business

Typeset in Sabon by
Pindar NZ, Auckland, New Zealand
Printed and bound in Great Britain by
CPI Antony Rowe, Chippenham, Wiltshire

British Library Cataloguing in Publication Data
A catalogue record for this book is available from the British Library

Library of Congress Cataloging-in-Publication Data
Rebuilding after disasters : from emergency to sustainability / edited by Gonzalo Lizarralde, Cassidy Johnson, and Colin Davidson.
p. cm.
Includes bibliographical references and index.
1. Emergency housing. 2. Emergency management. 3. Disaster victims—Care. 4. Humanitarian assistance. 5. Sustainable development. 6. Building—Superintendence. I. Lizarralde, Gonzalo, 1974- II. Johnson, Cassidy, 1975- III. Davidson, Colin H.
HV554.5.R42 2010
363.34'83—dc22 2009006691

ISBN13: 978-0-415-47254-8 (hbk)
ISBN13: 978-0-203-89257-2 (ebk)

ISBN10: 0-415-47254-7 (hbk)
ISBN10: 0-203-89257-7 (ebk)

Contents

Preface

Hernando de Soto

For most of us, the massive poverty that exists in the developing world is a distant statistic – until an earthquake, a hurricane, or some other kind of 'natural disaster' strikes a poor region of the globe, and the media brings the images of poverty and suffering into our living rooms. Genuinely moved, we reach for our checkbooks and then return to our relatively comfortable lives, until Nature strikes back again. What impressed me most about this book – a myth-busting effort that brings together diverse opinions on how to reconstruct such devastated settlements – is that the authors have moved beyond the obvious charitable solutions to make the case that natural disasters are often so deadly and long-term due to very human mistakes in construction, exacerbated by socio-economic inequities.

The authors make it clear that their book is not built on theoretical discussions about an ideal world but based on 'empirical research and experience from "the field."' As such, *Rebuilding after Disasters* has positioned itself as a necessary handbook for international organizations, governments, NGOs, and anyone else serious about helping the billions of people around the world for whom just one natural disaster turns into a human catastrophe from which they will never recover.

As I read sections of this book, I found myself often nodding in recognition as well as agreement based on my own 25 years of experience in the shantytowns of the developing and post-communist world. The authors set out to challenge several 'myths' about reconstruction efforts after a disaster, and what resonated most for me was the clarity of their case that even before any natural disaster strikes, there are already a series of man-made problems in place that are likely to make the disaster worse and reconstruction harder. The authors also forcefully argue that the 'sustainability' of reconstruction strategies must include social and economic responsibility. I could not agree more. As a professional myth-breaker, let me contribute to their impressive brief for helping victims of disaster some of what I have learned about life – and suffering – among my fellow inhabitants of the developing world.

When asked about strategies to confront natural disasters in developing countries, I am inclined to point to two recent natural disasters that grabbed our hearts – the hurricane called Katrina that flooded the city of New Orleans in 2005 and the tsunami that ravaged 11 countries on the shores of the Indian Ocean just eight months before. The media images from both regions were tragically similar: demolished buildings, floating corpses, stunned survivors, and water, water everywhere. There was, however, one decisive difference: in New Orleans, to guarantee quick and efficient reconstruction, authorities salvaged the city's legal property records that would quickly determine who owned what and where, who owed what and how much, who could be relocated quickly, who was creditworthy to finance reconstruction, whose property was so damaged that they needed help, and how to give energy and clean water to the poor.

In the Asian countries ravaged by the tsunami, there were no such records, because most of the victims lived and worked outside the law. In Banda Aceh, Indonesia, 200,000 homes were washed away, most of them built without property titles. When the water receded from Nam Khem, Thailand, a well-connected tycoon rushed in to grab the valuable beachfront. The survivors of the 50 families that had occupied the shore for a decade protested, but they did not have legally documented property rights to back up their claims.

Building houses and tracing roads and parks at the margins of the law and without a registered property title not only delays and thwarts the reconstruction of a region devastated by a natural disaster, it also adds to the level of vulnerability of the population who have no alternative but to live in buildings that are constructed with little attention to existing safety codes. In 2006, an earthquake rocked Pakistan, leaving an estimated 73,000 people dead. When a similar-sized quake hit the Los Angeles area in 1994, 60 people died. The difference? As seismologists like to say, 'Earthquakes don't kill people, houses do.' It is inadequately constructed housing, that is, built outside the law, ignoring construction codes, that kills people.

In the developing world, natural disasters not only turn cities into rubble, they lay waste to entire economies. That is why I have long argued that a system of widespread legal property rights is a *sine qua non* in the fight against poverty – and a vital factor for any rational strategy for decreasing the devastation and death from a natural disaster and reconstruction. What poor homeowner – never mind developer, bank, credit bureau, or government agency – has any incentive to invest in safer housing and reinforced concrete without evidence of secure, legal ownership and the possibility of getting credit? Also, when property is clearly established, the concept of community participation acquires a whole new meaning. If the members of a locality are aware of who owns what, solidarity and collaboration will replace the tensions and confrontations that multiply in the midst of devastation. No one will dispute a property, and everyone will be advocates of reconstruction.

A stable legal property system also helps determine the collaborative relations between individuals and the community, between individuals and NGOs, between the community and local, regional, and national government. And for anyone committed to the 'sustainability' of reconstruction reforms – as the authors of this book clearly are – reforming the legal system so that it protects and empowers the poor majority is essential. As devastating as they always will be, neither hurricanes nor tsunamis can destroy the hidden infrastructure of the rule of law. When Nature challenges man's ingenuity, one tool that everyone, including the poorest of the poor, should be able to reach for is legal property, essential for the creation of harmonious towns and communities capable of standing up to the forces of nature – and rebuilding afterwards, quickly, efficiently, and fairly.

Hernando de Soto
President of the Instituto Libertad y Democracia

1 Rebuilding after disasters

From emergency to sustainability

Gonzalo Lizarralde, Cassidy Johnson and Colin Davidson

There are various misconceptions in both the theory and the practice of reconstruction after disasters. First, natural disasters are not really natural (in the sense that they are not exclusively the result of natural phenomena; they are the result of the fragile relations between the natural and built environments). Second, contrary to common belief, evidence shows that effective rebuilding does not necessarily depend on the speed of construction, and it does not always benefit from the usual separation into three different phases: emergency housing, temporary housing and permanent reconstruction. Even more surprising, this evidence shows that the most important contribution of architects and other specialists does not come from where it is commonly believed to (design and construction) but instead from a proper understanding of the roles and capacities of the multiple actors involved.

From emergency …

> In the earthquake I was with my wife, Rubiela, in the town, and we were surprised to see the houses falling down. … we almost had to walk back to the farm as there was no transportation. When we arrived, I felt happy to know that my family was alive, but at the same time very sad to see the house totally destroyed … We thought we could not rebuild our house again because we didn't have any resources …
>
> Oscar Bermudez, citizen and farmer of Calarcá, Colombia, when asked about his experience in the earthquake.[4]

The experience lived through by Oscar Bermudez is repetitively shared by millions of people worldwide. Sadly, it is probable that – in the next few years – there will be another disaster in the Andean region of Latin America, on the Pacific coast of Central America, in Europe, in southern Asia, in Central Africa and in many other regions of the world. The majority of the most devastating of these disasters will occur in cities of the developing world. Houses, infrastructure and public facilities will probably have to be rebuilt quickly and in a situation of emergency. Certainly they will have to be built amid a period of stress and disorder and with limited resources. Hopefully they will be built in a way that provides sustainable environments with improved conditions for this generation and for those of the future.

This is a major challenge for the professionals of the building industry, particularly in developing countries. This book deals primarily with the actions required after the disaster has occurred, but it is based on an understanding of the complex relations between post-disaster interventions and pre-disaster mitigation and prevention. We emphasize the role of the built environment (particularly the provision of housing) in the rebuilding of lives and sustainable livelihoods after disasters. The contributions in this book concentrate on the principal challenges facing the professionals and practitioners of the building industry, but they also highlight the relationships between the building industry and other areas of intervention, including humanitarian aid, medical assistance and economic reconstruction. The contributions bring into focus the complex and dynamic relations between societies, space and urban development.

The arguments in this book are based on empirical research and experience "from the field." This book is not built upon theoretical discussions and guidelines of how things *should be* in an ideal world (i.e. how people *should* participate, how governments *should* react, how professionals *should* perform, etc.) but rather upon how things *are actually done* and *how doing them can be improved* within the real constraints and challenges that are common both to the building industry and the humanitarian/development sector. The contributors to this book recognize the links with other areas of intervention, but they respond with straight answers to questions that frequently arise among the professionals of the building sector, such as: How can we, as professionals, react to a disaster situation? How can we improve post-disaster reconstruction? What are the roles of architects, engineers and development practitioners after disasters? What are the roles of government actors and non-governmental organizations (NGOs)? What is the role of local communities and how can it be respected?

In order to answer these questions, it is very important to distinguish common misconceptions or myths from factual realities of reconstruction. This book challenges, among other subjects, the following myths:

- the fact that disasters are natural (though they do follow natural events);
- the common belief that effective rebuilding depends on the speed of construction;
- the notion that housing reconstruction should be separated into three separate types – emergency, temporary and permanent;
- the idea that there are two dominating paradigms – bottom-up and top-down;
- the belief that community participation holds the key to successful reconstruction;
- the preconception that prefabrication and industrialization should be avoided;

- the idea that centralized decision making is the key to effective housing provision.

The field of reconstruction – both theory and practice – is filled with concepts that together amount to evolving paradigms; they sometimes help to clarify the real problems and assist the search for systemic plans of action, and sometimes their effect is exactly the opposite.

Reconstruction after "not-really-natural" disasters

It is commonly accepted by international organizations that a disaster is "a serious disruption of the functioning of a community or a society involving widespread human, material, economic or environmental losses and impacts, which exceeds the ability of the affected community or society to cope using its own resources."[36] Even though there is little controversy about this definition, it does not sufficiently explain why disasters happen. In other words, why is there a limit of destruction beyond which societies cannot cope with their own resources? To explain this limitation and explain the causes of disasters, geographers, anthropologists and other specialists in social sciences have developed the concept of vulnerability.[3,10,23] They examine the various physical, social, economic and environmental factors that lead a community to a certain level of "weakness" such that a hazard leads to a level of destruction from which the community cannot recover without external intervention.

The United Nations International Strategy for Disaster Reduction defines vulnerability as the "the characteristics and circumstances of a community, system or asset that make it susceptible to the damaging effects of a hazard."[36] The concepts and definitions of vulnerability are still evolving. One well-regarded vulnerability model, the "pressure and release model" developed by Ben Wisner, Piers Blaikie, Terry Cannon and Ian Davis, describes how vulnerabilities correspond to unsafe conditions originating from existing dynamic pressures (caused by social, political, economic and cultural factors in the system).[3] Very often, these dynamic pressures originate in political, economic or social circumstances, which are called "root causes." According to this approach, when unsafe conditions meet with a natural hazard (earthquake, floods, landslides, etc.), a disaster occurs. Figure 1.1 shows – as a way of exemplifying this argument – the vulnerability model applied to the 1999 earthquake in Turkey.

This understanding of vulnerability is useful for identifying the macro-scale causes of disasters through the accumulation over time of unsafe conditions (Lee Bosher further discusses this issue in Chapter 12). However, models of vulnerability indicate very little about what type of actions are required to overcome the disaster once the natural event coincides with the accumulated vulnerability. In this book, we look at the concept of vulnerability from the perspective of post-disaster recovery. Vulnerability can be understood as a

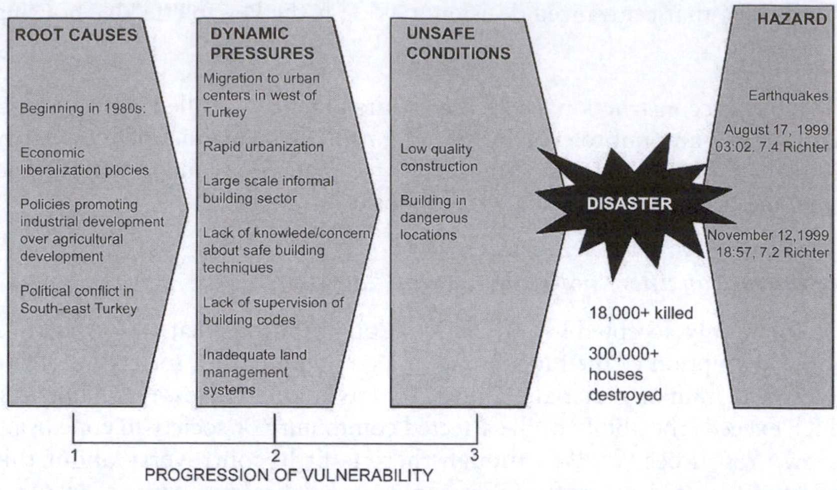

Figure 1.1 The disaster "pressure and release" vulnerability model (proposed by Wisner, Blaikie, Cannon and Davis[3]) adapted – by way of example – to the Turkish disaster in 1999. Economic liberalization and political turmoil prompted rapid migration to cities and thus uncontrolled urbanization in which there was little control over respect for the building codes. This favored shortcuts in construction techniques, which increased the vulnerability of inhabitants to earthquakes. The result: more than 18,000 people killed and more than 300,000 houses destroyed.

lack of access to resources (either material, such as finance, housing, roads, infrastructure, public services, etc., or organizational, such as insurance and the individuals' decision-making capacity, education, information, etc.). Thus inherently unsafe conditions and dynamic pressures in the social and physical environments also correspond to inappropriate or insufficient access to the resources that permit a community to deal with the effects of hazards.

Approaching reconstruction in this way not only builds upon the concepts and ideas elaborated by previous research but also permits taking a step forward in identifying what the role of reconstruction is after a natural hazard.[3,10] It is very often believed that reconstruction is "[the group of] actions taken to re-establish a community after a period of rehabilitation subsequent to a disaster. Actions would include construction of permanent housing, full restoration of services, and complete resumption of the pre-disaster state."[34] This concept has frequently been accompanied by the idea that the reduction of the vulnerabilities and sustainable reconstruction are *only* achieved through the reinforcement of local strengths. "The key to success ultimately lies in the participation of the local community – the survivors – in reconstruction" argued the United Nations Disaster Relief Organization (UNDRO) in a paramount publication in this field published in 1982.[35]

It is usually recognized that there are two types of resources that determine the "level of development" a community has: (i) "hard" resources (this describes tangible and physical resources such as housing, infrastructure, public services, etc.) and (ii) "soft" resources (this describes non-tangible or non-physical resources such as employment, education, information, etc.). However, if one considers that vulnerability is the lack of access to resources, and that the disaster reduces that access to resources even more (since banks, offices, housing and commerce will have been destroyed), one begins to understand what the process of reconstruction is for: improving people's access to resources that have been lost and developing access to the basic resources that people probably did not even have before the disaster. Only through the improvement of these two levels of resources will risk be reduced and the community be prepared to face the next natural hazard. Fulfilling this condition is a requirement to facilitate the long-term sustainability of the reconstruction and all the associated interventions.

Consequently, post-disaster reconstruction is defined as the *process* of improvement of pre-disaster conditions, targeted to achieving long-term local development and disaster risk reduction through the pairing of local and external resources, thus giving residents increased access to both "hard" and "soft" resources. This definition is represented by Figure 1.2, which illustrates in a vertical scale the level of access to resources (that is to say, the reciprocal of the level of vulnerability) and has a horizontal scale of time. The level of access to resources is affected by the hazard (earthquake, flood, storm, etc.). If the hazard is strong enough and the pre-disaster access to resources of the population is low, the community cannot cope with the losses and damages exclusively with its own resources. This particular case, where external aid is required, is called a disaster. The process of recovery (represented by the

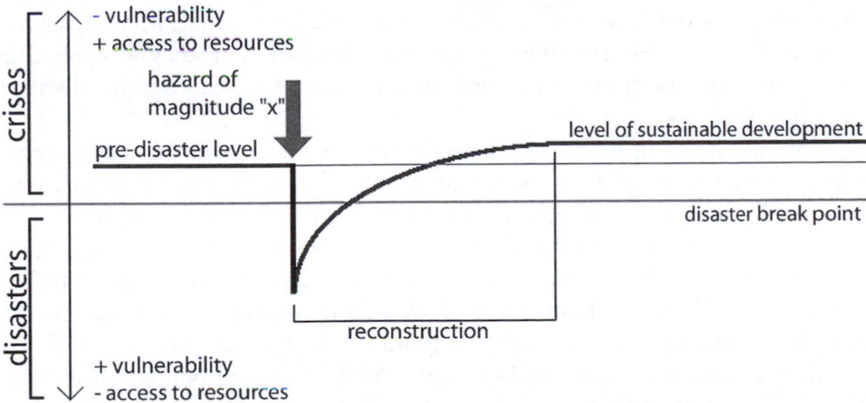

Figure 1.2 Model illustrating the concepts of vulnerability and post-disaster reconstruction.[17]

curve) corresponds to the reconstruction process, leading to an increase over the pre-disaster level of access to resources.

The notion that the success of a reconstruction project depends on the speed of the construction of houses

This notion is false for two reasons: (i) because it is not construction activities but the acquisition of land and the development of legal and administrative procedures that often delay housing reconstruction most, and (ii) because houses, alone, are rarely the first priority of affected populations.

Very often, images and testimonies of disaster survivors and newly homeless families in newspapers and on the television inspire well-intentioned architects, industrial designers and engineers to propose emergency shelters (often produced by industrialized methods) that seek technical efficiency for rapid mass production. However, evidence provided by empirical research in this field demonstrates that the principal delays in post-disaster rebuilding come from obtaining safe land for housing (at a reasonable price and in convenient locations) as well as from developing the legal and administrative procedures to obtain and transfer subsidies and loans. In reality, those two activities often require long procedures at various political and administrative levels.[17] For example, political lobbying and administrative and legal procedures delayed rural reconstruction in El Salvador for more than 10 months after the double earthquakes of 2001, and they delayed for more than 12 months the post-Mitch reconstruction of Choluteca in Honduras in 1998.[18]

Contrary to what most building professionals would like to believe, rebuilding housing is not necessarily the first priority of disaster-affected populations, and some forms of housing are simply not acceptable even in dire post-disaster conditions. The rural reconstruction project conducted in Colombia in 1999 showed that the construction of infrastructure and buildings for income generation had as much or more importance as the reconstruction of housing units per se. Chapter 2 shows that, in many cases, affected families preferred to invest the subsidies and loans they were eligible for in building sewage systems, small industries, access roads and production facilities, etc.

More evidence illustrates this argument. In fact, sufficient cases demonstrate that it should no longer be assumed that affected families will necessarily accept and occupy housing units that are provided to them after disasters (even if they are offered for free). Examples in Honduras, Nicaragua, El Salvador and other countries show that sometimes beneficiaries abandon the houses offered to them due to lack of infrastructure and services or simply because they do not really respond to their needs and local ways of living (see also more examples in Chapter 8). Research in Nueva Choluteca, Honduras, showed that many houses built by international NGOs after hurricane Mitch on a piece of land located a few kilometers away from the original town were abandoned.[18] This is not really surprising, considering that the unemployment rate in the new settlement was almost 50 per cent and the infrastructure was not finished for many years after the construction of the houses. However, it also shows that it was not the houses that really motivated the choices of residents but rather other variables (employment opportunities, closeness to relatives and friends, access to health services and schools) (Figure 1.3).

Restoring income generation, instead, is a common priority for affected residents. As explained in the following chapters, housing in developing countries (post-disaster or not) requires, in reality, an integrated approach to solving problems – a "systems approach" (see the Conclusion) – in which domestic solutions are combined with income-generation activities (Figure 1.4).

The notions that there are three types of housing and two dominating paradigms

Building affordable housing is a complex process that – even in regular circumstances – consumes great amounts of time and resources and requires complex logistics, administrative innovation and careful management (an argument that has been extensively studied by Keivani and Werna[15]). Unfortunately, this complexity is often underestimated. Touched by the dramatic images of devastation and homelessness, architects, designers and engineers constantly explore innovative forms of emergency shelter: light structures, foldable units, improved tents, etc. These are temporary solutions that aim at providing shelter while permanent rebuilding takes place. Research conducted by Cassidy Johnson (Chapter 4) has shown that these rapid constructions are used by decision-makers and politicians to show that actions are being taken and decisions are being made during the times of chaos after the disaster.[13] However, common practice has led to the belief that rebuilding must utilize three distinct types of housing: emergency shelters, temporary houses and permanent houses. While it is necessary that families have a place to call "home" and go about their daily activities during the period when permanent rebuilding is happening, it does not mean that different types of buildings are necessary for emergency, temporary and permanent housing phases.

According to Quarantelli,[27] *emergency sheltering* and *temporary sheltering* correspond to the immediate protection of the survivors against natural elements during the emergency and for the first few days after the disaster. This type of sheltering often includes tents, plastics, corrugated iron sheets, etc. provided to affected families by international agencies of disaster aid such as the Red Cross or by national bodies such as the army and the civil defense organization. These sheltering stages are – by their very essence – provisional, and the agencies that assume this responsibility do not usually build houses. Therefore, their intervention is limited in time; once the emergency assistance phase has been completed, the problem of housing is still present but permanent solutions often seem far away. A second temporary solution is thus used.

Aware of the effects of these delays in starting permanent housing

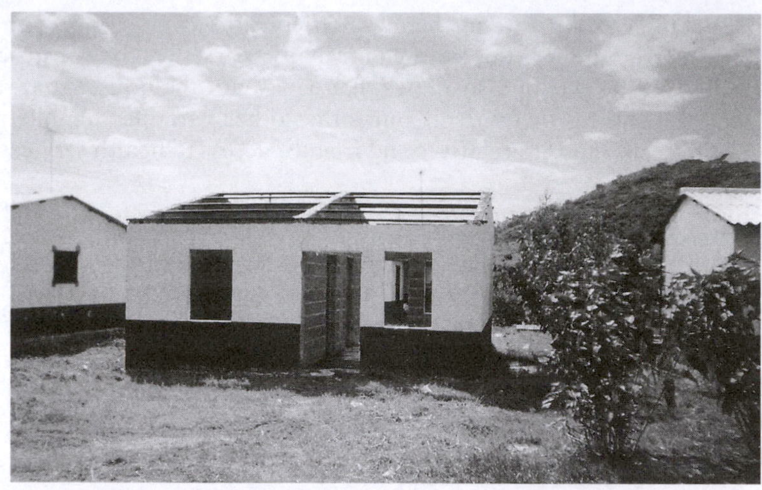

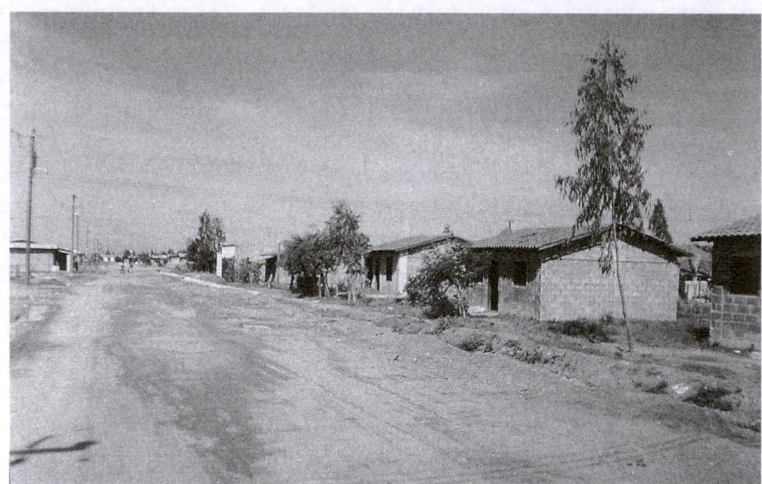

Figure 1.3 Post-disaster houses in Honduras. Houses that are ill-adapted to local needs and lifestyles represent a second disaster (sometimes as dangerous as the original one). **Top:** Beneficiaries dismantled the roof, doors and windows and abandoned this house built as part of a post-Mitch reconstruction initiative in Nueva Choluteca (Honduras). **Bottom:** Without proper infrastructure and with little sensitivity for lifestyles in hot weather, this housing settlement in Nueva Choluteca had a low economic recovery and led to increased criminality and major public-health problems.

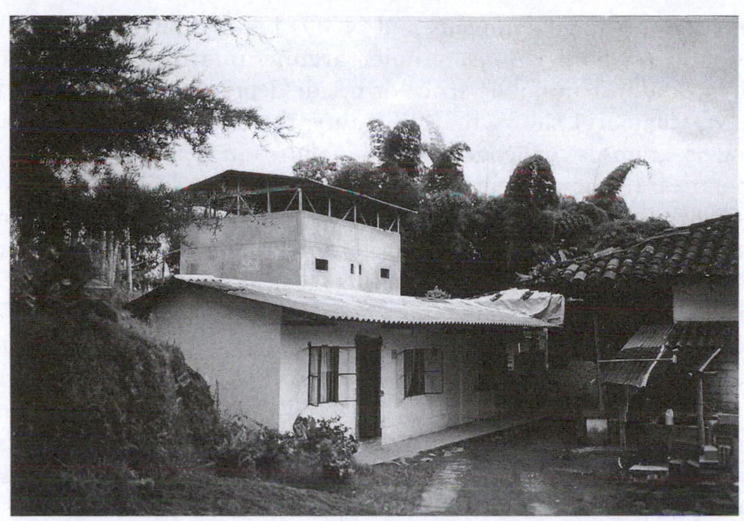

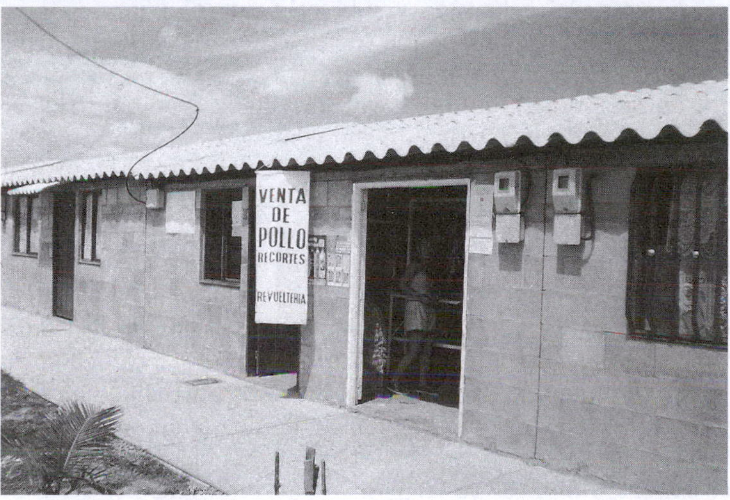

Figure 1.4 Post-disaster houses in Colombia. Domestic and income-generation activities often merge in low-cost housing in developing countries. **Top:** Having the option of deciding how to invest their own subsidies, beneficiaries of this rural reconstruction project in the coffee-growing area of Colombia decided to build infrastructure for coffee production (as in this picture), in this way boosting their economic recovery. **Bottom:** Thanks to proper public services, informal commerce quickly appeared in post-disaster urban residential projects in Colombia after the 1999 earthquake, demonstrating the crucial links between income generation and domestic activities (the sign reads "chicken for sale").

construction, many governments and NGOs become involved in the mass provision of *temporary housing* units, arguing that they can be installed on public land, urban public space or beside debris and affected buildings. However, Chapter 4 shows that, in reality, the effectiveness of temporary housing programs is challenged by two main realities particular to developing countries: (i) the mass-produced units (often largely prefabricated and industrialized) are disproportionably expensive compared to permanent housing solutions built with traditional materials; and (ii) in contexts of constant demand for affordable housing, temporary units tend to remain longer than expected and sometimes they even become permanent. These obstacles have been largely reported by Johnson, *et al.* in the reconstruction process of Turkey in 2001 and of Colombia in 1999[14] and have also occurred in many other locations, as reported by UNDRO.[35] During the seventies and eighties, this form of housing was often delivered by special contractors that sponsored innovative shelter solutions produced with high-tech industrialized methods. These shelters usually implied standardization and resulted in repetition of a "universal" unit that rarely responded to the specifics of climate, topography, local customs and local forms of living.

Most recent practices include the construction of shack-type temporary units made of timber and and/or corrugated iron sheets. Usually located in public or vacant land and built with perishable materials, this form of housing has primitive infrastructure and is made by organizations that are not permanent (regular) housing builders. Even worse, the providers of this form of housing rarely anticipate and plan for a natural transition to permanent housing. In the case of temporary housing built in the city of Armenia, Colombia, after the earthquake of 1999, large amounts of timber and corrugated sheets that were used to build the 6000-unit temporary camps was neither transferred to users nor used in any useful manner. Instead, it was stored, lost or trashed. In a remarkable example of lack of coordination between organizations and of political absurdities, a public university that was responsible for managing the publicly funded temporary camps found that a national law bans the delivery of goods that belong to the state to individual citizens without a special permission from Congress. Unfortunately, this included used wood, nails and corrugated iron sheets, even after they were no longer needed for temporary housing.[14]

Permanent housing is usually the last step, and this step is often conducted by regular organizations of the building industry (contractors, planners, etc.) that are often constrained by two preconditions: centralized provision and the use of a single technology. This responds to the fact that, after bidding processes where multiple companies compete for the contract, contractors and governments alike believe that they have found the "optimum" solution, which needs to be widely exploited and optimized. Furthermore, affordable housing produces slim profits per unit, and thus it is often considered that gains can only be obtained from economies of scale, where standardization and repetition are prioritized.[20]

Internationally accepted guidelines for reconstruction produced by UNDRO in 1982 tend to perpetuate this fragmentation into three modes of housing.[35]

In other cases, permanent housing is organized by agencies, contractors or NGOs that implement self-help and participatory programs. Readers could expect that these types of initiatives might allow for much more variety and multiplicity of technologies, materials, housing layouts, etc. Strangely, this is rarely the case. First, working with low-skilled labor (typical of self-help programs) implies that the housing types must be simplified as much as possible. This often results in the building of single-storey detached units, and it does not facilitate building alternatives that would probably be better for optimizing scarce and expensive land (such as mid-rise multi-family buildings or two-storey units). Second, for a strange reason, agencies tend to consider that a fair distribution of resources implies giving the same product to each beneficiary (instead of the more sensitive approach to fair distribution resulting from giving to each beneficiary what she/he really needs). Third, agencies resort to the repetition of a basic unit after realizing that training unskilled labor is difficult and therefore training in one single technique is simpler than training in a variety of operations (more arguments on this issue can be found in Chapter 9). Finally, designs usually lack the architectural imagination and creativity that are required for producing alternative uses of standardized materials and components.

Current research has found that most of these interventions are also characterized by two extreme approaches that have now become the two main paradigms of reconstruction: the bottom-up approach, placing exclusive emphasis on community participation, self-help and local solutions, or the top-down approach, claiming the advantages of easy-to-assemble prefabricated or industrialized techniques.

A great deal of optimism about technological developments and the application of industrialization to mass housing characterized post-disaster interventions during the seventies and eighties. This is not surprising, considering that it was precisely during the sixties and these two decades that the most important work on industrialized and prefabricated methods of construction was accomplished in Europe and North America. However, this optimism was quickly overtaken by the negative social, technical and cultural effects that those industrialized units caused in developing countries. In fact, opponents of high-tech prefabrication and industrialized solutions gathered considerable evidence of the multiple failures of standardized solutions in Turkey, Peru, Nicaragua and Africa. The peak of this opposition came when UNDRO claimed that reconstruction initiatives should avoid "designing, manufacturing and stockpiling prefabricated emergency shelter units (other than tents), as this solution is too costly and a waste of resources for developing countries."[35]

Following the frustration caused by this form of top-down approach, a general consensus has now emerged on the advantages of using local resources and different forms of self-help, encouraging local residents to participate in the rebuilding process. Trying to clarify forever the controversy around imported technologies, the report *Shelter after Disaster*[35] emphasized that post-disaster housing should be considered in the same way that John Turner perceived housing in general in developing countries in his book *Housing By People*.[32]

Housing By People claims that beneficiaries should be encouraged to work on their own solutions to the housing problem as it impacts on them, and that local materials and traditional technologies should be prioritized over imported technologies and foreign solutions. By now, the principle has been largely adopted by NGOs and decision-makers that repetitively emphasize the importance of community participation in post-disaster interventions. This does not mean that the optimism that accompanied high-tech solutions has completely vanished. Instead, various companies still promote ready-to-use housing units, such as the Italian "Armadillo" (a shell-shaped modular unit of steel), under the belief that they can greatly contribute to post-disaster rebuilding – if not in all developing countries, at least in some transition and developed economies.[11]

The concept that community participation holds the key for successful rebuilding

The problem surrounding community participation is that, as sound as the bottom-up approach might be, this principle is hardly put into practice and its implementation suffers from major obstacles. Chapter 9 shows that surprising behaviors on the part of the participants were found by the Canadian anthropologist Alicia Sliwinski while studying a self-help post-earthquake housing project in El Salvador. Contrary to common belief and official rhetoric, Dr Sliwinski found that the community participation scheme implemented in La Hermandad by different agencies of the Red Cross was far from being the "good neighbor" friendly environment that theory leads one to expect.[6] Instead, she found social tensions and hostile behaviors in the community, contradicting the previously held view (published in *Shelter after Disaster*[35]) that associated project performance directly with community participation.

Similarly, the comparison of four cases of reconstruction in Colombia, Honduras and El Salvador, conducted between 1999 and 2004 by Gonzalo Lizarralde, demonstrated that the performance of housing projects does not depend solely on the participation of the local community, but instead on the careful coordination of different participants (which is called the "organizational design" in Chapter 5). Success lies with the development of strategic planning and management – instead of tactical (i.e. project-focused) planning.[18] In reality, these studies showed that, very often, the participation of the community ends up being a mere involvement in construction activities, with little decision-making responsibility over design, planning, management and financing of the project being assumed by the participants.

Despite the fact that the term "community participation" has been largely used in ways that often do not really reflect the initial principle of responsible, democratic and fair involvement of users, it keeps on being the official rhetoric of NGOs involved in low-cost housing almost worldwide. However, recent research proves that "community participation" can also have side effects that are not necessarily positive for the city nor for the community itself. In fact, while keeping track of three low-cost housing projects in the townships (historically, the segregated slums) of Cape Town, South Africa, Lizarralde and Massyn found that communities can sometimes make short-term decisions that can have mid- and long-term negative results for the built environment at large and for the economic and social development of the community itself.[21] In one remarkable case, a local community that had achieved an appropriate level of autonomy and self-governance yielded a great deal of decision-making power to an external NGO in order to take advantage of additional funding for the project. The dynamics of the project quickly changed, and the community accepted a series of "suggested" solutions that now threaten its capacity to enhance its social integration with neighboring areas and also the possibility of economic development for a significant number of self-employed residents.

This argument does not imply by any means that community participation is not important or desirable (an argument that is amply developed in Chapter 9). Instead, it means that real decision-making power over design, planning, financing and management of the project for individual users (and through collective arrangements) must form part of that participation. More recently, this has developed into what is termed an "owner-driven approach" or a "user-driven approach" in which agencies provide housing finance and technical expertise and the rest is up to the owners to manage (see Chapter 8).

The idea that prefabrication should be avoided to give priority to traditional technologies

The design of imported industrialized units used in reconstruction projects during the seventies and eighties was often ill-adapted to local needs and expectations. Not only were the technologies difficult to adapt to accommodate specific local requirements (culture, climate, etc.), but also the materials and parts were not easily available to residents after the reconstruction projects were finished, should they wish to add more onto their houses. As has previously been shown, all of this has generated increased skepticism and lack of confidence in prefabrication for post-disaster housing (the recommended policy was to avoid "Designing, manufacturing and stockpiling prefabricated emergency shelter units"[35]). It is not surprising then that most NGOs acting after Hurricane Mitch in Central America or in the post-tsunami reconstruction in southern Asia relied on labor-intensive construction methods and rejected prefabricated technologies (in both these cases, builders were hired and local residents were engaged in self-help).

However, arguments in favor of a systematic rejection of prefabrication in developing countries do not stand up to a careful analysis of costs and benefits. In fact, recent studies show that the decentralized prefabrication of light components (contrary to the centralized heavy industrialization adopted in various projects during the seventies and eighties) already plays a fundamental role in low-cost housing in many developing countries.[7] This observation was also confirmed by Stallen, Cabannes and Steinberg[31] and by Kellett and Franco[16] in many countries such as Mexico, India, Colombia and the Philippines. This form of decentralized prefabrication of "light" components cannot be ignored, because it already accounts for an important part of the construction sector. A recent study of the informal construction sector conducted by Lizarralde and Root also confirms this fact.[19] The study concludes that decentralized prefabrication of light components already plays a major role in the informal construction of slums in South Africa (the post-apartheid suburban townships). Building professionals have much to learn from the way in which construction is carried out in informal settlements in poor countries – and in Chapter 2 Lizarralde argues that it is precisely the informal business sector that is the only one that has been capable of providing housing solutions for the bottom tier of poor (Figures 1.5, 1.6 and 1.7).

Not only have the technical aspects of prefabrication, emergency housing and the rhetoric of "community participation" diverted attention from the crucial issue of strategic planning and real user-based decision-making, they have also diverted attention from another crucial issue of housing reconstruction: financing and project management.

The concept of decentralization and its impact on financing and project management

During the late eighties and the nineties, post-disaster low-cost housing was influenced, like many other aspects of public involvement in developing countries, by the waves of decentralization and reduction of the public sector. According to this so-called neo-liberal approach, housing was better handled by local administrations than by central governments. It then became desirable to limit the influence and size of national agencies involved in housing and to transfer as much autonomy as possible to small municipalities to deal with housing delivery. This thesis maintained that the ideal role of central governments in housing was to "enable the markets to work," a strategy that simultaneously allowed the transfer of responsibility to the private sector while reducing the size of the public agencies and thus of the state.[39]

The principle may be sound; indeed, centralized and largely bureaucratic governments – even in developed nations – were not efficient housing builders, and local municipalities could more easily deal with local infrastructure, local patterns of land tenure and local modes of housing provision.[37] However, Ben Wisner and other researchers have found that, when double

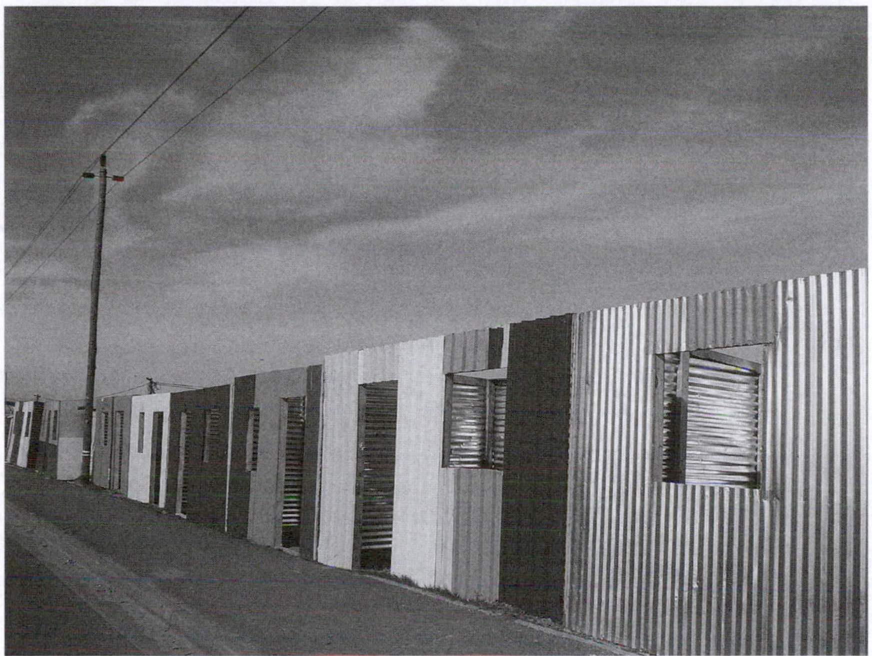

Figure 1.5 Prefabricated informal housing. Architects and urban planners interested in reconstruction have much to learn from the way in which the informal sector produces buildings for the poor. This informal sale of prefabricated shacks in the townships of South Africa delivers prefabricated housing solutions that can be customized and installed in 30 minutes. Using recycled materials and a simple technology, these solutions are well adapted to the needs of a sector of the population for which no architect has been able to produce a viable, large-scale solution.

earthquakes struck El Salvador in 2001 and Hurricane Mitch hit Honduras in 1998, the effects of decentralization and the reduction of governmental responsibility over housing had negative effects on the ability of any public body to effectively undertake post-disaster rebuilding.[39]

This is exactly what a study conducted by Lizarralde in Central America also revealed.[18] Just after the earthquakes of 2001, the municipality of San Salvador, the capital city of El Salvador, had the responsibility for rebuilding housing for thousands of families. Having assumed that responsibility, but being in constant tension with the right-wing party in office in the central government, the left-wing government of San Salvador started an ambitious plan of housing delivery. However, being such a poor city, the planning unit for human settlements of the municipality was composed of very few senior officers and a few enthusiastic but inexperienced junior planners; it was equipped with only a few computers and possessed a couple of old printers and plotters. Furthermore, the political tension between the two parties (which

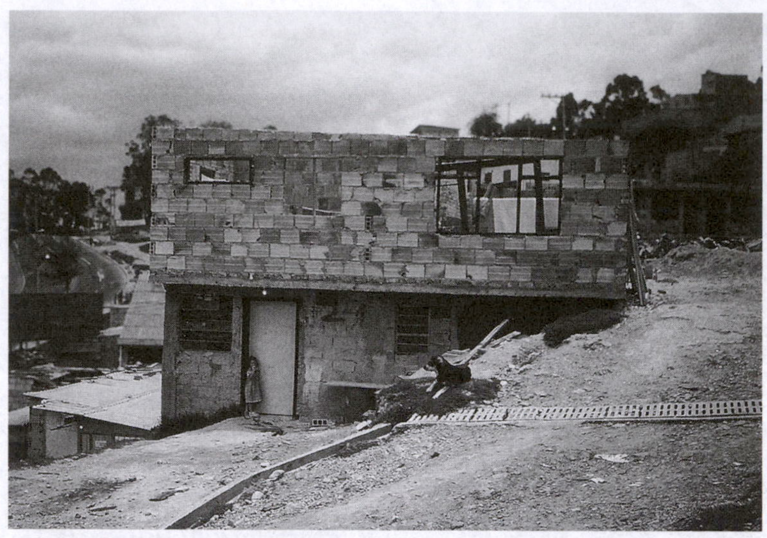

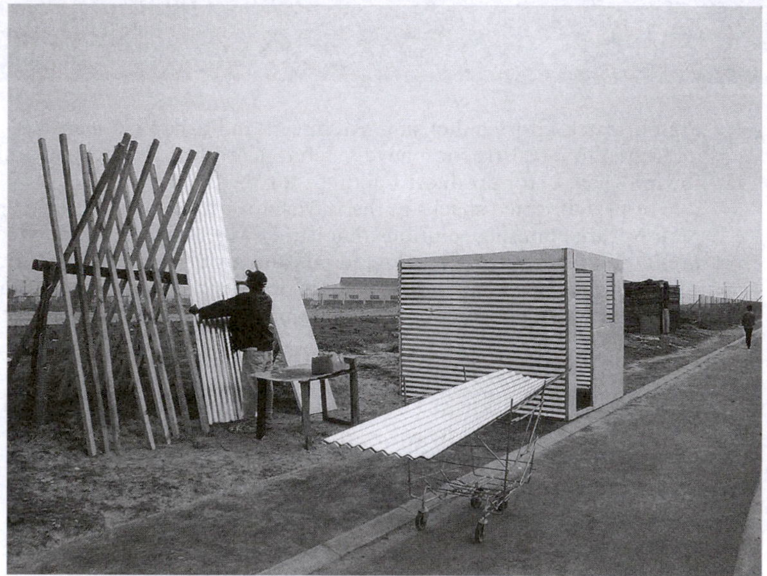

Figure 1.6 Informal housing. Architects interested in humanitarian and social causes must understand the progressive (and sometimes spontaneous) way in which cities are built. Thousands of small and medium-sized construction companies contribute every day to that process in a formal or an informal way. **Top:** An informal construction optimizing recycled materials (doors and windows) in Bogotá, Colombia. **Bottom:** A "sales point" of informal prefabricated shacks in the townships of Cape Town, South Africa.

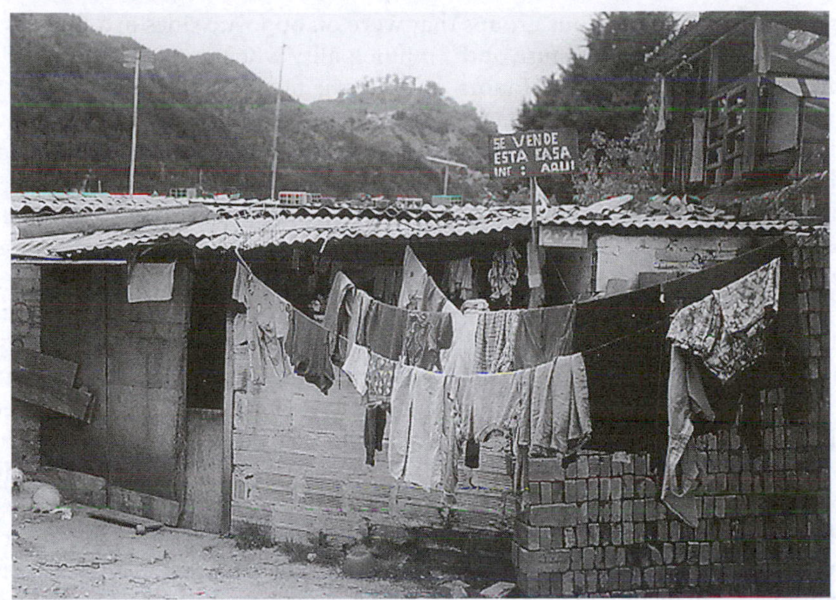

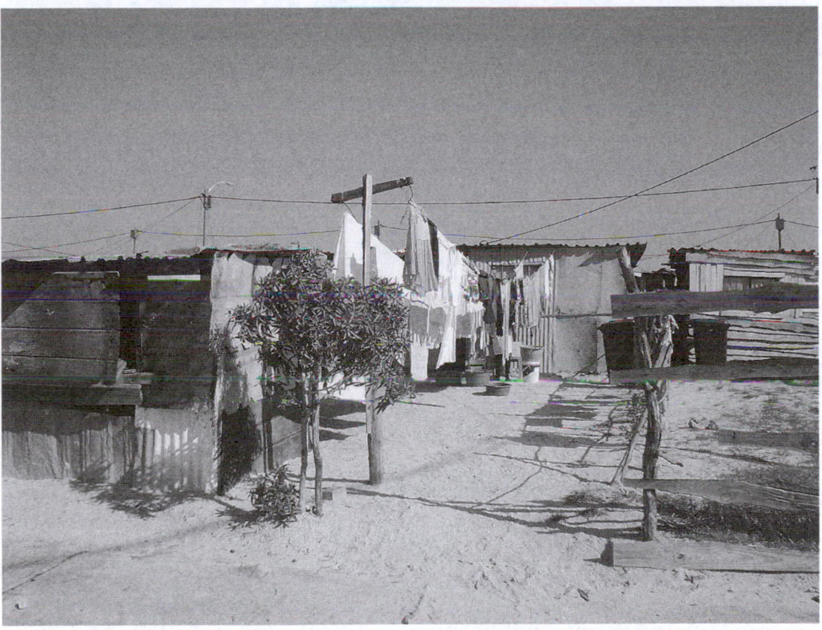

Figure 1.7 Houses-in-progress. Housing in developing countries is a process of construction based on the progressive improvement of both units and outdoor spaces. **Top:** A house-in-progress in the slums of Bogotá, Colombia (the sign reads "for sale"). **Bottom:** Another house-in-progress in Cape Town, South Africa.

evolved from two previous groups that were on opposite sides in a long civil war) did not benefit the cause of the municipality when it was trying to seek funding from international donors. Despite the fact that some international meetings for funding were organized, the lack of experience and know-how of the municipality resulted in a failure of fund-raising. The municipality was ultimately unable to attract international funding or loans and was forced to abandon – only a few months later – the principal housing project that had been developed for it by a committee of specialists and scholars, and, a short while later, the advisory committee itself was disbanded altogether.

The municipality of Choluteca was one of the poorest in Honduras before Hurricane Mitch flooded half of the town, leaving thousands of homeless and a significant loss of jobs. The disaster drew considerable international attention, and more than 13 NGOs gathered to produce what was soon called "Nueva Choluteca," a 2000-family settlement 15 kilometers away from the affected old city. The group of NGOs (the majority of them international) produced more houses than permanent jobs, infrastructure and services. Therefore, it is not surprising to find that four years later, an evaluation of the project conducted by Lizarralde showed that the settlement suffered from high unemployment and crime rates as well as increased problems of public health.[18] Unable to manage the settlement and provide adequate infrastructure, the municipality of Choluteca was found in 2004 to have little control over Nueva Choluteca. By then, all the NGOs had left the area, leaving behind a few churches and more than two thousand detached houses that were not well adapted to the extreme heat of the region. With very limited financial means, a reduced and ill-equipped staff and little know-how and expertise in urban management, the municipality was well aware of the problems of the settlement but unable to act upon them.

Unfortunately, a lack of financial, legal and administrative means is frequent in small municipalities in developing countries, and it affects their capacity to build not only the post-disaster housing that is required but also regular housing projects targeted to reducing disaster vulnerabilities and exposure to risk.[17] This does not mean that officers and decision-makers in towns and small cities are lazy or negligent; instead, it suggests that those officers and decision-makers (and their work) require adequate integration and coordination with national agencies and with the private sector. At least this is what seems to be demonstrated by an analysis of the 1262-unit housing project "Juan Pablo II" in Facatativá, Colombia. In this initiative, conducted in 2007 after the urgent need to reduce disaster risk in the city was identified, 103 families were successfully relocated from disaster-prone areas into a safe, compact and green neighborhood with easy access to jobs and the city center. In this model, an efficient partnership between the local and national government, private companies that administer social benefits and a residential developer was created. The partnership managed to successfully channel public subsidies and create the administrative means to use public funds and transform them into core houses, ultimately transferring them to an ongoing process of progressive construction managed by individual beneficiaries. Even though some mistakes were made in the urban and architectural designs, this strategy of partnership between local administrations and national agencies can be held up as an example for future municipality-based initiatives of disaster prevention in developing countries.

Misplaced attention

Evidence shows that existing approaches do not really tackle the main problems of reconstruction. Instead, attention has been misplaced onto aspects that guarantee neither better performance of post-disaster housing projects nor long-term development for the beneficiaries. For example, the emphasis on providing the three distinct types of housing (emergency shelter, temporary housing and permanent reconstruction) has resulted in redundancy, lack of coordination, fragmented distribution of aid and wasteful use of resources.

As another illustration of the misplaced approaches, the emphasis on industrialization and high-tech buildings unnecessarily led to supposedly universal and repetitive modules that were ill-adapted to the singularities of climate, culture, social habits and individual needs of the recipient communities. This launched a reaction in which it was argued that community participation was the key to the success of housing projects, an approach that – although important – also proved not necessarily to lead to the best overall project performance. In the meanwhile, financial and project-management concerns received little attention. The result has been a well-reported list of unsustainable rebuilding projects in El Salvador, Turkey, Nicaragua, Honduras, Peru, India, Sri Lanka, Colombia, Bangladesh, Iran, Ecuador, the United States and many other countries. It appears then that the main challenge for decision-makers is to integrate and balance the needs of the emergency with long-term requirements of sustainability.

From emergency ... to sustainability

> In the earthquake I was with my wife, Rubiela, in the town, and we were surprised to see the houses falling down. ... we almost had to walk back to the farm as there was no transportation. When we arrived, I felt happy to know that my family was alive, but at the same time very sad to see the house totally destroyed ... We thought we could not rebuild our house again because we didn't have any resources ...
>
> Thanks to God and the Coffee Growers' Committee we found the way to rebuild. With my brother who helped me, we provided the labour force; we worked really hard but it was worth it. It was a process of four months but now we have a better house than the one we had before ...
>
> The complete testimony of Oscar Bermudez, a quotation from which was partially transcribed in the beginning of this chapter.[4]

Evidence shows that not all the beneficiaries of reconstruction projects are as lucky as Oscar Bermudez. This is particularly because, rushed by the urgency of attending to immediate needs, reconstruction projects rarely develop into sustainable solutions in the long term. But the next question is: Which type of sustainability?

The term "sustainability" has been so widely used that it rarely means anything significant anymore. The objectives of sustainability (reduction of pollution or economic feasibility, for example) are very often described in parallel with design approaches to achieve them (increasing densities, for example) and with tools to operationalize them (community participation, for instance). As a result, the term is very often arbitrarily used in both regular construction and reconstruction to describe energy efficiency, pollution reduction, environmental protection, social involvement, green building, etc.

For the sake of clarity concerning ways to improve post-disaster rebuilding, it is crucial to discuss the issue of sustainability in terms of its three dimensions:

1 social responsibility;
2 economic responsibility;
3 environmental sustainability.

These three dimensions will take different forms, as described in the following section, where 14 objectives of sustainability and some tools and methods to achieve them are suggested. This approach is based on the definition of sustainable development proposed by Stephen Wheeler,[38] in which he condemns the difficulties caused by the more popular definition provided by the Brundtland commission, which stated that it is "development that meets the needs of the present without compromising the ability of future generations to meet their own needs." In order to avoid the debate about the needs of each generation, Wheeler proposes that sustainable development corresponds to "development that improves the long-term health of human and ecological systems."

First dimension: social responsibility

This dimension concerns the important relations between the built environment and the consolidation of social values. Seen in this way, the design professional (architect, designer, urban planner, etc.) has the responsibility of identifying his/her own role in the pursuit of solutions for social problems (particularly those related to social vulnerabilities). It is implicitly assumed that the designers must then develop the expertise required to respond to those problems, linking ethical, functional and esthetic considerations. This approach reflects the definition of the role of architecture as proposed by Ian Low: "The establishment of order, far more than the creation of form describes the labor of the architect; order(s) that seek to participate in and contribute to the work of democracy in a globalizing world."[22] In this regard, sustainable interventions in the built environment before and after the disaster are those that respond to the following objectives:

1 Social development. It includes developing the "social capital," as defined by Robert Putnam: "the meaningful human contacts of all kinds that characterize communities."[26]
2 The development of autonomy for social groups and individuals. This objective includes the reduction of dependency of marginalized and vulnerable groups.[24]
3 Social integration. Defined by opposition to social segregation on age, race, religion, etc.,[8] this objective often includes citizens' participation in decision-making and political responsibility, expressed as a commitment regarding redistribution of power and empowering of the poor and vulnerable. Various tools have been proposed for achieving this objective; for example, a ladder of participation for stakeholders based on active decision-making was proposed by Sherry Arnstein for the North American context[1] and by Gualardo Choguill for developing countries[5] (also explained in Chapter 9). More recently, the concept of design management (and various models for the insertion of the design process in the construction project) has been developed to clarify the role of stakeholders in architectural and urban design.
4 Transparency in decision-making. This objective also demands the involvement of stakeholders in active decision-making and is linked to the concept of citizen participation.[1] In this book a careful approach to community participation is proposed, together with an observation of the secondary effects it can bring at regional and urban levels (accompanied by the approach to decision-making that was developed by Lizarralde and Massyn[21]).
5 The preservation of values and cultural heritage. Without assuming dogmatic approaches to conservationism, the following notions (among others) should be considered: (i) collective memory;[28] (ii) the capital concentrated on traditional construction know-how;[12] and (iii) the common tension between local values (identity) and global tendencies in architecture and urban planning, as discussed by Tzonis and Lefaivre through the concept of critical regionalism.[33]

Second dimension: economic responsibility

Sustainable rebuilding includes considering the long-term economical and social consequences of the interventions, in particular the consequences on:

6 Economic development. This objective includes the increase of family income in a globalizing economical system – a "system of cities," as it has been recently called by Saskia Sassen.[29] This often includes the careful

spatial integration of residential and commercial uses (an argument that was extensively developed by the architect Norbert Schoenauer[30]) and the creation of incentives for external investment.

7 The reduction of maintenance costs and the expenses associated with later transformations and adaptation to buildings. In this regard, architect and urban designer Clément Demers has classified some principles that must be considered in every construction project:

- building "the right way" the first time: buildings that respect principles of quality will probably not have to be rebuilt (reducing later costs associated with rebuilding);
- recognizing that lower quality often represents important additional costs in the long run and negative effects in the environment;
- recognizing that exaggerated quality might also represent important additional costs and negative effects in the environment;
- targeting "zero mistakes" and "zero delays" in project management;
- recognizing that quality is also associated with productivity.[9]

8 The reduction of costs related to later modifications to the building caused by changes in the functional program (that is to say, in the definition of what the building is to accommodate). This is an objective that has been largely proposed by the Task Group 57 on Industrialization in Construction of the International Council for Research and Innovation in Building and Construction (CIB).

9 The optimization of local available resources – in particular, the optimization of infrastructures and existing buildings – including, of course, the option of recycling buildings and infrastructure for new uses (an argument also discussed in Chapter 4).

10 The reduction of construction waste in materials, equipment and services (transportation, energy, labor force, etc.) and the increased use of recycled materials.

Third dimension: environmental responsibility

It is important to remember that the "green" aspects of sustainable development correspond to only a fraction of the overall ethical responsibility of post-disaster interventions, and they must accompany the complex relations that link them to social and economical considerations. In this regard, post-disaster sustainable interventions properly balance multiple objectives, including:

11 The optimization of resources used in the project, particularly non-renewable resources. In a paramount article titled "Green urbanism and the lessons of European cities," Timothy Beatley[2] defined some principles of intervention that include:

- favoring cities that "live within their ecological limits," reducing their ecological footprints and thus the use of land (a basic resource for building). In this respect, the argument for appropriate densities and the concept of "compact city" have been largely discussed, and their advantages have been largely demonstrated. Interventions must therefore recall what Michael Porter has called "the competitive advantage of the inner city";[25]
- the optimization of used energy. This objective targets responsible use of energy in buildings for lighting, heating, cooling, etc;
- the optimization of local resources, including (only when appropriate) the preference for local labor force, local knowledge, local technology and local materials.

12 The minimization of risks associated with possible future effects of the natural environment over the built environment (notably for the prevention of future disasters).

13 The reduction of negative effects on the natural environment over a short, medium and long term. In "Planning sustainable and livable cities," Stephen Wheeler describes nine main directions for urban sustainability, which directly or indirectly include:

- less automobile use, better access (less and more efficient transportation of residents and construction components);
- the reduction of emissions related to the creation and use of energy;
- the reduction of emissions related to technologies used;
- the reduction of other forms of pollution (noise, visual pollution, etc.).[38]

14 The preservation and restoration of natural resources and ecosystems.

Economic recovery, wellbeing and long-term development: what is the designers' role?

The principal difficulty of reconstruction is not so much that of building houses (which in most contexts is relatively easy to solve from the technical point of view) but of creating – through the built environment – the conditions for economic recovery, wellbeing and long-term sustainable development. However, presented in this way, this is a statement of the solution as much as a statement of the problem, because how do we know what those conditions are?

The following chapters attempt to answer this question. The underlying argument is that organizational design (the design of the team that will conduct the project and the proper distribution of roles and responsibilities within that team) must embody a proper balance between the technical, social, cultural and administrative issues that need to be considered for responding to economic recovery, wellbeing and long-term development.

Building professionals and other decision-makers have the responsibility of determining the "rules of the game" that are required for developing sustainable housing solutions that respect the environment, the culture and the society. It is the responsibility of these professionals to interpret the ways of living of affected residents and the housing typologies of disaster-affected areas, to analyze those ways of living and those typologies and to translate them into technical, organizational and design solutions capable of promoting long-term development. Various examples show that it is precisely the absence of competent decision-makers and designers in disaster-affected areas that has favored the development of inappropriate solutions that are – often – as dangerous and problematic as the disaster itself.

Chapter 2 introduces the main challenges of housing reconstruction and explains innovative ways of improving housing programs by learning from the informal sector, particularly using new examples from Latin America and South Africa. In Chapter 3, Rohit Jigyasu argues for a careful understanding of technological choices and traditional technologies while presenting the case of Gujarat, India. Chapter 4 explains the main challenges and difficulties found in temporary housing, with surprising examples from post-earthquake rebuilding in Turkey. Chapter 5 explains the importance of organizational design and project management and argues for a systems approach to the design of the project team. In Chapter 6, Isabelle Maret and James Amdal explain the major difficulties encountered in the post-Katrina reconstruction in New Orleans. Chapter 7 presents the issues related to land, drawing important lessons from the post-tsunami reconstruction in Asia, as studied by Graeme Bristol. In Chapter 8, Jennifer Duyne Barenstein compares different procurement strategies and theories to explain the advantages of owner-driven reconstruction. Alicia Sliwinski takes a critical approach to community participation in Chapter 9, while Nese Dikmen, in Chapter 10, argues for a better understanding of rural forms of living in Turkey. In Chapter 11, Roger Zetter and Camillo Boano use post-tsunami examples to demonstrate the importance of place-making and understanding how people use space. Finally, Lee Bosher argues in Chapter 12 that post-disaster reconstruction is closely related to pre-disaster resilience.

2 Post-disaster low-cost housing solutions

Learning from the poor

Gonzalo Lizarralde

Governmental and non-governmental organizations alike often lead reconstruction programmes that include direct planning, design and management of housing projects. Even in cases in which some form of consultation with beneficiaries is accomplished, these initiatives are too often based on concentrated decision-making aimed at obtaining a unique housing model that is repeated and offered to residents. The common failure of these practices suggests that decision-makers (and some researchers) are failing to look for answers where they can, realistically, be found – namely in the informal housing sector.

Concentrated decision-making – why and why not

Trying to identify the conditions that need to be considered for economic recovery, wellbeing and long-term development in a regular low-cost housing project is a major challenge, and without any doubt it is even more difficult in the disruption of a post-disaster situation. Governmental and non-governmental organizations alike often tackle this complexity by attempting to plan, design and manage post-disaster housing through a process that brings a considerable number of responsibilities into the hands of one entity (and few people) that collects and uses the available information. In this chapter I refer to this attempt as 'a concentrated decision-making process' to remind readers that decisions made under this approach are made upon the information collected by one or a few organizations (in contrast to a decentralized individually driven approach, which I describe later in this chapter). The natural response is, most often, designing a unique housing model that responds as well as it is reasonably possible to the problems that have been identified, considering the limited information that is available.

Before being studied in the context of post-disaster reconstruction, this approach to design was largely studied by Nobel economics prize-winner Hebert Simon in his milestone work *The Sciences of the Artificial.*[14] According to Simon, organizations confronted with complex 'artificial' problems (problems in which human artifices are at stake, such as housing) are interested in how things *ought to be*. However, the complexity and dynamics of variables and information required to design how things *ought to be* make it virtually impossible to create the 'optimum' solution. That is why – not having found any other useful word in the English language – Simon proposed the term 'satisficing solution' to define the response to a design problem in which limited information is available and computable.

In common post-disaster reconstruction practices, the supposedly satisficing solution often corresponds to creating a model unit; that is, the unit that best responds to the variables, challenges and needs that have been identified during the process of obtaining and computing the available (often limited) information. Being the result of a cost-benefit analysis, the model unit is often considered 'optimal' (in fact contradicting the use of language and the very first principle proposed by Simon) because it is often considered to provide most of the advantages with the minimum use of resources. Once this model unit is identified, organizations proceed to build it repetitively to be offered to as many beneficiaries and affected families as resources allow. The exercise often implies repeating the model at large (based on the argument that economies of scale are obtained this way), and thus its application requires obtaining large portions of land. The problem is that large portions of land are often scarce and expensive in city centres and in well-located areas where jobs, services, infrastructure and transportation are available. Often the result is rebuilding in peripheral or low-demand areas, in which land has a lower impact on the overall budget (this is usually land that is less attractive for residential development).

It is therefore not surprising that residents dislike the housing units provided through this model unit scheme – to the point that sometimes they do not even occupy them. In reality, this unit approach is often the satisficing solution for NGOs and organizations leading the project, and it is rarely satisficing for the needs and expectations of the users (Chapter 5 dwells on the issue of satisficing, in the context of wicked problems and optimum solutions). As I will show later, too often unemployment rates increase, public services are insufficient or too expensive for both beneficiaries and municipalities, maintenance costs are unsustainable and commercial activities do not recover easily.

In fact, it is naïve to believe that even a disciplined group of decision-makers can – in a state of emergency – design, plan and manage a unique solution for solving the overwhelming problems of post-disaster reconstruction within a *concentrated* decision-making process. Recent studies in this area demonstrate that there are just too many variables and too much information required to properly respond to post-disaster needs. The group of experts attempting to design the model unit need to consider, evaluate and balance, among other issues, fluctuating information about economic investment and management options, land prices, complex cultural desires, unexpected social attitudes, controversial traditional values, day-to-day behaviours, political limitations, administrative needs, logistical considerations, fuzzy legal procedures, interrelated infrastructure costs, recycling needs, maintenance costs, environmental considerations, political pressure and so on. This information has proven to be too large and too dynamic to compute, and thus it is almost impossible to obtain the housing solution that would 'satisficingly' fulfil all needs. When built, those supposedly optimum solutions instead rarely fulfil the needs and expectations of anybody.

Consequently, promoters of community participation often encourage NGOs and public agencies to consult residents and beneficiaries about their own housing needs and expectations. They usually consider that the final answer ultimately lies with the residents themselves, who should provide the major input to the design and planning of the project. However, rather than decentralizing decision-making altogether, they usually advocate for conducting some types of consultation processes in order to obtain additional information about the beneficiaries' needs and expectations. The logic is simple: who would know better what is best for beneficiaries than the beneficiaries themselves?

The logic is simple but not necessarily right. Most experienced researchers know that even though it is very important to ask residents and disaster survivors about their needs, expectations and hopes, this is not enough to provide a clear answer – even less to provide a housing plan or the model of a 'satisficing' housing unit. Three constraints often affect the quality of the information provided in such consultation processes.

First, used to being neglected by social services and public attention, low-income residents might exaggerate their needs and expectations about the built environment – particularly if some stranger (who, just for being a stranger, might automatically be mistaken for a public officer from the government or an NGO) wanders around asking about the type of environment users would like/expect to live in.

Second, beneficiaries might not be aware of all the long-term consequences of some immediate desires (for example, having a larger plot front represents, over time, additional costs of maintenance of roads for the municipality).

Third, it is very unlikely that residents are able to compute – by means of a questionnaire or during a consultation session or interviews – all the possible alternatives and possibilities (and their consequences) that, as we have just discussed, are part of the post-disaster housing equation, particularly because most of those possibilities have counter-effects on each other. For example, having a bigger house represents higher costs of heating over time; installing all the infrastructure lines at once might be initially more expensive, but it is certainly cheaper and easier than installing different networks over time; and separating the houses from each other – at least with a 1.5 metre gap – might make them 'look nicer' than row housing (of course, in the eyes of users) and they might become more independent, but the expensive land that is left between them is wasted, as it cannot have any real use.[3,11]

Unfortunately, many PhD students reveal, while doing their doctorate research, that they are unaware of this issue, conducting large-scale surveys asking residents about their needs and expectations in housing. They quickly realize that their findings are of little use, particularly when they receive answers such as 'I would prefer to have two extra rooms', 'we would prefer to have more trees', 'the size of the plot we received is too small' and so on. The reason is that, in reality, most of these answers respond to different forms of the same vague question: 'What type of environment would you like to live in?' This is very different from the more useful and precise question 'What type of environment are you ready to have, can afford and will be able to maintain?'

In reality, performance requirements have to be filtered through the sacrifices required to attain them. What are often considered higher performance requirements (larger plots, detached units instead of apartment blocks, larger houses, etc.) have a cost that – of course – has to be balanced with other priorities and needs (schooling for children, furniture, health, etc.). This does not mean that all the decisions that people make about their built environment are purely economic. Some households might have an unfenced front yard because they prefer this, not because they cannot afford a fence. In the case of reconstruction in Nueva Choluteca, Honduras, for example, the fences that were promptly built by the beneficiaries around the new post-disaster houses reveal quite a lot of information about their needs and priorities in housing (in fact, residents in Nueva Choluteca were very afraid of losing the few belongings that they kept after the disaster, and they were afraid of escalating crime caused by unemployment that was caused in turn by the difficulty of finding work near the new settlement). Having used this logic in their research, architect and researcher Regan Pontagaroa and his students have stated, 'People might lie, buildings don't'[5] (in a reference to the work of Stewart Brand[2]).

Interestingly, it is very likely that key approaches to obtaining housing solutions that are well adapted to the needs and expectations of low-income residents already exist but decision-makers have not been able to see them or recognize them as such (in part because these solutions are highly dispersed and in part because they are undervalued). This is the central argument of this chapter.

The formal versus the informal sectors

If it is true that pertinent approaches for obtaining this information and these solutions already exist, the consequences are profound and profoundly disturbing. First, it would mean that it is no longer necessary to 'invent' or to completely design the solutions for post-disaster reconstruction from scratch – for they would already have been identified and created. Second, it would imply that an approach based on a concentrated decision-making process (that often seeks to invent an 'optimum' solution as suggested above) can be substituted for by simply looking at, and selecting from, the available approaches to the multiple and dynamic challenges of reconstruction.

The underlying argument is – of course – that responding to the qualitative and quantitative deficit of housing in the developing world requires a trained and sensitive eye that is able to perceive the many small (often spontaneous) innovative solutions where they already abound: in the slums. A number of researchers have, for some time, been supporting this search for promising sources; they include John Turner,[15] Vikram Bhatt and Witold Rybczynski,[1] and Peter Kellett and Graham Tipple.[7] More recently another group, including Colin Davidson, Cassidy Johnson, Dave Root and myself, used this principle in an innovative approach to research on low-income housing.[4,12,13]

Slums, according to this approach, are not as hopeless, disorganized, spontaneous and chaotic as external observers usually think. Instead, they are created by a sophisticated 'industry' and a complex system that almost nobody recognizes but which is capable of building shelter for millions of poor families worldwide: this is the informal sector.

The informal sector, unlike the formal sector, is not composed of professionals of the building industry nor of formal companies; nonetheless, it is responsible for building about half the housing stock in developing countries (Bhatt and Rybczynski's work, mentioned above, was correctly called 'How the other half builds'). This informal construction sector is, instead, composed of small and medium informal companies that work without legal recognition or status, that do not necessarily follow acceptable standards and that accompany a share of self-help construction. In a hostile environment that usually neglects its presence, this sector has been the only industry capable of providing housing for the poorest sectors of society. Worldwide, it develops millions of housing units every year, providing shelter for families that otherwise do not have access to any of the products of the formal construction industry.

With no access to the formal financial system, to regular legal means or to orthodox administrative structures, this industry has been forced to adapt itself to a very hostile economic, political and legal environment. It has been forced to innovate and to produce affordable solutions for those who have little or virtually no financial resources. The obvious premise is, therefore, that the informal sector must be doing quite a lot of things right. It also has – of course – deficiencies and limitations (probably nobody would like to be forced to live in a slum or a shack), but it appears clear that its adaptive response to the day-to-day struggle for providing housing has given this sector the necessary information about poor people's needs, capacities, priorities, modes of living and expectations. For decades, its products (the individual shacks, the patterns of land use, the form of informal settlements, etc.) have embodied all this information. However, it is to be postulated that researchers and professionals concerned with reconstruction should be able to garner this information, interpret it and ultimately use it for developing better housing projects, policies and initiatives.

Learning from the informal sector

Buildings respond to a sum of information about the needs, expectations and priorities of their residents and their projected capacity of investment. Houses and apartments represent – at every stage – the amount of investment that households are willing to put into their housing, given the income and resources they possess or the ones they think they will possess in the future.

A series of research projects were conducted by my team during the period 2002 to 2008 in order to validate this argument. This required studying various informal settlements in various contexts, and thus, after considering several alternatives, the following cases were selected:

- The barrio El Paraiso in Bogotá, which was built by low-income residents along the 'Circunvalar' highway (an expressway in the east of the city). The houses, which range from cardboard shacks to three-storey masonry houses, have been – and still are – constantly consolidated; indeed, the settlement was recently 'legalized' and the infrastructure was upgraded. A number of houses built by the informal sector in the city of Armenia in Colombia were also studied (all the cases from Colombia are represented by letter 'a' in Table 2.1).
- Three settlements in South Africa were also included in the study: Guguletu, Mfuleni and Mitchel's Plain (all in the city of Cape Town). These settlements contain thousands of spontaneous constructions built mostly by black residents in illegally occupied land or on formal lots provided by the government (letter 'b' in Table 2.1).

These cases shared multiple similarities with informal settlements in Indore, India (letter 'c' in Table 2.1), as studied by Bhatt and Rybczynski,[1] and with informal housing in New Delhi, India (letter 'd'), as studied by Kellett and Tipple.[7]

Various formal solutions for post-disaster housing and regular affordable housing were also studied as a control group, to be able to identify patterns and compare the different strategies that are used by the informal and the formal sector. The selected cases included:

- The case of Choluteca, Honduras ('e' in Table 2.1), a post-Mitch reconstruction project developed in 1999 to relocate about 2000 families of the Choluteca region. More than 13 local and international NGOs participated in various projects of single-storey detached units.
- The case of La Paz, El Salvador ('f' in Table 2.1), a post-earthquake reconstruction project of detached 36 m² houses developed in 2001 and 2002 by the Salvadorian NGO FUNDASAL.[8]
- The case of El Cantarito in the town 'La Tebaida' in Colombia ('g' in Table 2.1) in which 972 houses were built by the Colombian NGO Corporación Antioquia Presente. The 72 m² masonry units were built

as a relocation project for families affected by the 1999 earthquake.[8]

- The case of Calarcá, Colombia ('h' in Table 2.1), a post-earthquake (1999) housing project developed by Colombian NGO Fenavid using a prefabricated system of cement panels developed by the company Servivienda.[8]
- Two projects of affordable housing targeted to reduce disaster vulnerabilities: a 1262-unit project launched by the Municipality of Facatativá in Colombia for subsidized housing ('i' in Table 2.1) and a 192-unit community-based project of subsidized housing in Netreg, Cape Town ('j' in Table 2.1).

Finding patterns

The comparison of all these cases, plus observations of the multiple dynamics that occur in informal settlements, discussions with residents and a number of interviews with officers responsible for the formal projects, allowed fourteen patterns to be identified. They provide some surprising findings.

1. Flexible use of enclosed and open spaces

Informal housing solutions transfer a great variety of domestic activities to the highly interconnected use of indoor, outdoor, enclosed, open and semi-open spaces. Income-generation activities, bathing children, laundry, eating, playing and a great variety of social activities occur very often in semi-open or enclosed (but not roofed) spaces outside the house. Particularly in all-year-warm climates (India and Colombia, for example), an increased integration of indoor and outdoor spaces facilitates the development of these activities. Spaces delimited by walls but without roofs and by roofs but without walls help the development of these activities. In the informal sector, the projection of domestic activities outdoors helps reduce the demand for built (roofed and enclosed) area, thus reducing construction costs.

Formal solutions often make a clear distinction between interior domestic activities and the 'outside'. This lack of integration between indoor spaces and the exterior creates what I call the 'box effect': users are inside or outside of the box, with little options in between (Figures 2.1 and 2.4).

2. Combination of one-, two- and three-storey units

The informal sector takes full advantage of the possibilities for the evolution of the house. Informal units grow over time, following the availability of resources and the dynamics of family needs (Figure 2.3). When units are erected on small plots (increasing affordability), later additions require the construction of a second level. Informal settlements in Bogotá, for example, often include three-, four- and five-storey units built on 6 m-wide lots.

Formal reconstruction, on the other hand, tends to follow a single-storey pattern, a type that (as we discussed in the section "Rebuilding after disasters:

Table 2.1 Occurrence of patterns in the settlements studied

		Informal housing				*Formal projects*					
	Patterns found	*a. Colombia*	*b. Cape Town*	*c. Indore*	*d. New Delhi*	*e. Honduras*	*f. El Salvador*	*g. El Cantarito*	*h. Calarcá*	*i. Facatativá*	*j. Netreg*
1	Flexible use of enclosed and open spaces	Y	Y	Y	Y	N	N	Y	Y	N	N
2	Combination of one-, two- and three-storey units	Y	Y	Y	Y	N	N	N	N	N	N
3	Priority given to interior comfort and quality of the interior spaces, with limited interior subdivisions	Y	Y	Y	Y	N	N	N	N	N	N
4	Unclear distinction between the original core and later additions/ modifications	Y	Y	Y	Y	N	N	N	N	Y	N
5	Unclear distinction between temporary units and permanent houses. Progressive approach, with quick first construction and no clear end to the building process	Y	Y	Y	Y	N	N	N	N	NA	NA
6	No uniformity in façade. Variety of textures and colours	Y	Y	Y	NA	N	N	N	N	N	N
7	Great variety between housing units	Y	Y	Y	Y	N	N	N	N	N	N
8	Intensive use of recycled materials and components	Y	Y	Y	NA	N	N	N	N	N	N

	Patterns found	*Informal housing*				*Formal projects*					
		a. Colombia	*b. Cape Town*	*c. Indore*	*d. New Delhi*	*e. Honduras*	*f. El Salvador*	*g. El Cantarito*	*h. Calarcá*	*i. Facatativá*	*j. Netreg*
9	Combination of different materials and technologies. Progression from 'light' to solid technologies	Y	Y	Y	Y	N	N	N	N	N	N
10	Variety of functions and uses. Mixture of residence and income-generation activities	Y	Y	Y	Y	N	N	N	N	N	N
11	Strong emphasis on safety from theft and robbery. Delimitation of the land and fencing are priorities	Y	Y	NA	NA	N	N	N	N	N	N
12	Variety of open spaces	Y	Y	Y	NA	N	NA	N	N	Y	N
13	Hierarchy of streets and paths	Y	Y	Y	NA	N	N	Y	N	Y	N
14	Variety of plot sizes and forms	Y	Y	Y	Y	N	N	N	N	N	N

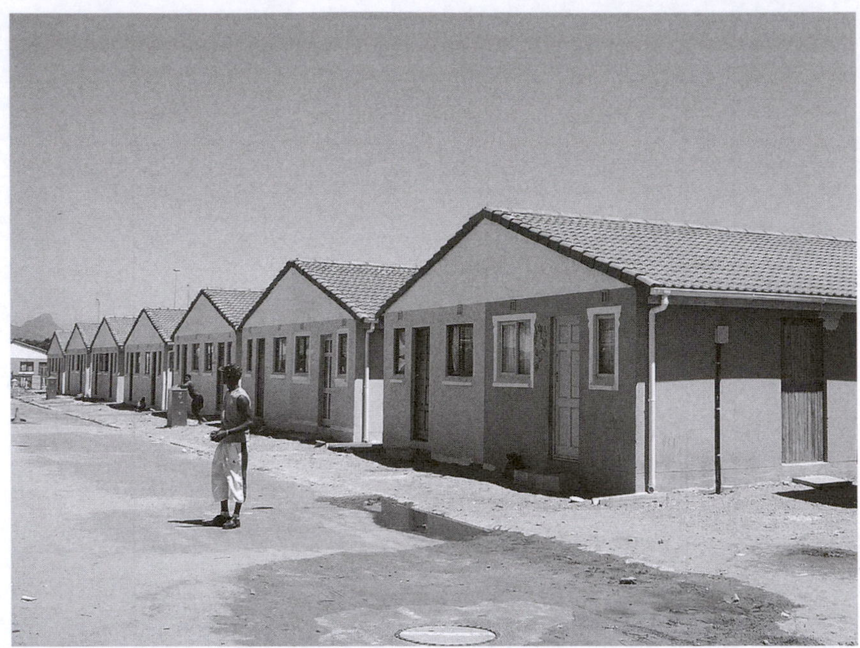

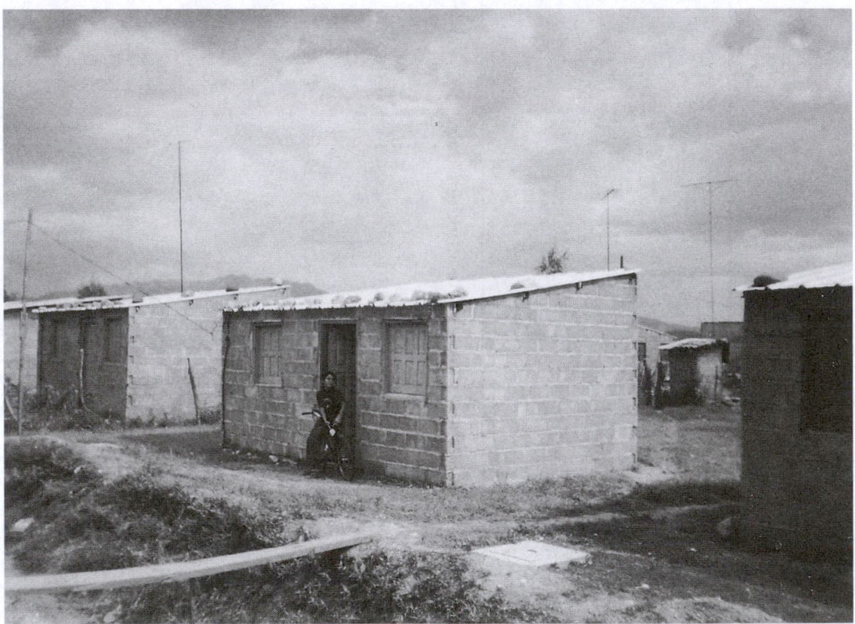

Figure 2.1 Formal housing. **Top:** Repetition and uniformity characterize this project in Netreg (South Africa). **Bottom:** Unit in Choluteca, Honduras. The design dramatically separates indoor and outdoor space, creating the 'box effect'.

From emergency to sustainability) is associated with ease of construction and efficiency for mass production through mutual-aid programmes targeted to unskilled labour (a well-known exception to this pattern is the formal four- and five-storey-high post-disaster buildings often built in Turkey).

3. Priority given to interior comfort and quality of the interior spaces, with limited interior subdivisions

Even in cases where the exterior façades of informal housing seem 'unfinished' (by formal standards), the interior often exhibits particular care put into the interior comfort and the quality of indoor spaces (Figure 2.2). Sometimes equipped with TVs, DVD players, stereos and refrigerators, these interior spaces tend to have minimum subdivisions and to serve various uses during the day.

Following conventional developed-country standards, formal units demonstrate an effort to classify and subdivide interior spaces; thus bedrooms, kitchens and living rooms are separated. This can be seen as an effort to prioritize 'conventional' standards of functionality over the informal perceptions of comfort.

4. Unclear distinction between the original core and later additions/modifications

In the progressive evolution of informal units, the original core and later additions and modifications tend to merge into a unified unit. The use of light materials (wood and corrugated iron sheets) and recycled components plays a fundamental role in the flexibility of the units.

Formal solutions, on the contrary, rarely anticipate later modifications and additions, reducing the possibilities of properly articulating them to the original core. Underestimating the importance of housing evolution leads to the need to demolish brick walls or concrete slabs to attach the additions, and it reduces the possibilities of having structurally sound joints between the core and the additions.[9]

5. Unclear distinction between temporary units and permanent houses. Progressive approach, with quick first construction and no clear end to the building process.

In the progressive evolution of informal units, the temporary shelter – frequently used for land invasion in the early stages of the settlement – is smoothly transformed into a permanent or 'solid' solution. This evolution increases affordability, for an improvised shelter (illegally built overnight) can become a house in the lapse of a few years (Figure 2.3 and 2.4), thus spreading out the need for financial and other resources.

Despite the fact that this pattern is found in almost every informal

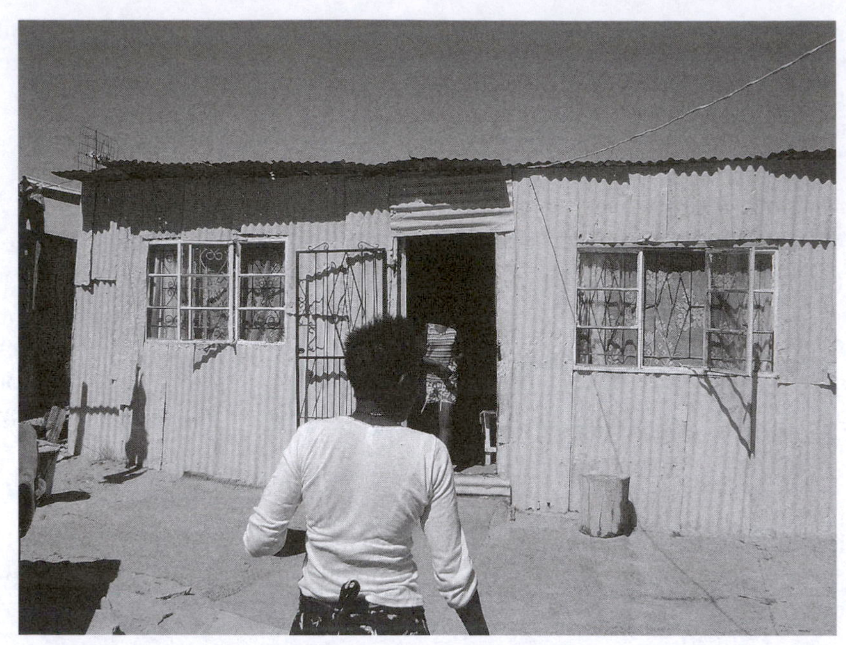

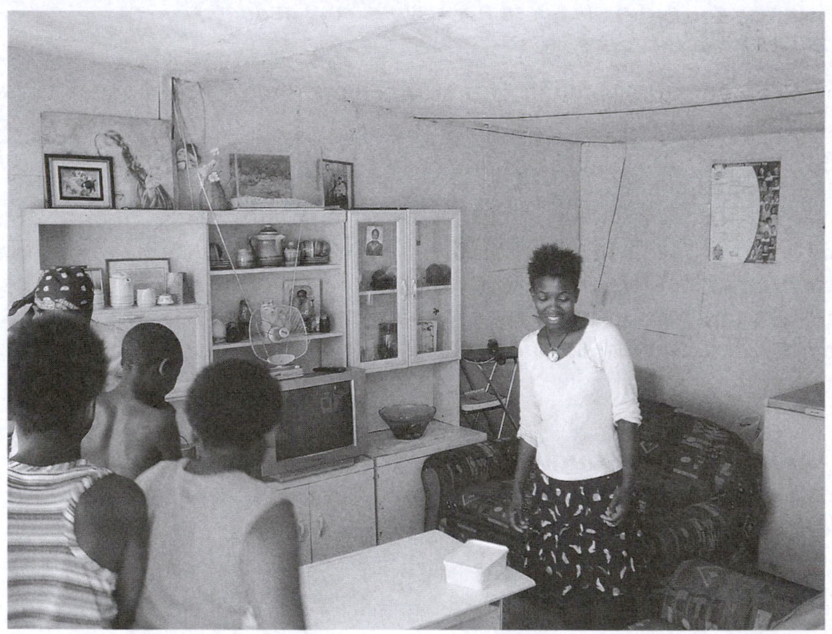

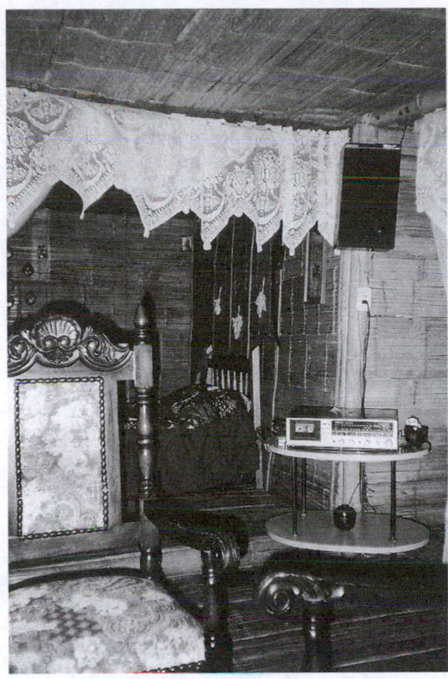

Figure 2.2 Interior of informal housing. **Above:** Interior of an informal unit in Armenia, Colombia. Despite the fact that the house is built on illegally occupied land, the interior demonstrates care for comfort and quality of space. **Opposite page:** These two images of the same unit in Cape Town, South Africa, show the difference between interior and exterior finishing.

settlement in developing countries,[6] formal reconstruction still follows a two- or three-step process in which emergency, temporary and permanent sheltering are unnecessarily fragmented.

Timescales also differ in the formal and informal sectors. In order to succeed in the illegal occupation of land, the informal sector relies on quick construction through the use of improvised units made of recycled and unfinished materials. These units act as 'seeds' that are then improved upon over long periods of time; in other words, these constructions do not follow the traditional definition of a project, with a clear beginning and a clear end (thus with a limited duration), that is typical of the formal sector.

6. No uniformity in façade. Variety of textures and colours

Despite common misconceptions about informal settlements, they usually are a tangible proof of the importance that households attach to the aesthetic appearance of their homes. The use of vibrant colours, façade decoration and careful choice of textures demonstrates that not everything in informal sectors is about lack of choices (this pattern was also found by Jennifer Duyne

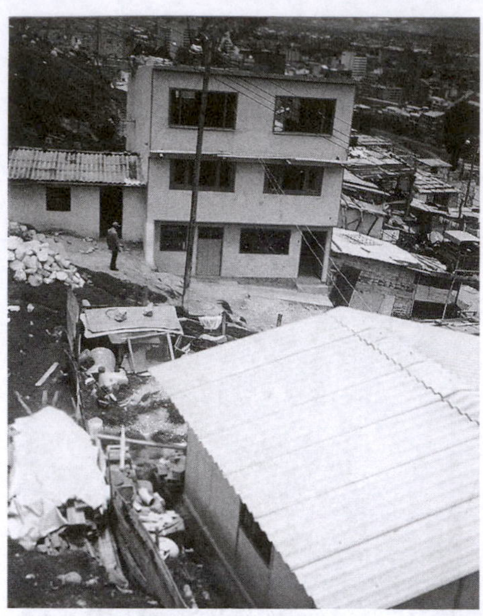

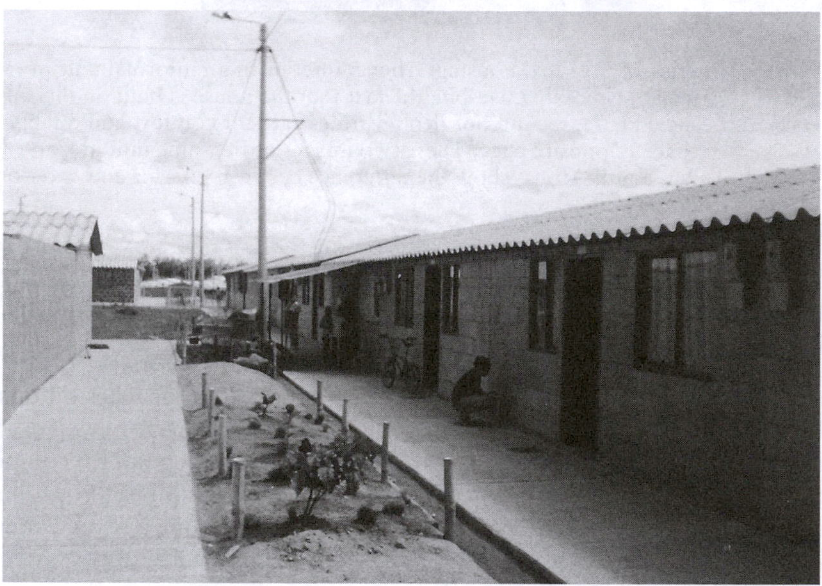

Figure 2.3 Formal and informal houses-in-progress. **Top:** Informal settlement in Bogotá showing four different stages in the housing evolution process: from a shack made of scrap wood to a three-storey unit made of concrete and masonry. **Bottom:** One-storey units in El Cantarito. Although higher densities were obtained by adopting the row-house approach and infrastructure could be provided, a few months after the project was finished, users had already modified the rigorously standardized façades to personalize them with colours and finishes.

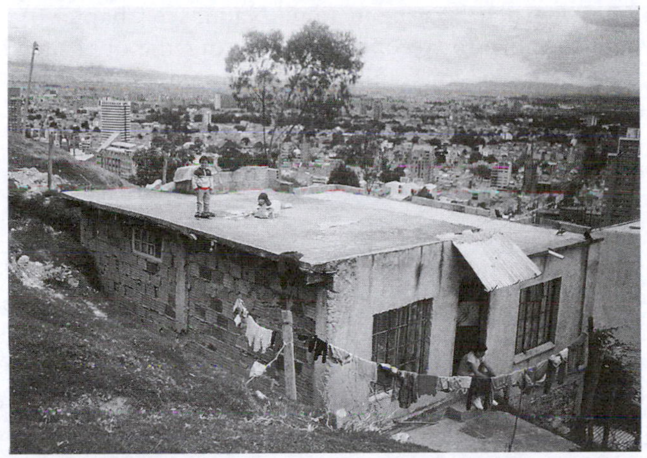

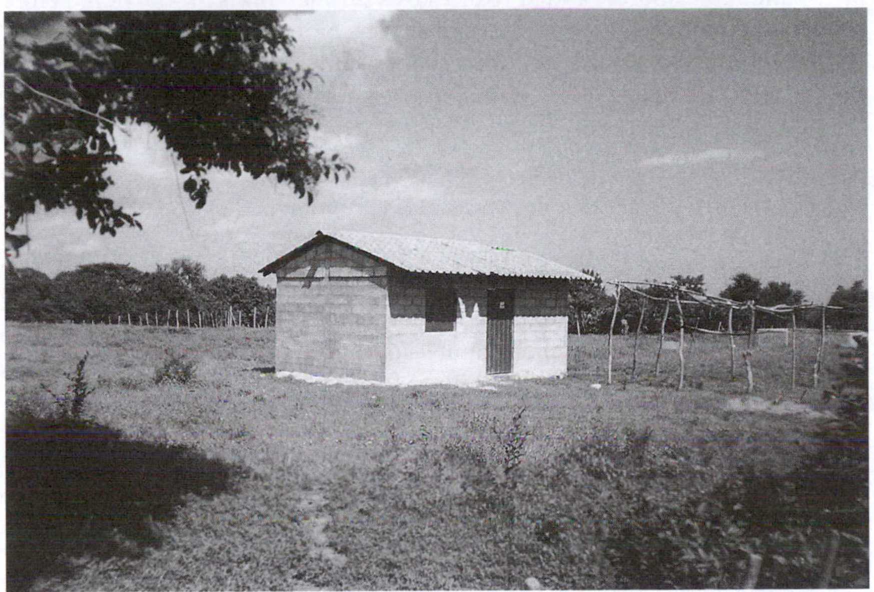

Figure 2.4 The progressive unit vs. the 'box effect'. **Top:** Informal dwelling in Bogotá. The progressive improvements in materials and technologies increase the value of the property (the concrete slab for the roof allows for the later construction of a second level). **Bottom:** Free-standing unit in La Paz, El Salvador, characterized by the 'box effect' and total uniformity in technology and materials.

Barenstein in vernacular housing in Tamil Nadu; see Chapter 8).

The formal solutions for reconstruction favour the opposite strategy for aesthetics and cost reduction, opting for homogeneous facades with a minimum variety of materials, finishes and colours (Figures 2.2 and 2.3).

7. Great variety between housing units

Variety in housing forms, sizes, finishes and technologies is an important strategy for cost-reduction in the informal housing sector. This allows every family to have – at each stage over time – exactly the amount of invested capital it can afford. In this way, each household slowly evolves at its own pace from rough and precarious materials to more expensive finishes. This naturally becomes a powerful way of personalizing each of the units.

By adopting the opposite approach, the formal reconstruction sector emphasizes uniformity among housing units in order to guarantee equality in the distribution of resources and to reduce costs through mass production. Before residents actually personalize their units with colours and modifications, this formal approach often builds boring rubber-stamp settlements that advertise the poverty and the 'receiver status' of the beneficiaries and that contradict the basic notion that every family is different.

8. Intensive use of recycled materials and components

The recycling of materials and construction components is one of the most efficient cost-reduction strategies adopted by the informal sector. It is therefore not rare to find an aluminium window, a ceramic toilet, an industrial truss or a prefabricated kitchen counter in a spontaneous shelter. This reuse of components saves energy and capital for the households, allowing them at the same time to increase the value of their property. In South African townships, for example, Dave Root and I found a sophisticated informal industry that uses recycled materials to produce prefabricated shacks that are easy to transport and assemble.[12]

It is always surprising that, despite the fact that disasters rarely completely destroy all the components and materials of the affected houses, very little recycling is applied to formal post-disaster reconstruction strategies. This is probably due to the fact that governments and NGOs feel uncomfortable with allowing exceptions to construction standards; however, such a strategy obviously contradicts all the common rhetoric of sustainability as largely publicized by development and humanitarian NGOs.

9. Combination of different materials and technologies. Progression from 'light' to solid technologies

The combination of construction technologies (masonry, prefabricated panels, concrete, etc.) is an important solution for cost reduction in the informal sector.

This variety allows each family to progressively invest capital in their house and to increase its value through later modifications – at a pace that matches additional resources as they become available. Besides, very often 'light' technologies such as timber frames and corrugated metal sheets are slowly replaced by 'solid' technologies such as masonry and concrete structures.

Minimum variety in construction technologies is adopted in formal reconstruction. Once again, standardization and uniformity are prioritized over variety and individual multiplicity of choice.

10. Variety of functions and uses. Mixture of residence and income-generation activities

Informal housing solutions provide for an inseparable interdependence of domestic and income-generation activities in low-cost housing. During the day, spaces might change their use, and thus domestic spaces might serve for storage, workshops, stores or small manufacturing in the informal sector (Figure 2.5). The interdependence of their activities facilitates both housing affordability and income generation for households. Very often, this is the only choice for women who need to engage in a productive activity as well as take care of children and domestic chores.

All of this is often neglected in formal reconstruction projects that artificially distinguish between commercial and residential uses. This distinction is worsened by the 'box effect', which limits the possibilities of interaction between the interior and the exterior. In the informal solutions, the possible link between indoor and indoor-outdoor spaces and the street is crucial for the delivery of income-generating services (ironing, clothes repairs, haircutting, etc.) and for the productivity of stores and retail outlets (Figure 2.5).

11. Strong emphasis on safety from theft and robbery. Delimitation of the land and fencing are priorities

The widespread use of bars for windows and doors, fences around the plot and locks demonstrates the importance that informal dwellers give to prevention of theft, robbery and break-ins. The common use of exterior fencing or even low walls is also interpreted as an effort to clearly delimit the acquired property.[10] These priorities are rarely considered in the solutions provided by formal housing reconstruction.

12. Variety of open spaces

Spontaneous settlements have a great variety of open spaces, including small plazas, irregular squares and open areas between units. These public or semi-public spaces play a fundamental role in community building and in social interactions between residents. It is therefore not rare to find in informal settlements a cluster of units around an open area (featuring a tree,

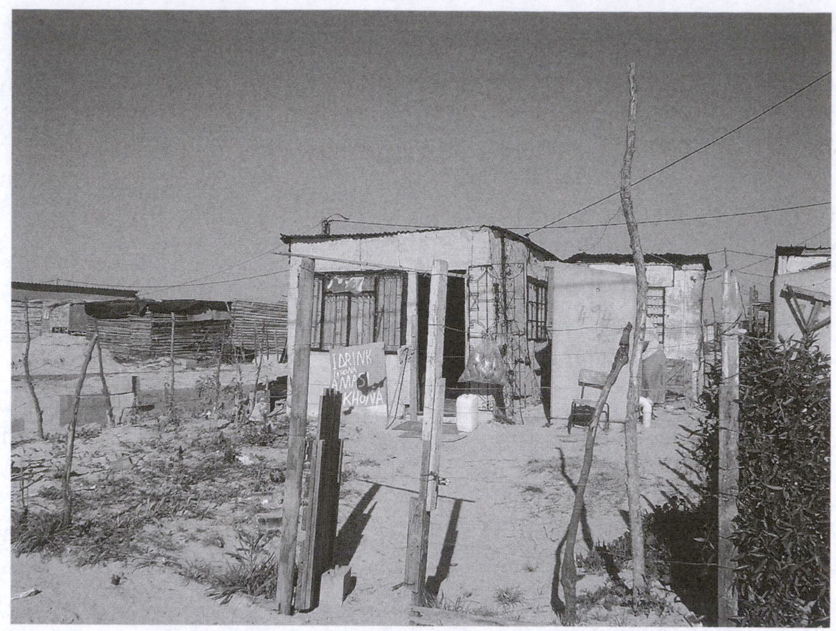

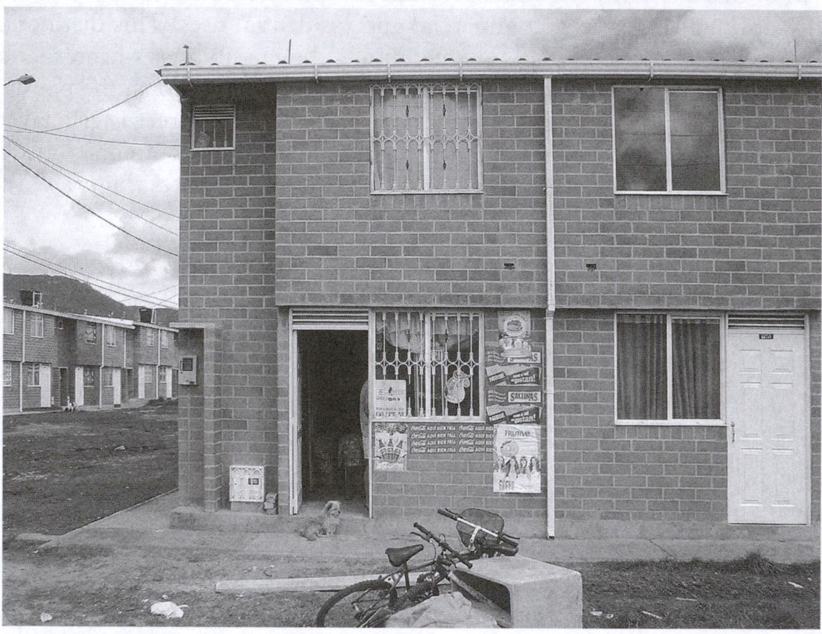

Figure 2.5 Examples of productive uses of space in housing. **Top:** An informal unit in Mfuleni, Cape Town, South Africa. **Bottom:** This formally built house was transformed into a house-shop by residents in Facatativá, Colombia, three months after occupation.

a water tank, a shaded area or a parking place). In the settlement layout, these open areas vary in importance and functionality, providing for a multiplicity of interactions between dwellers.

Post-disaster formal solutions often distribute housing units among a standardized pattern of streets. Public spaces provided in Nueva Choluteca, for example, consist of large public parks, but very little attention was paid to small-scale clustering of units.[10]

13. Hierarchy of streets and paths

Streets and paths in informal settlements also follow a hierarchy of different widths, finishes and public importance. Narrow streets and paths that might not provide access for cars are land-efficient and also serve for the ventilation and lighting of the units. In many cases, narrow alleys also permit double access to the units, which is particularly useful for units that combine residence and income-generation activities or for units that house an extended family (by providing an independent access for the family of the married children, for example). In cases of insufficient land availability, this solution permits increasing densities and therefore allows more affordable solutions for the majority. Higher densities also help reduce infrastructure costs (for building and maintenance) and consolidate the settlement as a whole.

Even when resources are extremely scarce, formal standards of infrastructure (wide roads accessible to vehicles, sidewalks separated from the street, double-lane roads, etc.) frequently influence post-disaster reconstruction projects, challenging densities and thus challenging the long-term sustainability of infrastructure and public services (Figure 2.1).

14. Variety of plot sizes and forms

In the informal sector, an increased variety of plot sizes and forms allows families of different sizes and with different incomes to provide themselves with a housing product that closely accommodates their own needs and possibilities and matches what they can afford. This feature is often ignored in formal reconstruction projects in which standardization of products and services (including lot sizes and forms) predominates over variety of choice.

Better post-disaster housing by learning from the poor

Substantial evidence shows that despite contextual differences, various common patterns can be identified among informal housing solutions. This might be surprising if one considers that housing is largely affected by contextual characteristics. However, it also confirms the notion that, despite the fact that no two final products (for example two informal houses or two informal settlements) are identical, a limited number of variables appear to recur in the informal housing process concerning cost-reduction, phasing of construction, choice of technology and adaptation.

Common patterns also exist among formal post-disaster reconstruction projects. However, the formal post-disaster reconstruction projects studied do not follow the same priorities and patterns as those found in informal settlements (see Table 2.2). One of the main differences between informal construction and professionally designed projects lies in the strategies used for reducing costs and increasing affordability. The formal reconstruction sector emphasizes standardization and uniformity in materials, forms, sizes, technologies and layouts (at both the level of the house and the plot). The informal sector relies on, and takes full advantage of, important competitive strategies: (i) recycling of used components; (ii) progressive construction; (iii) variety of house sizes and forms; (iv) variety of plot sizes and forms, according to the different economic possibilities of each household; and (v) combination of residential use with income-generation activities.

The use of recycled materials, light technologies (timber, corrugated metal sheets, etc.) and progressive construction contributes to the initial speed and ease of construction in informal settlements. There is much to be learnt from the way the informal sector responds to the issues of temporariness, sheltering, fast and efficient construction, commerce and production. The 'poor' teach us that low-cost housing is a progressive activity based on the development of a basic unit over time. Most often, this unit hosts not only domestic activities but also productive activities that are required for economic recovery and development. Finally, the informal sector shows that solutions obtained through concentrated decision-making processes do not enjoy the advantages of decentralized light prefabrication for low-cost housing.

Best practice example: post-disaster reconstruction in rural Colombia

If the informal sector and the households (responding to their own environment and their own needs through individual choices) are capable of spontaneously using large amounts of tacit information about real users' needs and expectations and devising solutions that respond to them accordingly, it could be expected that a reconstruction project that transfers decision-making to the beneficiaries and the informal networks they fit into should lead to positive outcomes. If this is so, it would reinforce the validity of the argument proposed in this chapter, namely that organizations and professionals must learn from (and properly integrate) the solutions provided by the informal sector to meet its own requirements. A reconstruction programme conducted in the Andean region of Colombia after the 1999 earthquake does exactly that.

The earthquake most affected the rural coffee-growing area of the country, disturbing the main export. Concerned about local residents but also about

Table 2.2 Comparison of the patterns found in informal housing and in post-disaster (formal) projects

	Patterns in informal housing	*Patterns in formal projects*
1	Flexible use of enclosed and open spaces	Box effect: clear distinction between indoors and outdoors
2	Combination of one-, two- and three-storey units	Predominance of one-storey units
3	Priority given to interior comfort and quality of the interior spaces, with limited interior subdivisions	Subdivided interior layouts and clear subdivisions of spaces
4	Unclear distinction between the original core and later additions/ modifications	Lack of coordination between original core and later additions or modifications
5	Unclear distinction between temporary units and permanent houses. Progressive approach, with quick first construction and no clear end to the building process	Clear distinction between temporary units and permanent houses. Two- or three-step approach. Project with clear end
6	No uniformity in façade. Variety of textures and colours	Great attention to façade uniformity, finishes and colours
7	Great variety between housing units	Uniformity and standardization between housing units
8	Intensive use of recycled materials and components	Little use of recycled materials and components
9	Combination of different materials and technologies. Progression from 'light' to solid technologies	Uniformity in the use of materials and technologies
10	Variety of functions and uses. Mixture of residence and income-generation activities	Clear distinction of uses. Oriented towards residential use
11	Strong emphasis on safety from theft and robbery. Delimitation of the land and fencing are priorities	Strong emphasis on structural safety. Delimitation of land and fencing are not priorities
12	Variety of open spaces	Uniformity in open spaces
13	Hierarchy of streets and paths	Homogeneity in streets and paths
14	Variety of plot sizes and forms	Uniformity of plot sizes and forms

the earthquake's impact on the national economy, the central government launched an ambitious programme of reconstruction procured by a nationally administered fund. The fund targeted individual projects in different cities, villages and areas, particularly the coffee-growing region in the mountains.

Knowing that the coffee-growers had been badly affected by the disaster and recognizing the additional difficulties of reconstructing in the rural areas, the fund called upon the help of the coffee-growers guild. The guild already had for many decades established a complex but highly efficient infrastructure of committees working in the area for matters regarding coffee production and exports. Their pyramidal structure consisted of a national committee in charge of regional committees that supervised local committees. Even though the structure allowed the guild to have large amounts of information at various levels (from national statistics to comprehensive local knowledge about family values and traditions), the organization did not have the expertise to develop a housing project. And even though the organization had various engineers, managers and specialists in agriculture 'in house', it had no architects, builders or civil engineers with experience in housing. The guild opted then for an alternative approach, responding on the one hand to the mandate it had received from the government and on the other to this lack of local capacity to design, plan and build the houses. It decided to act only as a manager of funds, with a controlling power over the quality of the construction work undertaken by, or for, the coffee growers themselves.

The process was simple: residents could apply for the funds administered by the coffee growers' organizations by proposing an individual project of reconstruction. This individual project could be of any type: reconstruction of a damaged house, demolition and new construction, reconstruction of coffee-processing infrastructure or repairs to existing structures, other new infrastructure, infrastructure for coffee-production or spaces for income generation (stores, workshops, small industries, etc.). Residents were then free to design their individual projects themselves or to hire engineers or specialists. In all cases, engineers of the organization had to approve the plans and guarantee that the structures were structurally sound. In many cases, residents drafted by hand on scrap paper their own houses and repairs, and engineers completed the information with structural details and specifications.

The basic subsidy could be matched with additional resources: a loan given by the coffee-growers' organizations, private loans, individual savings, etc.

Once the subsidy and the loan were approved and the individual designs were also approved by the engineers (acting as auditors), residents were given a first payment. With this, residents had to accomplish significant progress with the project before a next evaluation (usually after completion of 25 per cent of the work). Beneficiaries were free to build however they preferred, with whatever materials and technologies they chose; they were also free to build by themselves, to hire the construction (as in a turnkey project) or to hire labour. In all cases, engineers inspected the projects before giving the second payment, which had to correspond to a significant advancement of the work (often 50 per cent of the total project). The process of evaluating construction progress and inspection was often conducted four times until total completion of the work.

Additionally, the coffee-growers' organizations promoted an exhibition of prefabricated housing. Sixteen companies were invited to promote their housing solutions in the exhibition; the coffee growers could even choose one of the prefabricated houses or, instead, choose some of the components or features of one of them.

The results were very positive. Aware of the fact that they could use their funds as they wanted (as long as they were related to reconstruction), residents assumed total responsibility for their own reconstruction and made important efforts to reduce costs and optimize the resources. This brought several positive consequences:

- Residents who had construction skills used self-help construction, while aging residents and some women opted for hiring labour or having relatives or friends help in construction.
- Residents optimized the use of resources by resorting as much as possible to recycling. Even in cases in which their original units had to be demolished, they recuperated useful components such as doors, windows, toilets, sinks, roof tiles, etc.
- All the constructions were seismically sound while responding at the same time to individual needs, tastes and priorities. Residents chose each element, each colour and each material they wanted to have. They designed, planned and managed their own project and assumed total responsibility for it.
- The freedom to match the subsidies with additional sources promoted an important contribution from the beneficiaries. They contributed to the project from their savings, with additional loans and with labour. The freedom to use the resources as they wanted stimulated residents to search for the best available prices in the market for construction components. This helped the local economy while reducing the price of construction significantly.
- The prefabricated housing exhibition had a surprising but positive effect. Most residents did not buy the finished units (as was initially expected), but instead they visited the exhibition in order to obtain ideas and copy construction details and layouts. Some residents then bought construction materials (even from the same companies that were exhibiting) and built their own houses by themselves, customizing the designs to meet their own needs.
- Conscious about the limitations of their resources, residents optimized their projects by creating flexible spaces that responded to various uses. As with the units frequently found in the informal sector, houses and units were built to mix domestic activities with income generation (storage of coffee beans, space for drying coffee beans, storage of equipment, convenience stores, etc.).
- Residents did not concentrate on one technology or housing model. Instead they combined different construction techniques and materials

according to availability, price, speed of construction, available skills, etc. It was therefore not rare to find a mix of steel structures with local masonry or a house made of local masonry but with prefabricated panels and corrugated roof sheets.

- Finally, as long as projects respected the evaluation process conducted by the engineers, they could propose to build them by phases, adopting the informal approach of progressive housing.

In conclusion, residents resorted to their own informal networks to obtain materials, labour, additional funding, etc. All of this allowed them to reduce costs, personalize their projects, optimize resources and respond to their own needs, expectations and priorities, while also promoting the local economy. The coffee-growers' guild completely decentralized the decision-making process.

Therefore, no complicated consultation process was required to support a centrally planned, designed or managed programme (nor to produce a unique housing model). There was no need to ask residents about what they wanted, needed or expected, since the process itself favoured the adaptive emergence of the best solutions. There were, in effect, many solutions, all of them exploiting the best opportunities, the available resources and the best local knowledge. It was a 100 per cent bottom-up project in which few architects and planners were actually required. Significantly, several earthquakes of different magnitudes have affected the region since 1999; no deaths, major injuries or relevant material losses have occurred since then.

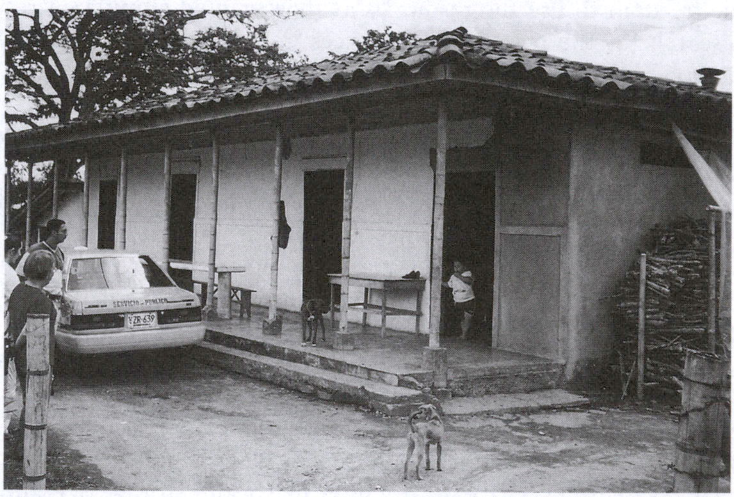

Figure 2.6 Reconstructed house in rural Colombia. The beneficiaries optimized the resources and subsidies to develop their customized projects (here a storage room was rebuilt in a partially affected house).

3 Appropriate technology for post-disaster reconstruction

Rohit Jigyasu

Reconstruction following disaster provides a unique opportunity to introduce appropriate technology that takes into consideration specific hazards to which the affected region is exposed. On one end of the spectrum are 'state of the art' techniques of construction, on the other end is a conservative approach that seeks to repackage and reintroduce traditional construction systems. Sustainability is the key determining factor for the success of technology.

Introduction

There is a strong belief that contemporary technology is superior and would serve as panacea for vulnerability reduction in the areas with 'poor' vernacular constructions, but there is also a convincing belief that traditional knowledge accumulated over time is best suited for reconstruction. However, the suitability of the introduced technology in disaster-affected areas depends not only on its disaster-resistant qualities but also upon several factors such as social and economic context, availability of material and other resources, local skills and aesthetic sensibilities. Traditional construction practices and delivery mechanisms often embody local knowledge accumulated over time through successive trials and errors. Therefore these cannot be rejected outright when deciding on the appropriate technology for reconstruction. The challenge is how to integrate positive elements of these practices into the proposed solutions. The true measure of the success of the technology introduced during reconstruction can be gauged by the extent to which it becomes part of the sustainable local building culture of the region long after the reconstruction process is over and all the external support is withdrawn. Longitudinal studies on post-disaster reconstruction in Latur, Gujarat and Kashmir following the 1993, 2001 and 2005 earthquakes bring to light many of these issues.

Disasters can initiate development

Overlooking the basic safety parameters in construction is one of the main reasons for the large-scale damage seen in disaster situations today. Any disaster, in spite of the havoc and destruction that it brings, presents the affected people with a chance to rebuild anew, rectifying the mistakes committed in the past. Thus, in a rather unusual way, disasters do lead to development. The post-disaster phase actually allows one to reconsider safer building technology in order to improve the resilience of the built environment and its communities in the next earthquake. Judging the success or failure of this technology would require considering the following questions:

- What kind of technology is more appropriate and why?
- How should this technology be introduced to maximize its effectiveness?
- Who are the key actors that need to be engaged in this process?
- How does one assess the performance of technology vis-à-vis the ground realities rooted in local contexts?

The choice of appropriate technology for construction is dependent on various factors that are embedded in the very fabric of the community where the reconstruction is being carried out. In fact, any construction is in effect a living, breathing piece of infrastructure, an inseparable part of the community into which it is being built. Therefore consideration must be given not only to the safety issue but to all seemingly unrelated factors, such as the cultural influences, societal structure and even culinary habits!

These challenges are investigated through the case of post-disaster reconstruction in Gujarat following the 2001 earthquake and its long-term implications for the building culture of the region. Some reference is also made to the reconstruction following earthquakes in Marathwada (1993) and Kashmir (2005) in India.

Gujarat rocks on its national day

26 January 2001 – the national day of India – was the dreadful day when an earthquake of intensity Mw 7.7 struck the Kutch and Kathiwar regions in Gujarat state in the western part of India at 8.46 am (local time). This was India's most damaging earthquake in the last fifty years.

According to the official figures, one month after the earthquake, the total population affected by the earthquake was a staggering 15.9 million out of a total population of 37.8 million (of Gujarat State). The numbers of dead and injured were placed at 19,727 and 166,000 respectively.[12] According to another report, 7904 villages in twenty-one districts of Gujarat were affected by this earthquake. 332,188 houses were destroyed while 725,802 house were damaged to varying degrees.[8]

In the aftermath of the earthquake, the Gujarat government was eager to bring some definite plans to the people before it was criticized for its lack of response. Accordingly, as early as 14 February 2001, the government embarked on a large-scale rehabilitation package, which had components covering urban and rural situations. Ironically, 'relocation' and full-scale 'village adoption' were the main highlights of this package, very much like the case of Marathwada, where a large-scale rehabilitation project was initiated by the Maharashtra government and financed by the World Bank following the 1993 earthquake. Even the criteria for relocation and house size were strikingly similar to the earlier case.[4]

However, in contrast to the Marathwada case, the government's plan for relocating villages in Gujarat was met with stiff resistance from the local people, who did not want to be uprooted. As a result, the Gujarat government finally decided not to press for relocation and advocated 'owner-driven' reconstruction as its primary approach, in contrast to the 'contractor-driven' approach that was followed in Marathwada (see Chapter 8 for a more in-depth review of owner-driven reconstruction in India). An owner-driven approach primarily lays the onus of responsibility and reconstruction of houses on the owner. It is essentially a community-led process in which the external agencies are the facilitators. Thus the government agreed to provide financial assistance to all those who did not want relocation and full-scale 'adoption'; such beneficiaries could undertake reconstruction on their own. As a result, owner-driven reconstruction on such a large scale turned out to be a pioneering attempt at post-earthquake reconstruction in India.

Under the owner-driven approach, the Gujarat government introduced a system whereby the families who chose not to be included in any NGO reconstruction programme received financial assistance from the government, depending on their entitlement. The compensation was released in three instalments, parallel to house-construction phases. The first, comprising 40 per cent of the total cost, was paid at the preparatory stage, the second (another 40 per cent) upon completion of walls and the remaining 20 per cent once the house was finished. The second and third instalments were only disbursed after verification and certification by government engineers, who were appointed for site supervision, overseeing the quality of construction and checking the use of basic safety features during the construction.[13]

With the adoption of the owner-driven approach, NGOs and international organizations came forward to help the local communities in deciding the design and technology of new constructions. Most of them promoted owner-driven construction by providing the beneficiaries with construction materials such as wood, bamboo, spreadsheets or concrete blocks and reinforcement bars, according to the structural design advocated by the outside organization. As part of public–private partnership policy, the government made the building materials available at subsidized rates. For example, UNDP, in partnership with local NGOs such as Abhiyan, initiated the 'transition recovery concept'. As part of this concept, the shelter programme was aimed at reducing vulnerability, building capacity, promoting sustainable recovery, demonstrating seismic safety in housing and providing alternative accommodation for the rural displaced.[11]

As reconstruction progressed, a significant gap emerged between the initial conception and the reality on the ground.[3] The owner-driven reconstruction in rural areas was mostly reduced to the involvement of owners as daily labour, carrying out tasks such as clearing the rubble, carrying the material, curing and blocklaying. In the urban scenario, professional builders took charge of the building activities, as was usual for any urban building project. Thus the role of the owner became that of doing all the paperwork to ensure that the grants and compensations were taken care of.

Therefore, in many cases, 'owner-driven reconstruction' was not, in its true sense, driven by the owners at all. This, as discussed later, had significant implications for the efforts made by various organizations to introduce safer technology.

Traditional or modern technologies and earthquake safety

The primary complaint made after the earthquake was the inability of traditional housing, with its designs and materials, to handle the impact of an earthquake. Total failure of stone masonry structures was observed all over the affected region. The towns of Bhachao and Anjar were completely devastated. The vulnerability of out-of-plane stone masonry walls could be discerned through the large amount of debris in the narrow lanes of these towns. The structures in the old city of Bhuj, within the fortification walls, were also badly damaged. There were many one- and two-storey stone buildings in mud mortar with poor bonding, of which hardly any survived without significant damage (Figure 3.1).

The most logical way out was therefore to introduce modern technology that had been scientifically tested and recognized worldwide for its ability to withstand the impact of an earthquake. It was mainly introduced in the form of reinforced concrete blocks using state-of-the-art construction techniques, such as pile foundations, and earthquake-resistant features, such as concrete bands at lintel level.[1]

On the other hand, several NGOs strongly advocated the use of traditional materials and technologies, such as timber-framed structures with brick masonry infill, wattle and daub, and adobe constructions. However, the use of stone – one of the main building materials before the earthquake – was completely rejected by everyone.

A few NGOs, most prominent amongst them being Abhiyan and UNNATI, introduced the use of alternative technology, which is basically an outcome of the integration of available local knowledge and scientific and modern innovations. Hunnarshala, a local foundation for building technology and innovations in Kutch, focused on devising new technologies and methods of construction by taking into account the available knowledge and materials, which are in tune with the social, economic and geographical factors of the particular region.

Hunnarshala, was founded after the 2001 earthquake to act as a technical knowledge bank for the local community, helping them to innovate, advise

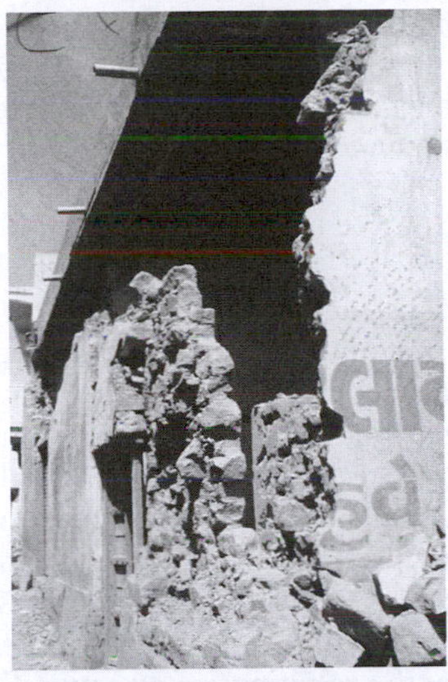

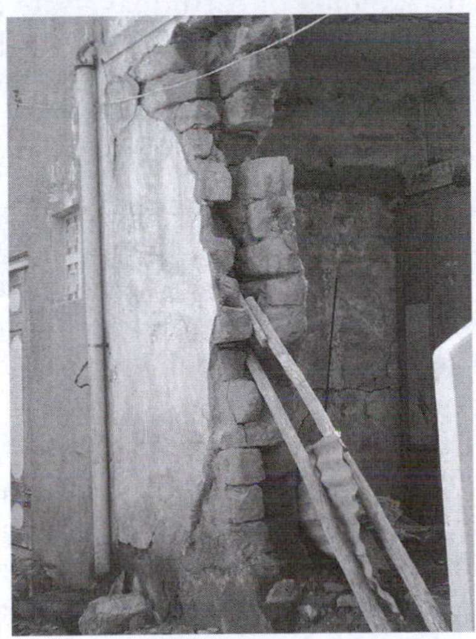

Figure 3.1 Poorly constructed stone masonry structures. This building in Limbdi collapsed during the February 2001 Gujarat earthquake.

and communicate various technical upgrades of available traditional technology.[3] With the involvement of traditional craftsmen and technical experts, traditional technologies are fused with modern ones. All technologies are scientifically tested for their strengths and weaknesses at their laboratory in Bhuj.

Hunnarshala has had a number of successful projects and innovations, amongst them compressed soil or clay blocks especially adapted for the local conditions and developed as ideal replacements for stones. The new material was tested by the Hunnarshala laboratory and found to be of superior quality to bricks, the other alternative available for the local people prior to the earthquake, apart from stones. This material has been used to great extent by various NGOs during the reconstruction phase.

Building culture in Kutch today

The main phase of reconstruction was finished by 2003–04. Since then, construction has been mainly extensions of the reconstructed structures that were provided or new constructions carried out by the people on their own. Interestingly, the technology that is apparent in recent construction is a mixture of all the available technologies and materials, including those that were developed and promoted by cement industries, such as concrete blocks, or by NGOs, such as compressed soil blocks or china clay blocks.

However, to increase their seismic resistance, the use of these new materials demanded various structural design improvements, which were alien to these people. Therefore, the resulting constructions, in most cases, do not demonstrate much understanding of earthquake-safe construction technology. In the absence of any technical understanding, such faulty constructions were brushed under the carpet by nicely plastering and painting from outside.

A few trends, however, are very prominent. For example, houses built of stabilized china clay blocks with thatched roofing are now having an extension done with brick walls and concrete roofing. The main problem is that the extension part does not have any reinforced concrete columns to support the concrete slab roof. Furthermore, around many such structures in the earthquake-affected region, new boundary walls are being constructed in rubble stone masonry (Figure 3.2).

An interesting case in this regard can be drawn from the example of bhungas. A traditional bhunga, the trademark settlement of the rural poor in some parts of Kutch, is usually circular in form with a sloping roof and has the inherent quality of earthquake resistance due to its shape, which allows the lateral force to dissipate. Post-earthquake, the bhungas made by an NGO were designed to be earthquake-safe by virtue of their circular form and concrete bands. But when the time and need arose for an extension to the house, the resettled families had to choose the technology and material that was affordable and readily available. Although many of them could get access to new materials like compressed soil blocks, they were not very conversant with good construction techniques using these materials. As a result, the extensions do not show any use of earthquake-safe features (Figure 3.3).

In another instance, villagers in Navagram, near Bhachao, used bricks to build new houses but did not install any earthquake-safety measures. For example, in this village, a shop of 9 by 9 feet was being constructed using a 3-inch-thick brick wall without any beams or columns – this was considered strong enough to hold a 9-foot rolling shutter! In the villages of Indraprastha,

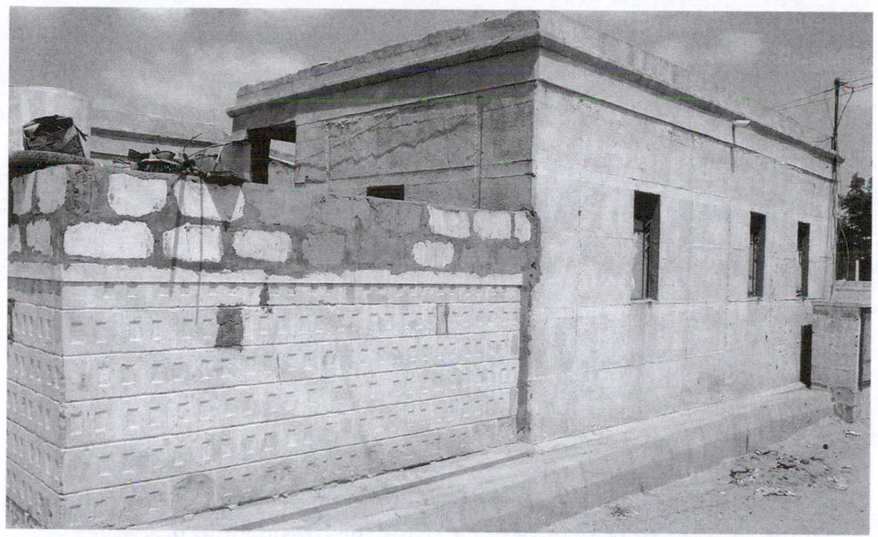

Figure 3.2 Piecemeal additions made to the reconstructed structures. These additions, using various materials such as clay blocks and stones, increase their vulnerability to earthquakes. Bhuj, Gujarat.

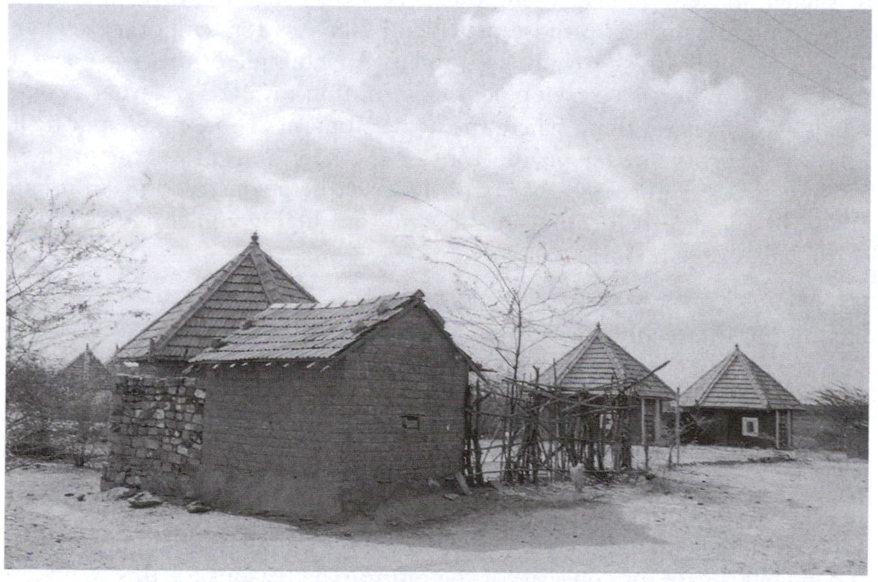

Figure 3.3 Bhungas reconstructed by an NGO after the earthquake. These bhungas are now being extended using stones and soil blocks, thereby increasing their vulnerability.

New Dudhai and Chandrani, similar cases of poor self-help constructions were observed.

In some cases, it was found that the new building materials and technology were culturally and climatically inappropriate. For example, in the village of New Dudhai, only eight out of the total 850 houses that were built by the state government were occupied. Most of the residents of the village chose not to resettle in the new site and instead renovated their original houses. One of the primary reasons was that the reconstruction at the new site was done using reinforced concrete. Though earthquake-safe and of much better quality, the new housing did not show enough consideration for the sweltering heat of the region, compared to the rammed-earth housing, which was economically affordable and climatically more appropriate. Another instance of inappropriate material was found in a village where marble tiles for flooring were provided by an NGO. The villagers, who were not used to this material, found it inappropriate and converted the main room in the reconstructed house into a kind of guest room, while making temporary structures in front of the house to cater for their residential needs.

In urban areas of Bhuj, Anjar and Bhachau, which suffered heavy destruction, a blanket ban was enforced on any new reconstruction until a master plan was executed, specifying the land use and building guidelines; a private firm was entrusted with this job. As a result of this, people in urgent need of shelter started reconstructing on their own, using whatever materials were available, including those provided by NGOs for temporary shelter. These structures are still being used today. An example of this was seen at the Gujarat Industrial Development Corporation's (GIDC's) Sardar Nagar rehabilitation site in Bhuj, where the owners of a new house have put their initial temporary shelter on the roof of the new house to cater to their growing needs (Figure 3.4). Many of these self-help constructions in urban areas are found to be of poor quality and thus highly vulnerable to future earthquakes (Figure 3.5).

Sustaining the technology

The biggest irony of the reconstruction process in Gujarat was that people continued to use old construction techniques/specifications and design forms, even in those instances where new materials were introduced. One of the underlying reasons for this was the loss of traditional knowledge, which is elaborated on later in this chapter. Furthermore, safe building practices were not assimilated into the general knowledge of the building community, which is definitely a case for concern for the future. The reasons for this trend are detailed below.

During the reconstruction phase, the problem lay with the abundance of foreign materials such as cement and steel, which were made available by the government at subsidized rates, thereby invading the market for traditional building materials such as stone, wood and mud. Concrete blocks achieved

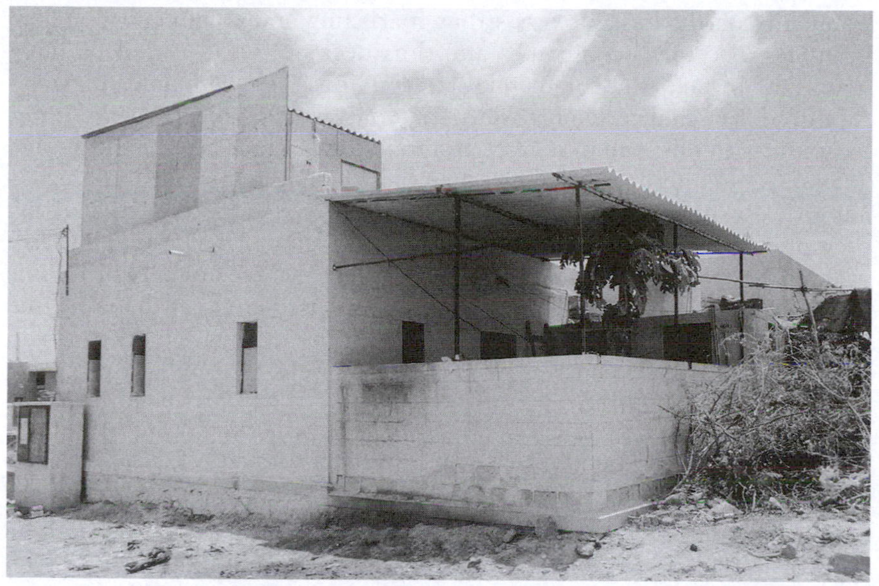

Figure 3.4 Temporary structures in Bhuj. A temporary structure has been added on top of a reconstructed structure in the relocated urban colony in Bhuj, along with other additions.

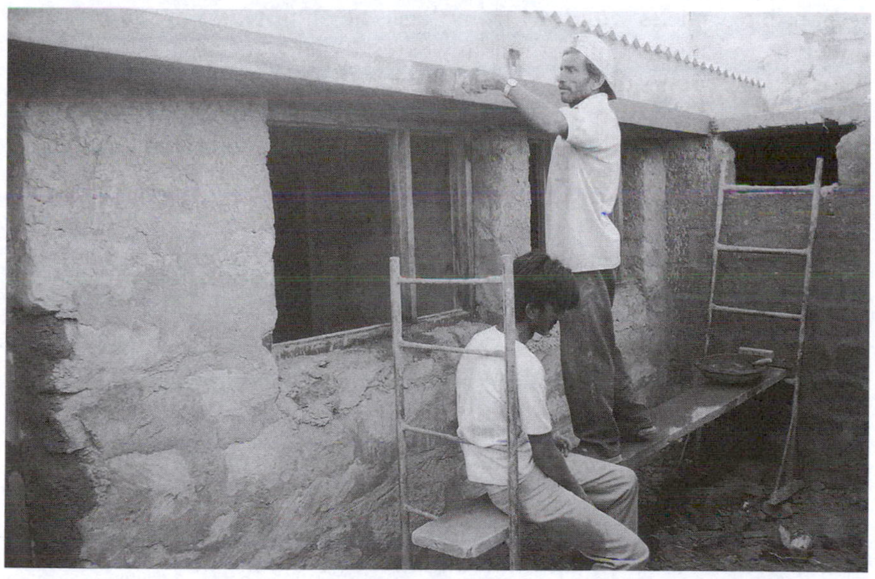

Figure 3.5 Self-help intervention. A self-help structure is being constructed in Bhuj using stones and concrete blocks, without employing any earthquake-resistant features.

popularity on the basis of very strong marketing and communication programmes of cement companies and thus became the favoured building materials. In fact, the commercial interests of these companies played a significant role in determining which materials were used.

Contrary to this, and in spite of promotion by various NGOs, the market availability of alternative building materials such as compressed soil blocks has gone down sharply since the initial phase of reconstruction, thus affecting their price. For example, a compressed soil block comes at a price of 8 Indian rupees (INR), according to 2008 rates. It is as big as three bricks, which come at 2 INR per piece. The concrete blocks being used come at the same rate as that of compressed soil blocks; however, due to aggressive marketing and better availability, the concrete blocks and the bricks are generally perceived as better building materials.

Recently there have been some efforts to promote entrepreneurial endeavours for alternative building materials such as clay blocks; for example the Chamunda Block Production Group is producing stabilized clay blocks for commercial purposes, promoted by UNNATI in Bhachao. However, these sorts of endeavours are still at a very nascent stage, and the number of such groups is very limited in comparison to the needs of the entire district.

Another problem is that the requirements of some of the building materials do not match the availability of resources. For example, Kutch is a semi-arid zone where water is very limited; concrete blocks, as well as compressed soil blocks, require strict quality control and proper curing. Once the responsible agencies withdraw from the scene and owners are supposed to undertake reconstruction without any external help, curing may turn out to be a difficult proposition in a drought-prone area, and the quality of these materials is thereby affected. For these reasons, it is highly doubtful whether such technologies would eventually take root within the building culture of the area.[4]

Communicating 'technology' – transfer or knowledge sharing?

One of the reasons why the earthquake-safe technology did not take root in the local building culture is that less emphasis was placed on the communication of the earthquake-safe knowledge at the grassroots level. This is due to the lack of real participation of the owners/residents in the reconstruction process; as mentioned before, in most cases they merely provided labour for the new construction. This resulted in an absolute lack of understanding about the basic properties of new materials and their proper and optimum usage.

Several notable communication initiatives were undertaken to instil safe building practices among the local communities. These included awareness posters, information booklets, training programmes and the construction of model houses. For example, Abhiyan, along with Setu, developed a handy booklet addressed to the mason community titled *Tome Koriyacho*, literally meaning 'Hey Builders'. The booklet was meant to introduce earthquake-safe features of buildings to the mason community. Several organizations, such as the National Centre for People's Action in Disaster Preparedness (NCPDP), carried out peer training programmes for senior masons on the basic principles and techniques for safe structures. These masons were supposed to communicate this knowledge further at the village level.

Technology-transfer initiatives largely followed the development communication process. Development communication, a term first coined in 1972 by Nora C. Quebral, means 'the art and science of human communication linked to a society's planned transformation from a state of poverty to one of dynamic socio-economic growth that makes for greater equity and the larger unfolding of individual potential.'[10] The problem with development communication stems from its very definition. The unfolding of 'individual potential' is often influenced by the fact that the knowledgeable do-gooder is usually an outsider, and thus can actually suppress the entire potential of the deprived group by causing complete destruction of the available knowledge base and loss of self-respect and dignity.

On the brighter side, though, there were some notable communication initiatives in Gujarat. One of those, performed by Setu, was to enable local people to make their own decisions under the guidance and advice of the professionals. Dhamadka Setu, in particular, set up a network of events that helped the community to integrate safe building practices into building. It organized regular meetings of the community and ensured that the knowledge interaction between the experts of various disciplines and the community continued throughout the reconstruction process. This initiative generated the necessary knowledge capital that would help to prevent a future earthquake from becoming a disaster.

Loss of traditional knowledge

Kutch has historically been an earthquake-prone zone; therefore, the repository of traditional knowledge for earthquake-safe construction has always existed. This was usually in the form of orally dispensed knowledge, handed down to subsequent generations of craftsmen in an unorganized manner. The technology used in old construction was found to be quite efficient in providing safety from earthquakes. However, in recent years, the lack of town planning (leading to massively congested roads and alleys) and the rising cost of materials (the price of wood, one of the traditional housing materials, has skyrocketed during last few decades), among other factors, have led to recent poor-quality construction in the area. Furthermore, the unorganized manner of knowledge transfer did not help less-capable builders and eventually compromised the stability of the buildings. Thus, apart from the very old structures in Bhuj, which had the additional factor of a lack of proper preservation weighed against them, the old-technology houses that were properly built did survive the earthquake with élan.[4,7]

Local people are generally aware of the fact that Kutch falls in an earthquake-prone zone. As a result, earthquake-resistant construction systems have evolved over time in the region. The typical traditional dwellings of Kutch, the bhungas, have withstood the test of time for centuries and have also withstood earthquakes, thanks to their circular form, which, as mentioned, is very good at resisting the lateral forces of earthquakes. Moreover, wattle and daub construction, especially where wood is used as reinforcement for the wall, has proved to be very effective. In Gujarat, many structures built prior to the 1950s had floor joists extending through the rubble stone walls to support the balconies. They were more successful in stabilizing the walls than were joists terminating in pockets, and they therefore performed much better against the 2001 earthquake.[7] In fact, in Anjar, this kind of structure was one of the rare ones found standing amidst the debris of collapsed houses. Some traditional construction employing wooden frames with masonry infill also performed well against the lateral forces of earthquakes, due to their capacity to dissipate energy. Many traditional constructions also have earthquake-safe features such as tie beams, knee bracing, tongue and groove joinery, etc. (Figures 3.6 and 3.7).[4,6]

Traditional constructions have other strengths besides their earthquake-resistant qualities. For example, the material used by most of these constructions can be procured locally. Also, the materials and the traditional knowledge of house building have the ability to handle the various ambient issues such as the scorching heat, semi-desert climate and economic environment. Take for instance the case of bhungas, which are not only

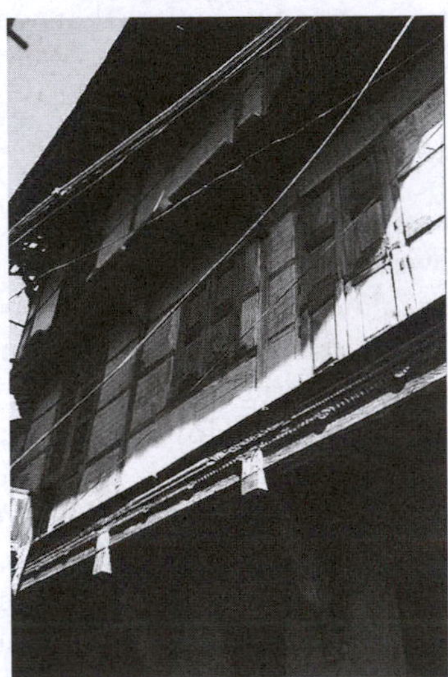

Figure 3.6 Traditional structures in Limbdi. One of the surviving traditional structures in Limbdi town has earthquake-safe qualities due to its timber-framed construction with masonry infill.

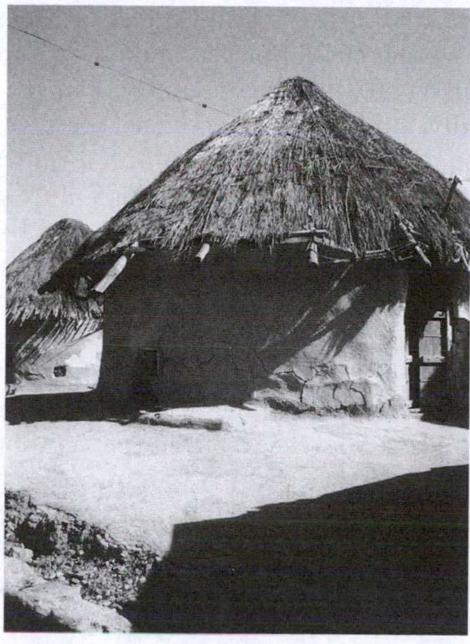

Figure 3.7 Traditional bhungas of Kutch. The traditional bhungas performed well against earthquake because of their circular form and wattle-and-daub construction.

earthquake-safe but also demonstrate a sensitive understanding of locally available resources, climatic conditions and people's spatial requirements. In fact, all these factors play an important role in the evolution of vernacular architecture at any given place. Similarly, rammed-earth constructions found in the region are acclimatized to the natural factors, besides being locally available, thus requiring minimal costs for construction.

Nonetheless, the initial reaction to the damage caused by the earthquake was to think that the traditional housing construction was not safe for earthquakes. The fact that traditional housing had its share of positive features was overlooked by most of the agencies concerned with reconstruction. Moreover, the introduction of new technologies and the enabling market mechanisms for these seem to have forced traditional technology somewhat into oblivion while, at the same time, the new technology introduced did not make its way into the building habits of the local people.

Misconceptions about 'technology'

A significant determining factor for the loss of traditional knowledge is the predominant perception of the local people, who favour the use of concrete as a symbol of progress. Therefore, introducing concrete slabs as roofing is considered good, even if they are made with poor reinforcement and mix and are not tied well to the walls. In spite of viable design alternatives proposed by various NGOs, most homeowners still prefer to replace traditional tiled sloping roofs with flat concrete slabs, even though the former are much safer compared to flat concrete roofs, which merely collapsed like cards after the earthquake. Ironically, similar processes were seen four years later after the Kashmir earthquake, where many reinforced cement concrete (RCC) constructions built after the earthquake did not follow even the basic rules of construction. For instance, rather than resting directly on the beams, the roof slabs of many structures were cast on two or three brick courses placed on the beams, which in some cases were not even at the same level.[6]

In a particular reconstruction site named Indraprashtha Nagar, the housing that was built by an NGO used a synthetic material for roofing that leaks during the rainy season. As a result, the residents have built a concrete slab without any reinforcement. So strong is the misperception against stones that even temples, which were originally built of stones, are being reconstructed in poorly mixed concrete but following exactly the same design as before (Figure 3.8).

One of the ironies of reconstruction after the Gujarat earthquake, as well as after the Marathwada and Kashmir earthquakes, was that stone, the main building material for the majority of the housing in rural as well as urban areas, was rejected outright by engineers as well as by the local people. Very few realized that the basic reason for heavy damage sustained by stone construction was not the stone itself but the way it was used as poorly bonded

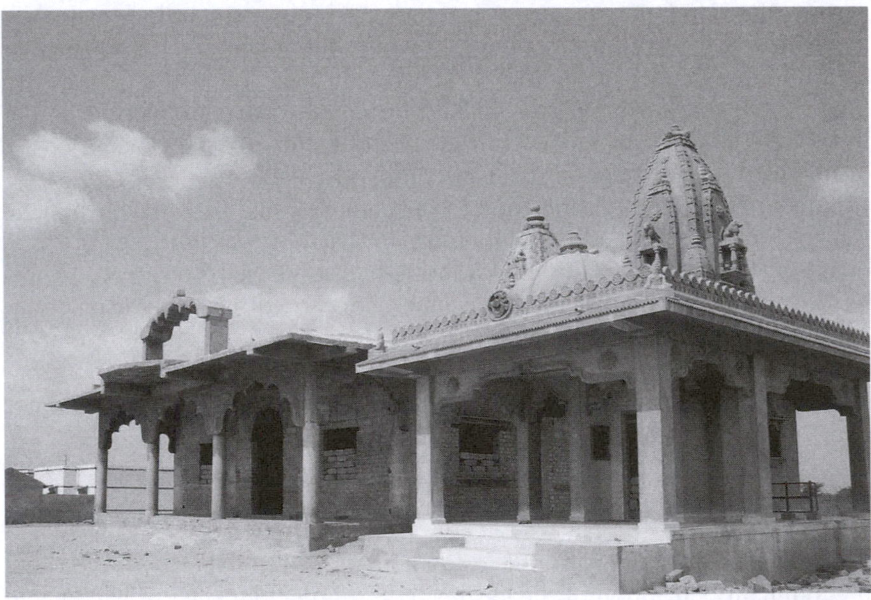

Figure 3.8 New temples in Chandrani. Due to widespread post-earthquake fear of the use of stones, replicas of traditional stone temples built with concrete can be seen in Chandrani village, Gujarat.

random rubble masonry. A good-quality stone construction following some basic principles of earthquake safety, such as use of well-cut stones from the right quarry, good bonding, the right mix of mortar and 'through stones' at regular intervals, could perform well against an earthquake. The issue is also linked to the thresholds of safety that one may accept for residential constructions; in the face of shortages of available resources, it might be acceptable to optimize (and not maximize) these thresholds so that there are more comparatively safer structures rather than fewer ones with very high factors of safety.

Therefore, instead of discouraging the use of stone, it would have been more effective to encourage good construction practices in stone constructions, since not only would these be readily available but also the services of artisans who are used to working with stone could have been better utilized.

General misperceptions abound for modern technology as well. In Bhuj, 'modern' multi-storeyed apartment buildings were considered unsafe after the earthquake, and new multi-storeyed constructions were banned. The residents of the existing buildings were supposed to be relocated. In fact, many of them continue to live in these unsafe buildings, as they do not have much income and also do not own land to build their own houses. Moreover, surrendering the land to the government in anticipation of financial compensation is a difficult proposition due to multiple ownerships. Thus they had to stick to the available buildings, fully recognizing the risk that they were taking. Rather than blindly condemning all the multi-storeyed/taller buildings as unsafe from earthquakes and totally banning their construction, the responsible agencies should have disseminated appropriate design and technology considerations to make these structures safer. The fact is that RCC-framed structures with solid brick infill on the ground floor are certainly much safer than the soft-storey structures that were heavily damaged in the earthquake (Figure 3.9).

Another example of misperception is the blind acceptance of earthquake as the culmination of the wrath of God, leading many people to accept it as an unavoidable event and thus overlook the need for earthquake-safe building technology. For example, in a reconstructed part of Bhuj, although the residents showed great concern over the possibility of a destructive earthquake in the near future, ironically these very literate people had invested all their savings into new unsafe constructions, considering the earthquake risk to be their destiny.

The economic factor: link with livelihoods

The 2001 earthquake had unforeseen and irreversible implications. For example, the rehabilitation packages, the new industries that came in after the earthquake due to agencies such as the Bhuj Area Development Authority (BhADA) expanding industrial benefits to them, various new technologies and materials that were introduced and the exposure that local people got all

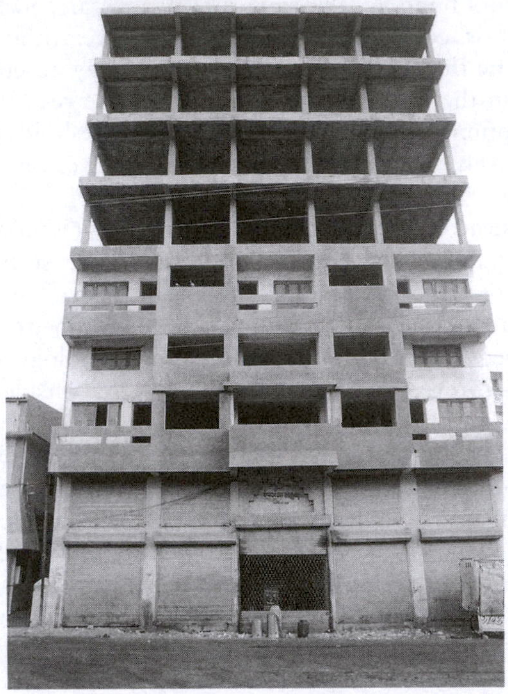

Figure 3.9 A multi-storeyed concrete-framed building in Bhuj. Due to widespread fear, a multi-storeyed concrete-framed building constructed just before the earthquake is lying abandoned in Bhuj, even though it did not sustain any damage from the earthquake.

actually changed life in Kutch in a unique manner. These changes resulted in far-reaching consequences for the previously underdeveloped urban and rural economy of the region. Unfortunately, the benefits of the new opportunities have not reached all sections of the community. In fact this dichotomy is most apparent when one takes a comparative look at the housing used by the rural and the urban today.

Different strategies were adopted for urban and for rural reconstruction. The difference has been apparent from the planning and strategy phases through to the execution stage. As mentioned before, in the urban areas such as Bhuj, the government announced a blanket ban on any construction until the master plan was ready, and no NGO or developmental agency was allowed to build post-earthquake. However, the preparation of the master plan took a considerably long time, although the financial package announced remained unchanged. Thus the package announced in 2001 became grossly inadequate when the actual construction started in 2003–04. Though the land was available at the same price as at the time of the announcement of the scheme, costs of all other components had increased considerably.

When the financial package was announced, the government pledged to provide the building materials at a subsidized rate. However, a quick check of the prices over time of the same materials shows the true picture. Cement pledged at 100 INR per cement bag at that time was, in 2008, at 220 INR; and steel bars, which were 17 INR per bar, cost 50 INR in August 2008 (one rupee equals 0.02364 US dollars as per interbank exchange rate on 3 August 2008).[9]

By a rough estimate, the mandatory 250-square-foot (approximately 25 square metres) construction, which was proposed at the rate of 120 INR per square foot (~1200 INR per square metre), is now approximately 400 INR per square foot (~4000 INR per square metre). Accounting for the high inflation rate, the goal of building earthquake-safe structures, at least in the urban areas, looks very grim.

Moreover, as mentioned before, the compensation for reconstruction was tied closely to the construction work. Therefore, the financial assistance was sanctioned against completion of a certain extent of the construction. The government's refusal to provide assistance for livelihoods in the urban sector hit the urban lower-middle-class and lower-class people very badly. The major grievance voiced against the entire relief package was that the programme did not take into consideration how livelihood options could have really made the process owner-driven. In fact, the common refrain remains that the Gujarati people, as industrious as people in any other part of the world, could have made the repair of their houses on their own had the government allowed them the easiest path to attain financial stability. The ability of the poor to undertake safer construction was severely compromised, in spite of the availability of technical expertise.

This policy stance made the situation of the urban poor really deplorable, as they were forced to reside in unsafe housing. In fact, many people were left with houses that had parts severely damaged due to the earthquake; they often shut down the damaged part and continued to live in the existing unsafe section of the house after sprucing it up from outside.

The towns had a high percentage of tenants. Some of these people have been residing in the houses they have occupied for several decades. Post-earthquake, they found themselves in a worse situation, as the packages announced by the government – being linked to buildings – had no place for this segment of the population. Also, in many cases, they did not have documents supporting their tenancy and subsequent rights to be compensated. In some instances, the owners whose houses were damaged decided to opt for relocation by surrendering their damaged property in the old town to the government, even if that meant further damaging the buildings to avail themselves of better compensation in return. This left the tenants, who had been residing in those houses, homeless. In fact, in certain localities of Bhuj, people are still living in the initial tent provided by various relief agencies (Figures 3.10 and 3.11).

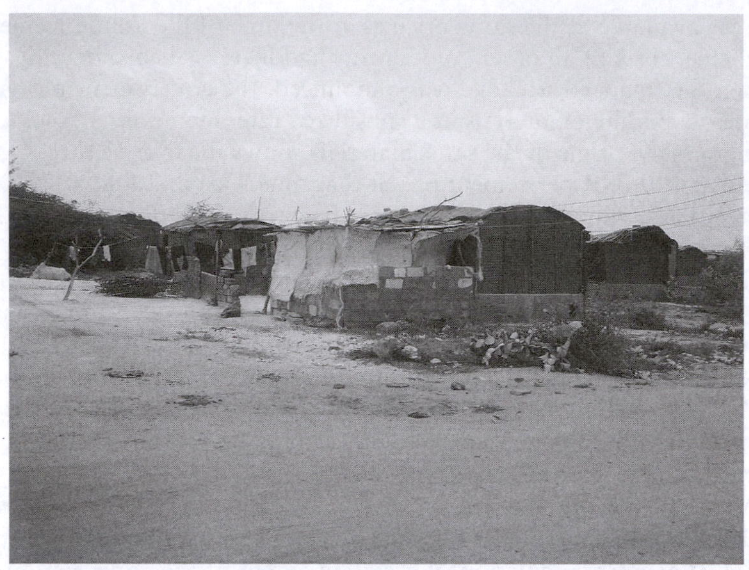

Figure 3.10 Temporary structures in Bhuj. Urban poor in Bhuj are still residing in temporary structures, even after seven years. The additions have subsequently been made using a variety of materials.

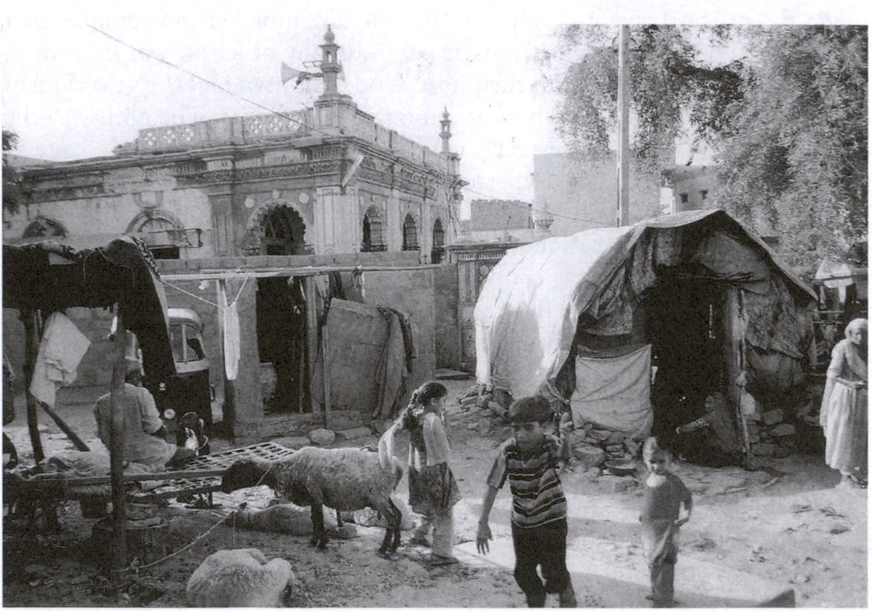

Figure 3.11 Temporary structures built by urban squatters in Bhuj. These structures use a variety of materials such as stones, mud blocks and canvas, and are highly vulnerable.

Similar issues were confronted in Bhachao, where not only did tenants continue to stay in damaged houses, but vacant lands and houses that were acquired by the government were encroached on by people migrating from rural areas in search of the better livelihood opportunities that became available during reconstruction. Due to the lack of secure tenure, these constructions are understandably of poor quality.

In rural areas, due to better economic opportunities, the rural poor have largely benefited from the various interventions and economic packages announced by several organizations and by the government. For example, although the initial days were bad for the craftsmen engaged in handicrafts, the sector recuperated pretty fast, since it was not infrastructure intensive. Also, the exposure to the outside world actually helped these craftsmen market their skills and various products to an international client base much more easily. For example, a village namely Bhujouri consists of several national-award-winner weaver families. The youngsters of this village now often participate in various international trade fairs by learning about them through the Internet. Also, the rural folk can get back to their traditional occupations of agriculture and animal husbandry.

As stated before, most of the constructions that are going on in the rural sector are basically expansions of the existing structures. Though some rules of safety are being violated, the massive loss of life that the 2001 earthquake created may not be the case if another earthquake happens in the future.

Lessons learnt

Any technology can be considered successful only if it gets internalized in the local building culture. However, this necessitates certain preconditions which go beyond its material and design aspects.

Technology introduced during post-disaster reconstruction should not be seen purely in the 'technical sense'. Rather, it should be based on certain basic parameters pertaining to the particular society in which it is used, thus allowing the technology to have a character that is specific yet adaptable, enabling it to undergo generic change from within rather than forced change from outside.

Technology, whether it is traditional, modern or alternative, will only be successful if it caters to multiple criteria. Of course, hazard safety is one of the primary concerns in disaster-prone areas, but equally (if not more) important are the considerations of economic viability, cultural compatibility and climatic suitability that govern the particular context. An appropriate solution would therefore involve necessary trade-offs between these factors to achieve viable alternatives, although this may necessitate optimization and not maximization of earthquake safety.

Moreover, technology should not be seen as a rigid design package to be provided on a palette to the affected communities. A technology is essentially a process for which appropriate design and delivery mechanisms need to be created and institutionalized to ensure its long-term sustainability. This means that technology introduced as a 'product' must be linked to this process right from the time of its conception. This is indeed a painfully slow process, and it requires mechanisms that support the local capacity to *innovate* and not merely *duplicate* what is provided to the beneficiaries.

The process of developing a technology should not be a one-way process in which experts develop 'appropriate' solutions for the local community. Rather it should be seen as a two-way communication carried out through equal engagement of experts and the local community, whereby the latter can contribute with their knowledge and skills that have been acquired over time through direct or indirect experience while the former contribute with knowledge developed through scientific research and experimentation.

Eminent Brazilian communication theorist Paulo Freire has shown in his book *Pedagogy of the Oppressed* how the poor and the deprived can actually use communication to empower their situation with no or minimal outside interference.[2] He talked about a new form of development communication process, namely 'development support communication', in which the goal was to provide minimal support from outside in the actual development task and to provide support related specifically to the communication part that is supplemental in bringing about the development itself. It ensures equal rights to the communicator and the recipient, allowing the message to have the required balance of *exchange* of information, in turn allowing the communication to actually support the overall development process.

It would be pertinent to mention here that rather than categorizing traditional and scientific knowledge into mutually exclusive domains, attempts should be made to recover 'scientific' aspects of traditional knowledge and the 'traditional' aspects of scientific knowledge. While the former will enable traditional knowledge systems to be easily understood by professionals, the latter would demand that larger scientific concepts get translated into modes of communication that are locally understood.[6]

The final outcome comes through comprehension based on sound knowledge rather than through perception based on the mere feeding of information. At present, there seems to be a deep division between the perceptions of what is 'modern' and what is 'traditional'. The former carries within itself the notion of progress of 'backward' traditional communities; the latter either implies outdated knowledge or nostalgic images to be romanticized. Unfortunately such misconceptions seem to have taken over the ability to understand what a good building is, as a result of which the ability of the local communities to engage in the creative evolution of safer and viable technology is severely compromised.[5]

It is important that the local community be sufficiently informed and empowered to take the most appropriate decisions on technology development and use. While the role of NGOs cannot be underestimated, it is critical to recognize the role of local governance in enabling a continuous transition from post-disaster to the normal development phase, which is when most of the external organizations retreat or shift their priorities to other areas. Active engagement of local government is therefore necessary right from the time key decisions for reconstruction are made in the immediate aftermath of the disaster. This was sadly lacking in the case of Gujarat.

Another important aspect noted in Gujarat is that the technological options that were introduced post-earthquake were essentially materials driven. Indeed, in many cases, the focus was on the development of technology for specific building materials. While this may be one of the essential components of a reconstruction programme, it is certainly not the only one. A comprehensive approach that integrates materials with construction systems as well as with architectural design is indeed necessary for technological success.

Finally, it is crucial to consider the inherent link between technology and the local economic situation, which is part of the larger developmental context in which the reconstruction takes place. It is important therefore to link physical reconstruction with the rehabilitation of livelihoods after the disaster. At the same time, it is important to create sufficient mechanisms to enable the poor to have access to safer technology that would reduce their vulnerability to future disasters.

Acknowledgement

The author acknowledges the technical support provided by Mr Sayantan Chakrabarti during the writing of this chapter.

4 Planning for temporary housing

Cassidy Johnson

In the aftermath of a disaster, temporary housing provides a place affected families can call 'home', a place where they can begin to recover from the tragedy while permanent rebuilding takes place. Forms of temporary housing vary from prefabricated units, provided in a top-down manner, to makeshift shacks erected on the roadside by families themselves. Strategic planning undertaken prior to the disaster can greatly improve temporary housing projects, both in the short and long terms.

Temporary housing projects are often criticised for being economically, socially and environmentally unsustainable. However, it can be argued that temporary housing provides an essential service to disaster-affected families, who need to recover their lives and livelihoods as soon as possible. In many post-disaster situations, the reconstruction of permanent housing takes several months to even start and probably a number of years to complete. So families need a place to resume their daily life, even if it's a temporary solution. Temporary housing takes on many different physical forms, from wooden shacks to more elaborate prefabricated buildings. Forms of provision are equally varied; housing may be provided through centralised top-down means or self-built by the affected families themselves.

This chapter offers an overall look at temporary housing and outlines key points about how to improve temporary housing. It is argued that the sustainability of temporary housing can be improved through strategic planning made upfront before the disaster. Specifically, the chapter proposes:

- a typology of temporary housing;
- key concerns in planning for temporary housing, as well as planning for its obsolescence.

The work draws particularly on the case study of the recovery from the 1999 earthquakes in Turkey, with additional information drawn from other international case studies.

What is temporary housing?

Temporary housing, sometimes referred to as transitional housing,[17] is both a stage in the social processes of recovery and a physical type of house.

After a disaster, housing recovery occurs in distinct stages; these stages may overlap, and not all affected families will pass through each stage. Quarantelli defined the housing recovery stages as follows: in the (brief) period during the height of the emergency, affected families are in the *emergency sheltering* stage; once the height of the emergency has passed, *temporary sheltering* is employed in the initial days after the disaster and is usually accompanied by provision of food and medical attention; third is *temporary housing*, where families can hopefully return to a semblance of normal daily living, albeit in a temporary place; fourth and finally is *permanent housing*, which may follow several months to several years later (see first chapter for a detailed discussion on the stages of post-disaster housing).[14]

In the *social* sense, temporary housing refers to being housed for a short time in a place where one can resume normal daily activities after the disaster. Temporary housing is meant to help people recover more because it enables autonomy in daily life to be established relatively quickly even though permanent reconstruction might barely be underway. In the temporary housing stage, families usually have a private living space and a place to cook their own meals so will feel better able to resume the activities of normal daily life.

Temporary housing in the *physical* sense can take on many different forms, depending on the particular country or whether it is in a rural or urban context. For example, a temporary house may be a prefabricated house, a mobile trailer, a shipping container, a rented apartment or a self-built shack.

Not all temporary houses are the same in terms of cost, level of comfort and accompanying services. Most importantly, temporary housing needs to be comfortable enough, with an adequate level of services, to enable people to live in dignity without 'breaking the bank' – either for the family, the state or the NGO (whoever is providing the houses). It is vitally important that the provision of temporary housing does not reduce the ability to provide good and safe permanent housing, as it is the permanent housing that will enable the community and its members to move towards full recovery.

From a survey of different forms of temporary houses employed after recent disasters, it is possible to consider a typology of temporary housing.[9] Some types require construction of new units, while others do not. While it is usually more cost-efficient to use existing buildings for temporary housing, there may be some social drawbacks to this.

Types of temporary housing that do not require new construction include:

- *Staying with family or friends*. The affected families stay with extended family or friends who live in or away from the disaster-affected area. Although this does not involve much resource expenditure, the families' recovery tends to suffer due to a lack of privacy and a feeling that they are imposing on their host. In most cultures this type of temporary housing is adequate for a short period but in most cases not for more than a few months.

- *Rented apartments*. If, after a disaster, there remains a stock of undamaged apartments, governments may lease or subsidise the rental of these apartments for affected families. In some situations, there may be an offer for families to evacuate to nearby areas, especially tourist areas in the off-season. Using rental apartments as temporary housing is economically sustainable, as it reduces the need for heavy resource expenditure in buildings and infrastructure. However, the numbers of such apartments are usually limited, and this approach is more an option for smaller-scale or localised disasters. One of the drawbacks is that the subsidies given to the affected families may have the effect of inflating the prices of rental housing generally and therefore may affect renters who may not be part of the programme.
- *Public facilities*. Families stay in public buildings that are retrofitted as lodgings. Due to the lack of privacy afforded in these spaces, they are only adequate for a short stay of possibly a few weeks up to a few months if absolutely necessary.

Types of temporary housing that do require new construction include:

- *Self-built shelters*. Families themselves build a temporary shack out of available materials. Self-built shelters may be located on the family's land (if they have it), in a public space or on vacant land in their neighbourhood. Depending on the context, this solution may be adequate if the house the family is capable of building responds to their basic needs. Authorities may try to discourage the use of pubic land for temporary housing or may work on the behalf of the affected people to negotiate temporary land leases. At the same time, the families may be involved in other government programmes for social assistance and permanent housing or, on the contrary, they may be outside of any government system of post-disaster assistance.
- *Tents*. Tents are quick to erect and cost-efficient; in the few days following the disaster, families are provided with tents by humanitarian organisations or the military. Families may stay on in these tents past the emergency phase and into the temporary housing phase; however, depending on the quality of the tents, they may not be suitable for extended periods of use. Winterised tents, which have flooring and more durable sidewalls, are more suitable for use through the temporary housing phase (Figure 4.1). Families may even add small private kitchens and make use of communal bathroom facilities.
- *Shipping containers or mobile homes*. Preassembled transportable structures are delivered to the disaster area, used as temporary housing and

then recuperated for use in future disasters. These may be placed on a homeowner's land or in settlements.

- *Temporary housing units.* Provided by governments, NGOs and aid organisations, these are small self-contained houses, often constructed with prefabricated parts, that are built in settlements in and around the disaster-affected areas. Units may be stand-alone (detached) or attached. Each unit usually includes kitchen and bathroom facilities, or facilities are shared between a few adjacent units.

Temporary houses can be *clustered* in mass housing 'camps', or units can be individually *dispersed* on or near the property of the affected family (Figure 4.2). When possible, it is preferable that temporary houses be located on or near the family's property, as this avoids further disruption for family members and allows them to use existing services and stay close to the former home, thus maintaining social networks. However, this is not always possible. In high-density urban areas where families are living in apartments, there may not be enough available land nearby. Or if the entire infrastructure is wiped out in an area, it may be some time before water and electricity can be restored to a dispersed setting, so clustering is necessary, whatever the disadvantages might be.

Why is temporary housing necessary?

Experts agree that considerable investment in temporary housing is a priori not wise, because the costs of building temporary housing and then permanent housing amounts to rebuilding twice over.[5,7,16] However, the reality

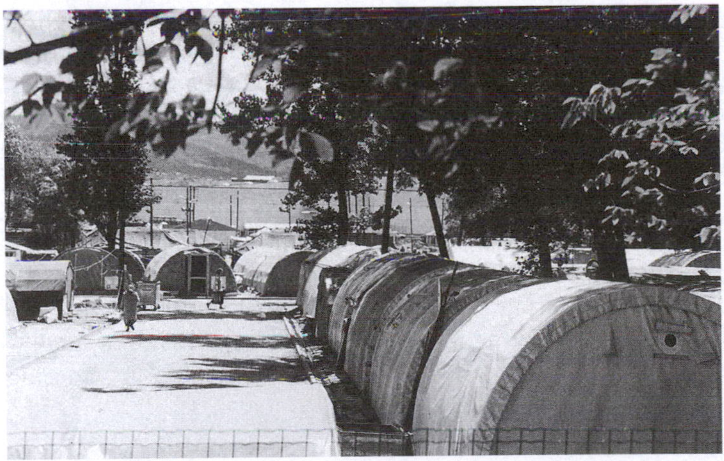

Figure 4.1 Winterised tents can be used as temporary housing. Kocaeli, Turkey.

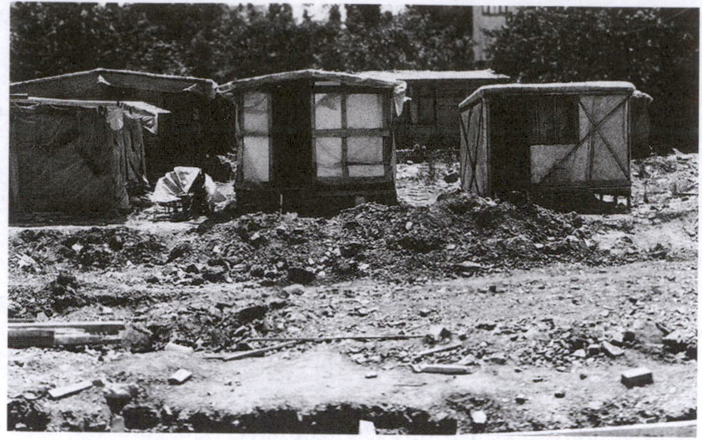

Figure 4.2 Self-built temporary housing units located on the roadway near the residents' damaged houses. Yalova, Turkey.

on the ground contradicts these expert opinions: some kind of temporary housing has been used after almost every major disaster in the last century. The most recent examples of temporary housing programmes are in the United States after Hurricane Katrina (2005), in Pakistan after the Kashmir earthquake (2005), in Thailand after the South-Asian tsunami (2004) and in Iran after the Bam earthquake (2003). Temporary housing is continually deployed after disasters so that families have a place to live, in dignity, until permanent housing is built. In a large-scale disaster, the numbers of people affected, the amount of damage to infrastructure and the overwhelming demand for building materials, contractors or even building permits can mean that permanent reconstruction takes time, at least several months and perhaps a couple of years. Furthermore, disputes over land rights, urban planning issues and obtaining adequate financing may delay operations, thus prolonging the permanent reconstruction period even further.

Even if the responding governments and NGOs adopt a policy of not providing temporary housing, families will often take it upon themselves to build their own temporary house. This is because disaster survivors do not wish to wait passively in tents or mass shelters for what may be at least several months for permanent housing to be rebuilt. For example, in Colombia after the 1999 earthquakes in Armenia, the government was slow in building temporary housing, favouring instead an accelerated permanent reconstruction programme; however, within months, the hillsides were full of small wooden shacks that families had erected for themselves as temporary housing.

The need for strategic planning

Temporary housing suffers from a major conceptual flaw – the fact that it may well turn out not to be temporary at all. While it is used to *temporarily* house families in the post-disaster period, the physical temporary housing units tend to become *permanent* fixtures in the community. Therefore, while temporary housing is required to meet the needs of families in the post-disaster period, it is also necessary to think about the long-term spectrum of temporary housing.

Empirical research on temporary housing programmes shows that strategic planning can greatly improve the outcomes of temporary housing, both for when temporary housing is used in the post-disaster period and in the longer term, after it is no longer needed as temporary housing.[11] Strategic planning is especially important for the temporary housing phase of reconstruction since decisions must be made extremely quickly, during the chaotic post-disaster period, about how to house homeless families. The time for adequate planning is so limited that there is a real risk that rushed choices will lead to problems later on. Put another way, quick decisions about *temporary* housing lead to *permanent* impacts on development.

Strategic planning, instigated by governments upfront before the disaster, can help to allocate resources for temporary housing (materials, land, financing) in case a disaster does occur (Figure 4.3). It can enable temporary housing to be available more quickly and to better meet the needs of affected families in the short term, as well as in the long term. As listed in Figure 4.3, part of the process of strategic planning requires knowledge of several key concerns, such as the possible types of temporary housing, how many people are likely to be in need of temporary housing for a given disaster, the time estimated for permanent reconstruction and the availability of sites for construction. These key concerns – which are explained in greater detail below – need to be understood before strategic plans can be drawn up. Once the strategic plan is created, it can be kept on hold, ready if, or when, a disaster occurs. If a disaster does occur, the plan must be updated tactically to meet the current situation, but it can draw on the existing information in the strategic plan.

1999 earthquakes in Turkey

On 17 August and 12 November 1999, two devastating earthquakes struck the Marmara and Bolu regions of Turkey, affecting the largely industrial areas to the east of the Istanbul metropolis. The two earthquakes reportedly killed over 18,000 people, injured over 45,000 people and rendered an estimated 250,000 people homeless.

In addition to immediate rescue operations and psychological, medical and nutritional aid, the government responded to this overwhelming emergency with a three-stage housing recovery strategy:

- Emergency shelters: tents, both canvas and winterised types, were provided in the early days after the earthquake and were set up in camps and along roadways.
- Planning for temporary housing began shortly after the August earthquake, and while the first units were made available within a couple of months, construction of temporary housing continued for several months, finishing in the summer of 2000. In total, 40,621 temporary housing units had been built, 9282 by NGOs and 31,339 by the government.
- The temporary housing was followed by an extensive government-initiated permanent housing programme, lasting over five years, which rehoused some 43,000 families in a range of different accommodations through a variety of procurement strategies. In addition to this, NGOs, community groups and individual families also built permanent housing.

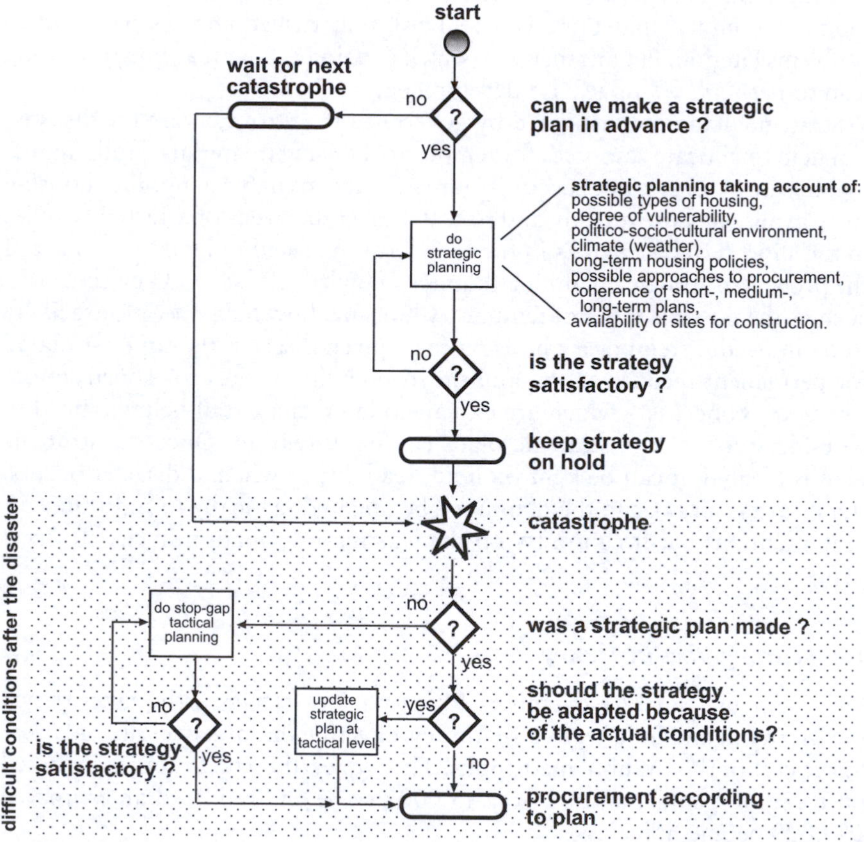

Figure 4.3 Strategic planning for temporary housing is better done before the catastrophe strikes (adapted from Johnson[11]).

I use the case study of the temporary housing programme after the 1999 earthquakes in the Marmara region of Turkey to explain the key concerns for strategic planning of temporary housing.[2,9,10,12] While the main case study is from Turkey, I also draw on findings from other case studies of temporary housing programmes in Colombia in 1999,[12] Japan in 1995,[3,8,13,15] Greece in 1986,[4] Mexico City in 1985[3] and Italy in 1976.[1,6,7] I make a distinction between planning temporary housing in the post-disaster period and planning for temporary housing in the long term, since a temporary housing programme needs to respond to both of these criteria in a clear manner.

Key concerns for temporary housing in the post-disaster period

In the post-disaster period, there are several concerns that a temporary housing programme must respond to and these are: timing of delivery, the approach to providing housing or enabling families to build their own housing, the cost and design of the temporary housing unit, the location, and access to services and maintaining social networks.

Timing

The most crucial factor for temporary housing is the speed of delivery; it must be available as quickly as possible after the disaster. Families need a secure and private place to regain their autonomy and begin recovery, and past experience shows that too much time spent in tents and receiving aid is detrimental to a family's recovery process.

In order to speed up the process for temporary housing, certain decisions can be planned for before a disaster occurs. For example, agreements can be drawn up for procurement of units with domestic or international suppliers, and responsibilities for temporary housing can be designated within local or central governments. Also planning for potential locations for temporary housing and planning for installation of the necessary infrastructure to support the settlements can save time in the post-disaster situation.

In the Turkish case, some temporary housing units were available in early November 1999; however, it took nearly ten months, until June 2000, to complete all of the settlements. While supply of the units and installation of infrastructure went smoothly, the main hindrance to making housing available quickly was the lack of suitable sites. Finding large tracts of empty land, preferably government-owned and located near the city centres, proved to be time-consuming. Learning from this experience, the Istanbul Metropolitan Municipality has, within its emergency planning process, already pre-designated locations for erecting temporary housing in the case of a disaster.

Striking a balance between providing and enabling

The organisational structure of temporary housing projects usually falls at the two ends of the spectrum: either they are top-down, and a turnkey solution is completely provided by the government or NGO, or they are totally bottom-up, and housing is built through self-help. Few temporary housing projects take a middle-of-the-road approach, such as an owner-driven government-financed model. Part of the reason may be the imperative to build temporary housing as soon as possible.

The temporary housing programme in Turkey after the 1999 earthquakes was, as most reconstruction programmes are in Turkey, facilitated through a top-down process whereby all necessary components for the temporary housing phase were provided by the government or, in some cases, by government/NGO partnerships. The residents had nothing do with the decision-making for temporary housing; they were simply allocated a house once the units were completed. This was not necessarily a negative point, since the units were built quickly and families were overall positive about the units.

However, once the settlements had been built, some of the NGO projects turned over the management of the settlement to a residents' association, which in at least one project turned out to be a success. Some people started small businesses to offer services, and even teenagers were charged with running the community drop-in centre.

Cost and unit design

One of the biggest problems with temporary housing programmes is that they are extremely expensive in relation to their lifespan. The cost for building the unit and infrastructure, the maintenance and finally the de-installation may amount to almost as much per square metre as permanent housing (as found by Geipel in his research on the Friuli earthquake).[7] Since costs for temporary housing are usually borne by the government or NGOs, expenditures on temporary housing can reduce the budget for permanent housing; obviously, every effort must be made to keep with cost per unit to a minimum.

The cost is very much related to the unit design and choice of materials. The most important aspect of design is that it provides a private and safe place for the family to go about their daily activities. However, what can be considered an appropriate design and level of comfort is very much dictated by local housing standards. In many countries, a basic wood unit, as long as it has access to a kitchen and a bathroom (preferably private), may be considered satisfactory as temporary housing. In more developed countries, high-quality prefabricated units are usually supplied after disasters, such as the trailers provided by the Federal Emergency Management Agency (FEMA) after Hurricane Katrina.

In Turkey there were several types of units employed. Basic one-room wood units, built by a local NGO, offered a private kitchen and bathroom and cost about US$1000, whereas government-supplied two-room units built from prefabricated panels and corrugated aluminium exteriors cost US$3300 per unit (Figure 4.4).

The large expenditure on temporary housing can be offset if the design of the unit allows for reuse for another function after the unit is no longer

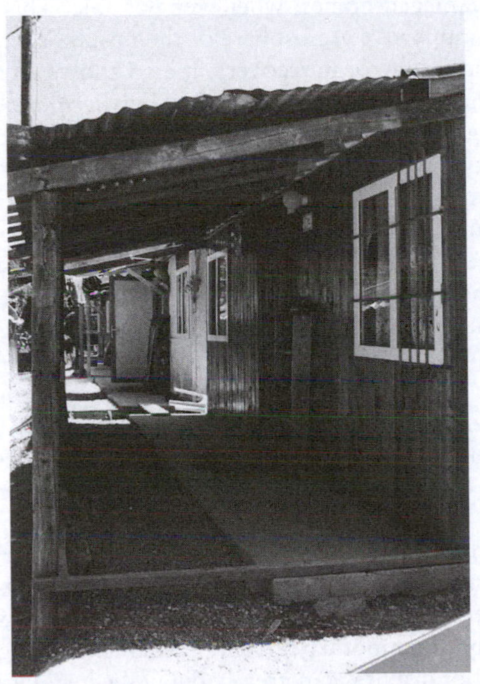

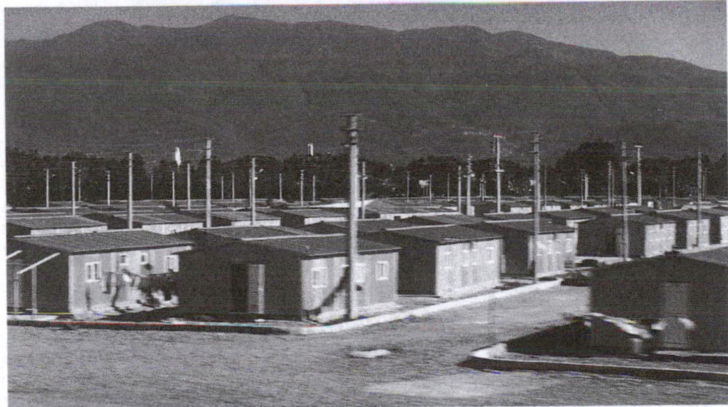

Figure 4.4 Temporary housing units. **Top:** Basic temporary housing units made of wood. **Bottom:** More elaborate prefabricated units. Düzce province, Turkey.

needed for temporary housing. This idea is explored later in the section on 'the second life of temporary housing'.

Location: access to services and maintaining social networks

Experience shows that temporary housing should be located in the city, near to the families' damaged homes, whenever possible. This allows people to benefit from the supportive atmosphere of their established social networks, which is an important factor in recovery. It also allows them to remain close to their jobs or income-generating activities. Furthermore, it reduces overall costs of the programme because it allows residents to draw on existing services in the city, such as schools, clinics, bus lines and garbage collection routes, rather than having to provide new services that are not established. Temporary housing may be clustered in small settlements on available tracts of land within the city or located along roadways if necessary.

On the other hand, it may often be quicker to build large settlements of temporary housing outside of the city, because land is more readily available and more houses can be erected at once. However, outer locations will also require a greater expenditure in services. Furthermore, moving inner-city families to the outskirts for temporary housing has been found to lead to social isolation and to problems in finding work. A frequent and inexpensive transport service is necessary if a periphery location for temporary housing is chosen.

In either case, residents of the local neighbourhood may resist a temporary housing settlement being located in their community. This was the case in several places after Hurricane Katrina in the United States, where families felt uncomfortable about temporary housing settlements being located close to them. These types of disputes can greatly delay the installation of temporary housing and create tension between communities.

In Turkey, temporary housing settlements were located both on the outskirts of the cities and in inner-city locations. Outer locations were for very large settlements, sometimes as large as 2000 units; these settlements were fully functioning communities, complete with schools, child care, medical clinics, cafés, markets, postal services, community centres and the like. Smaller settlements in the inner cities were mostly built by NGOs, who only needed small parcels of land for their projects. While some projects included a community centre, there were very few services provided in these smaller projects.

Key concerns for temporary housing in the long term

While the points above outline key concerns for temporary housing in the post-disaster period, there are also concerns for improving temporary housing in the long term. As is explored below, planning for temporary housing needs to consider the overall reconstruction strategy with a view to understanding how long families are expected to stay in temporary housing.

Furthermore, planning also needs to consider what will become of the units once they are no longer needed as temporary housing.

The need for an overall reconstruction strategy

Ian Davis, in his book *Shelter after Disaster*, advocates a strategy whereby the reconstruction of permanent housing is accelerated, thus reducing the need for temporary housing.[5] My research supports that proposition because, as stated earlier, if temporary housing consumes disproportionate amounts of the financial resources, it may limit resources for the permanent housing. In reality, however, accelerated reconstruction is often not possible because of complications with the permanent reconstruction.

Complications in permanent reconstruction are all too common, and sometimes it can take several years before permanent housing is built. For example, after the South-Asian tsunami, it took many months just to come to an agreement about how far permanent housing had to be set back from the shore. Furthermore, there were many issues with regards to evictions and tenure, which further delayed permanent reconstruction in some areas (see Chapter 7). In New Orleans, the urban planning process has been lengthy and has meant that many households (especially the poor) have not been able to resettle permanently, as of the end of 2008 (see Chapter 6).

Empirical research on temporary housing programmes reveals two different models of overall reconstruction strategy:

1 Relatively small investments in temporary housing – basic structures with little services – with the majority of government financing and organisational capacity going into permanent reconstruction right away (i.e. Davis's model).
2 Large investments in temporary housing – providing higher-quality housing and fully serviced settlements that will be inhabited for three or more years before permanent housing becomes available. Under this model, permanent housing may not even be started before two years have elapsed after the disaster, due to complications with planning for the permanent housing.

Model 1 was the case in Mexico City after the 1985 earthquake and in Colombia after the 1999 earthquake. In Mexico City, temporary housing was built, but it was very rudimentary and was located on the roadways next to the destroyed buildings.[3] In Colombia, the families mostly built temporary housing themselves, with some support from NGOs. These relatively small investments allowed for human and financial capital to be focused on the permanent housing right away. In these cases, temporary housing was only proposed as a stopgap to shelter families while works for permanent reconstruction were in progress.

This can be contrasted with what happened in Turkey after the 1999 earthquakes. The choice to make large investments in temporary housing (estimated at US$225 million) had many people worried that there would be little left over to finance permanent rebuilding. Due to the widespread damage over several urbanised areas, the government expected that permanent housing would take two or more years to complete; therefore appropriate loans were sought from the World Bank and the European Development Bank to help finance the permanent housing. In point of fact, families lived in the temporary housing for up to three years and in some cases for longer.

As is revealed here by both models and the cases they illustrate, *a strategy for the overall reconstruction is necessary at the outset and then planning for temporary housing can work within this strategy.* If permanent housing can be built relatively quickly (within several months) and there are few complications with regards to land rights or urban planning, then investments in temporary housing can be kept to a minimum and the emphasis can be on permanent reconstruction. However, if the extent of destroyed houses is very severe or if it is anticipated that there will be any delays with the permanent reconstruction, then more comfortable and well-serviced temporary housing will be necessary for longer occupancy.

The second life of temporary housing

The very fact that temporary housing is intended only for temporary use (i.e. a few months or a few years) suggests that it is worthwhile to think about a secondary function for it. However, in order to maximise efficiency, this 'second life' of temporary housing must be planned for from the outset of the programme.

There are five major options for the second life of temporary housing. These are: 1) rental housing; 2) reuse; 3) recycling parts; 4) temporary houses as 'cores' for permanent houses; and 5) refurbishment of the units and storage for the next disaster. Each one of these outcomes is explored in detail below.

RENTAL HOUSING

The case studies show that in post-disaster situations, there is always a shortage of affordable rental housing in the market. Rental housing is usually the last type of housing to be replaced, and the cost of renting most often increases in the aftermath of a disaster, pricing the poor out of the market. Temporary housing, especially if it is of decent quality and is well located, may be used as rental housing in its second life. Factors to consider in planning for this reuse are: management of the rental housing, transfer of ownership (if necessary, i.e. from the state to the local levels of government or to the private sector), ownership of the land or lease of the land for longer terms. Even if renting is not a formalised option, squatters may inhabit temporary housing. In Turkey, several projects, especially those located in the inner city, became rental housing for some families. Residents made an effort to improve their houses by adding gardens, exterior cladding and, if they were allowed, additional rooms (Figure 4.5).

REUSE

Units that were used for temporary housing may be reused for another purpose, even at another location. For example, in Turkey, in one temporary housing project, the used temporary housing units were donated to the local school by the sponsoring NGO. The units were disassembled, transported across town and reassembled as additional classrooms attached to the main school building. The design of the housing lent itself to this sort of reuse: 200 m^2, single-storey buildings made of steel structure with prefabricated sandwich panels contained eight 25 m^2 temporary housing units. The steel structure allowed the building to be easily transported, and the interior partitions could be removed or reconfigured to allow for flexibility in interior spaces. In another project, the local university purchased the used temporary housing units for use on its campus as student dormitories. The reuse of temporary housing in a new location of course requires more investment because there are costs associated with taking down the units, transporting them and reassembling them. Furthermore, the units must be designed with

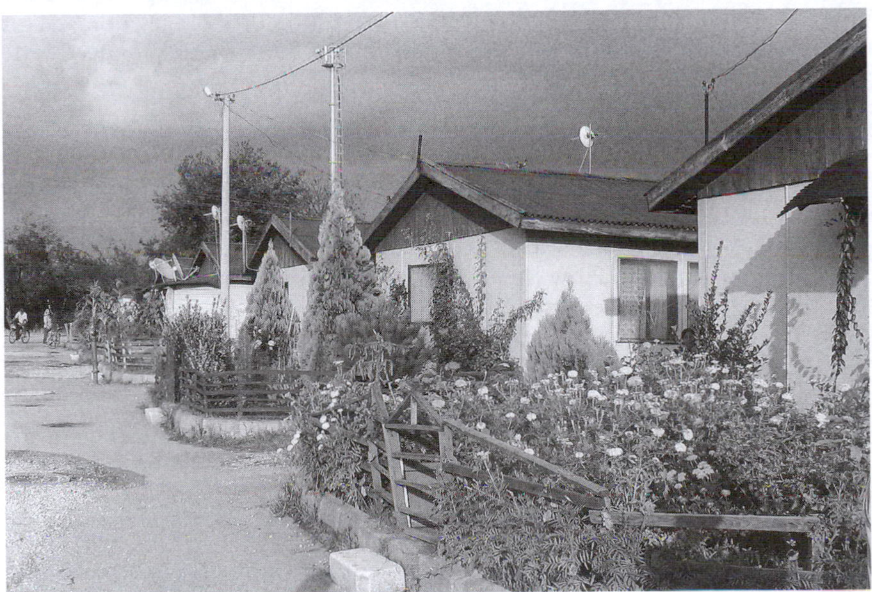

Figure 4.5 Rental housing. This temporary housing project has become rental housing, and residents have cultivated gardens. Düzce, Turkey.

flexible interior spaces to accommodate different functions and must be strong enough to withstand the move.

RECYCLING OF PARTS

Parts of the units may also be recycled into new uses. This can be a solution if the temporary housing units are, say, basic wood structures, since it might not be possible to reuse them as a whole. Indeed, the doors, windows, fixtures and pieces of wood can be extremely useful for permanent rebuilding. It is best if the parts can be donated to families or sold at very low prices; however, some legal mechanism may be needed to make this happen. As explained in Chapter 1, in Colombia after the 1999 earthquake, when it came time to dismantle the temporary housing, families wanted to take parts of the housing for their own use. However, this opportunity was missed, as the housing was the property of the government and therefore it could not be donated to private citizens.[12]

CORE HOUSES

One of the most sustainable ways to design temporary housing is through an approach in which the basic unit used for housing families in the emergency becomes the 'core' for a larger permanent house. The initial base unit may contain the plumbing and electrical services and a small amount of living space. Once resources allow, the family can add more living space onto the unit, as well as a more formal entrance, a veranda or storage rooms. This model works well in rural, peri-urban settings or anywhere where the family has their own plot of land on which to build. It allows the family to expand the house to meet their needs and within their budget.

This approach becomes more complicated if a family is landless; in some cases, the temporary house can be moved later to a plot of land where the family can stay permanently.

In Turkey, there was not a formal temporary housing programme using the core house model. However, many individual land-owning families did just this; they obtained a temporary housing unit, placed it on their land, and built a permanent house around the basic unit (Figure 4.6). Designs varied widely according to individual families' needs and tastes, but in my findings, the houses were all a source of pride for the family.

REFURBISHMENT AND STORAGE

Temporary housing units can be collected once the temporary housing phase is over, to be refurbished and stored away ready for use in the next emergency. This tends to be what most governments plan for in their temporary housing programmes. However, in reality, the costs of effectively storing temporary housing units for what might be many years can be extremely expensive.

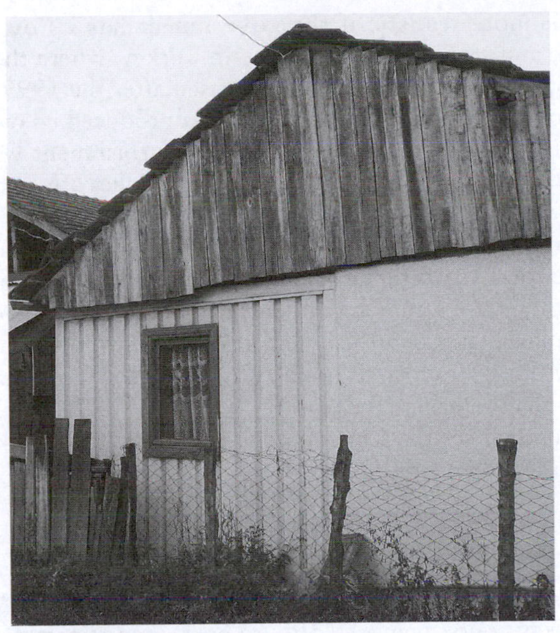

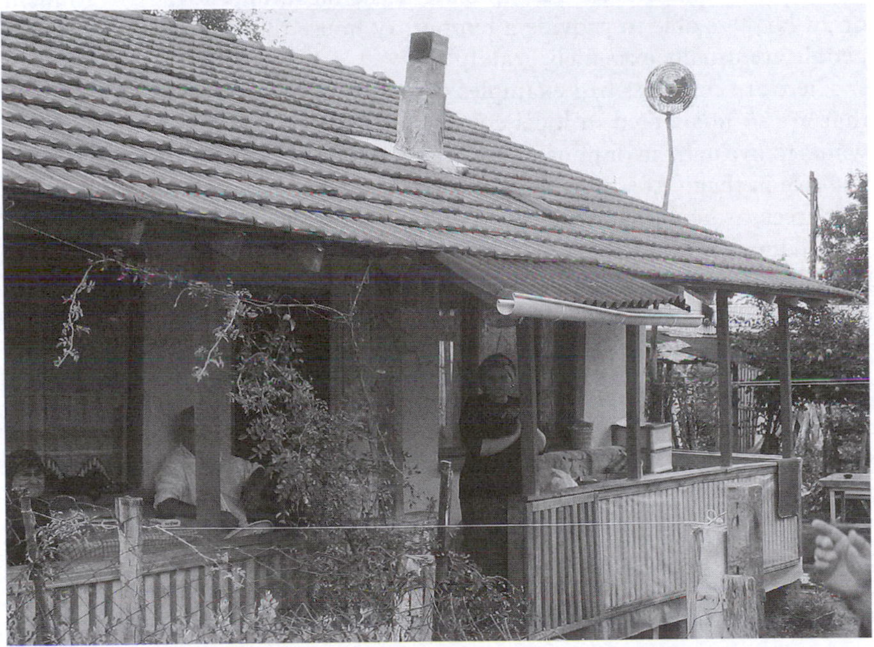

Figure 4.6 Core house. A shipping container was used as a temporary house and then additions were built around it to make a permanent house. **Top:** Side view of house showing shipping container. **Bottom:** Front view of house. Düzce, Turkey.

This option is more realistic if the government has its own facility for refurbishment and storage, as is the case in Turkey, where the government collected some of the container-type units used after the 1999 earthquakes. The facility, located in Ankara, had in the past produced its own temporary housing, so it was well equipped to do the refurbishment work. Some of the renovated units were sent to Bam to house families affected by the 2003 earthquake.

If the government has purchased units from a private manufacturer and plans to store them for future use, refurbishment work should be part of the contract, otherwise it may be difficult to obtain replacement parts years later. In the United States, refurbishment and storage was the common model used by FEMA for its trailers, although now FEMA is more likely to sell the trailers rather than refurbish them.

Table 4.1 summarises the key concerns for temporary housing, as raised above, and outlines some points for strategic planning.

Closing remarks

No one wants to, or plans to, lose their home in a disaster. When it does happen, people of course want their house back as soon as possible, but they also need a comfortable place to stay in the meantime. If the government or an NGO is able to provide a temporary house that suits people's needs, people are usually extremely grateful.

There are countless bad examples of temporary housing projects; designs that are so ill-adapted to local cultural or climatic conditions that no one wants to live in them or houses that are so inconveniently located that no one *can* live in them. At worst, temporary housing projects are a total waste of resources, as families completely abandon badly designed projects in favour of building their own shacks. At best, families are able to modify these units to meet their needs.

My argument here is that it is possible to make better temporary housing, that is, housing that is suited to the distinct needs of the disaster-affected families. However, in order to do this, forethought is needed on the part of the government and local authorities (or some cases NGOs) about how to best go about temporary housing. This includes thinking about what types of units are best suited to the cultural and climatic conditions, who can supply them and where they could be located. This also includes thinking about what services are needed to go along with the housing and what will happen to the units in the long run.

Table 4.1 Key concerns for planning temporary housing

What makes a good temporary housing programme?	*What needs to be planned in advance?*
Quickly available	Delegate responsibilities in advance Procurement agreements with suppliers Identify sites
Comfortable units	Appropriate design for the environment and culture Safe from dangerous materials
Not too expensive	Uses existing facilities if possible Offers basic accommodation; not overbuilt Possibility to recycle units into second use
Reuse	Identify potential reuses Integrate reuse potential into unit design and settlement layout Identify necessary policies, e.g. for donation
Maintains social networks	Locate as close as possible to damaged homes
Convenient location	Identify possible sites ahead of time and make arrangements for their use
Provision of services	Match with location; may be possible to use nearby existing services Include frequent, inexpensive bus service
Top-down provision of houses when necessary, while enabling residents to help themselves when possible	Consult people about needs and plan accordingly Decide what needs to be provided quickly, in a top-down manner Identify what could be managed by residents
Integrated within overall reconstruction strategy	Figure out how long temporary housing will be needed for Estimate a budget for temporary housing, including land, units, infrastructure and services

5 Multi-actor arrangements and project management

Colin Davidson

Some problems are so complex that you have to be highly intelligent and well informed just to be undecided about them.

Lawrence J. Peter[2]

One of the most difficult tasks in post-disaster reconstruction is organizing the necessary processes and procedures, particularly regarding the participants (beneficiaries, professional consultants, contractors, suppliers, public authorities, NGOs, etc.) and their roles; practical decisions have to be made, in a context of competing interests. Organizational strategies have to be "designed" and then implemented through contractually binding procurement procedures, adapted to local business customs and traditions.

Introduction

The success of post-disaster reconstruction depends to a large extent on the complex relationships between the multiple actors involved. These actors include the affected people, community-based organizations, local and central government, NGOs and international agencies and, of course, designers (who may be architects or engineers) and builders. The challenge is to "design" these relationships in the best interest of the recovery effort. To achieve the hoped-for success, two aspects are particularly crucial: (i) carrying out what can best be called systematic organizational design and (ii) choosing an appropriate procurement strategy – at the levels of both the reconstruction program as a whole and the individual projects that make it up.

In essence, *organizational design* and *procurement* are inseparable. Organizational design involves preparing for and consolidating the relationships between the parties who will be implicated with or affected by a program of work and its constituent projects; procurement translates this organization into a set of defined agreements with the participants. Conversely, adopting a particular procurement strategy (for whatever reasons – regulations, customs, habit, etc.) affects the nature of the organizational designs that are reasonable in the circumstances.

This chapter is in two main parts, preceded by a short prologue and followed by a postscript. The first main part examines the organizational design of the complex relationships between the parties involved in any construction or reconstruction work, leading to the creation of an organization (or, more properly, a *multi-organization*) that is to be responsible for the work. The second main part presents the realities of *procurement*, that is to say, the actual acquisition of the services (e.g. the participants in the program or project) and the goods (e.g. the systems of materials and products) that are available and/or are needed for effective recovery operations.

Prologue

Construction in general and reconstruction in particular are not simple operations to plan for, nor do they possess a linear decision path leading easily to an optimum solution. Recovery and reconstruction tasks fall squarely into the domain of "wicked problems," that is to say, problems that, according to Rittel and Webber,[11] have neither definitive formulations nor optimum solutions:

> The search for scientific bases for confronting problems of social policy is bound to fail, because of the nature of these problems. They are "wicked" problems, whereas science has developed to deal with "tame" problems. Policy problems cannot be definitively described. Moreover, in a pluralistic society there is nothing like the undisputable public good; there is no objective definition of equity; policies that respond to social problems cannot be meaningfully correct or false; and it makes no sense to talk about "optimal solutions" to social problems unless severe qualifications are imposed first. Even worse, there are no "solutions" in the sense of definitive and objective answers. (page 155)

Syarief and Hibino comment that there is no consensus on what these wicked problems are nor how they should be resolved; they do, however, provide a checklist of ten reasons for this, suggesting ten precautions that should be taken in initiating solutions, such as: coping with the "asymmetry of ignorance" between project stakeholders, demanding user participation, ensuring the transparency of process and recognizing the need for project leaders who act as problem *helpers* rather than problem *solvers*.[13] Conklin[2] expresses the characteristics of wicked problems in the following terms:

> The need or want is expressed in the language of what ought to be – what should be done, what should be built, what should be written. On the other hand, the process of design is constrained by resources – what can be done, given the available resources such as time and money and given the constraints imposed by the environment and the laws of science (page 15).

As Lizarralde explains in Chapter 2, this recognition of the constraints of what can be done – finding reasonable solutions to wicked problems rather than trying to optimize – led Herbert Simon to coin the term "satisficing" to describe the true goal of a project design team: finding at least a satisfactory solution from among a number of possibilities.[12]

Construction and *a fortiori* reconstruction fall into the domain of wicked problems for a number of reasons and have to be treated with particular care.

First, extending what Conklin wrote (quoted above), construction projects move from the verbal expression of needs (expressions of social opportunities) and demands (which can be contracted for at a given time)[14] to supposedly appropriate practical actions (preparing drawings and instructions, digging trenches, laying bricks, etc.). This process involves interpretation, weighing up of options and "translation" from the language of society to the language of building. It relies on discerned decision-making; it immediately raises the question of who is or are (or should be) responsible for the many decisions to be made.

This process, which is described in more detail by Katsanis and Davidson,[6] entails recognizing need, translating it into demand and setting the building activities in motion. It is cyclical: society's *needs* change and the *demand* follows; housing gets built and is occupied (reducing the demand for space); obsolescence continuously impacts on the occupied buildings, thus increasing the need for space (Figure 5.1).

In the post-disaster situation, where it is necessary to react to the disaster-induced destruction, this cyclical process breaks down; instead, many sources are mobilized to intervene, often in an uncoordinated way, with a minimum of continuity through which experience might otherwise be gained (Figure 5.2).

Second, one must not forget that construction is one of few activities where the purchaser or user agrees to acquire a building or an infrastructure *before* it exists (shipbuilding and film production are two other domains where this applies). Unlike purchasing a car or an existing house, where it is possible to inspect and evaluate the purchase before making a commitment, the decision to procure a new building (housing, community facilities, etc.) can only be based on informed trust – a trust in the competence of the agents to whom the work of analysis, design and production will be allocated. This is a trust that can be supported by an examination of their earlier work and that is protected by well-written contract documents. Under traditional construction conditions, the required *informed trust* is based on shared expert know-how; in reconstruction, there is little shared know-how and inconsistent levels of "expertise" – against the backdrop of very real and urgent needs.

The premise for the rest of this chapter is that construction and reconstruction problems are by their very nature *wicked* and that organizing for their "solution" is of itself a major design problem. However, it is a problem that can be tackled step by step and supported by certain systematic procedures, as will be shown.

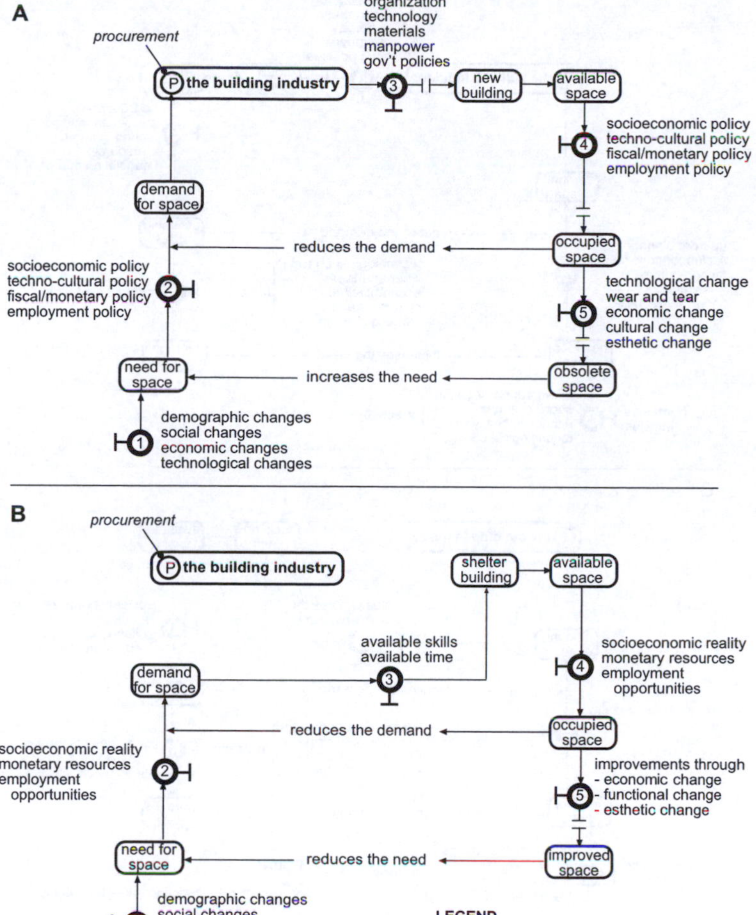

Figure 5.1 The habitual cycle of housing production. **A** by the formal sector and **B** informally.

A Changes/trends in society (1) create the *need* for space, which in response to policies (2) becomes a *demand* for space, which enters the building industry through procurement (P), mobilizing resources (3) to produce available space, which, in response to the same policies (4) becomes occupied, thus reducing the demand for space. However, this space becomes obsolete (5), contributing to increasing the need for space and to further cycles.

B Different changes (1) create the *need* for space, which in response to realities (2) becomes a *demand* for space, which is met by mobilizing individuals' resources (3) to produce available space, which in response to the same realities (4) becomes occupied, thus reducing the demand for space. Significantly, this space is continuously improved (5), decreasing the need for space; further cycles continue for other families.

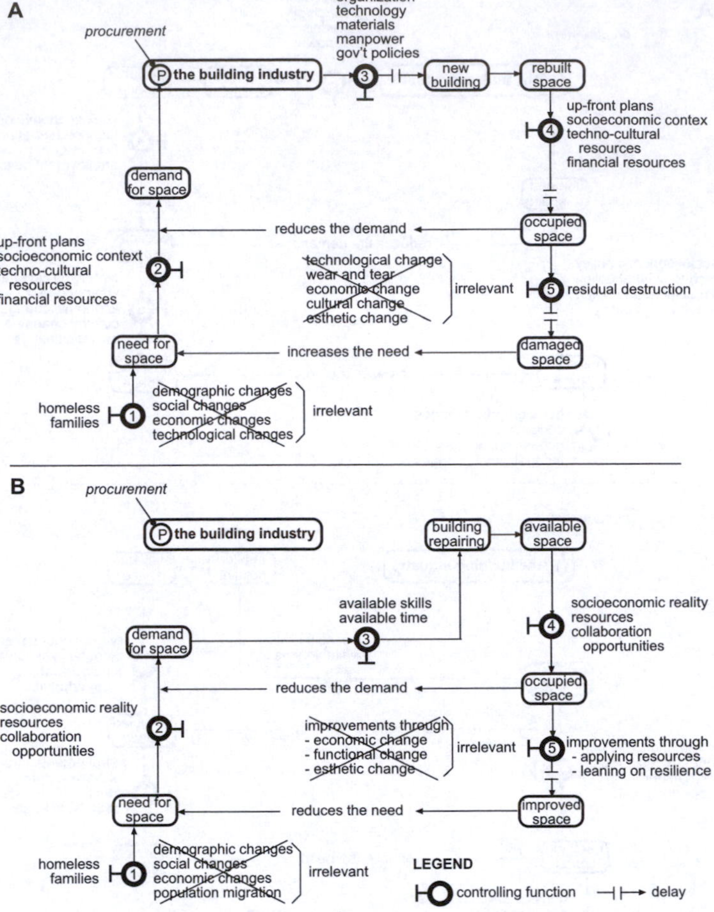

Figure 5.2 The post-disaster cycle of housing production. **A** by the formal sector and **B** informally.

A Changes and trends become irrelevant; instead, statistics about homeless families (1) create a great *need* for space, which in response to plans in their context (2) becomes a *demand* for space, which queue to enter the building industry through procurement (P), mobilizing resources (3) to produce available space, which in response to the same plans in their context (4) becomes occupied, thus reducing the demand for space. However, other space is still damaged (5), contributing to increasing the need for space and to further cycles.

B An identical reality (homelessness), felt first-hand, (1) creates a great *need* for space, which in response to realities and limited resources (2) becomes a *demand* for space, which is met by mobilizing individuals' resources (3) to produce available space, which in response to the same realities (4) becomes occupied, thus reducing the demand for space. Significantly, this space is improved as quickly as possible (5), decreasing the need for space (at least in principle); further cycles continue for other families who could not start quickly enough.

Organizational design

Organizing for construction – a design problem

Since construction involves the resolution of wicked problems, initiating a construction program or project requires a systems approach to establishing what the organization to be mandated to carry it out should be like. Who should participate and on what basis? Indeed, who should even decide who should participate? What principles should guide their participation and, particularly, the relationships between them?

Three questions have to be addressed: whether to build, how to organize and how to initiate a project. The organizational design for conventional construction projects is examined first, then the particularities of the reconstruction context are identified.

First question: whether to build?

There is an apocryphal story about the chairman of a major food retail chain who knew that his warehousing constituted a bottleneck in his enterprise, impacting negatively on the company's "bottom line." As was his habit, he played golf every weekend in summer, finishing in the clubhouse for chats with his guests and fellow golfers. One week, he discussed his warehouse problem with an engineer, who rapidly commented that it was an easy problem to solve – by building an addition to the existing warehouse. The following week, his guest, a dealer in materials-handling equipment, pointed out that it was easy to stack the merchandise to a greater height in the existing warehouse. The third week, discussions with a marketing consultant led to proposals to solve the same problem by better supply-chain management. Each weekend, discussion generated a new view of the problem and a totally different approach to solving it.

This story and the problem it reveals (as far from the world of reconstruction as it may be) does not seem to be particularly "wicked," yet its solution takes on completely different orientations depending on the available expertise and corresponding world view adopted by the principal protagonists.

In stable environments, a situation that is thought to require a construction project often turns out to be better resolved by redeployment of existing resources through rehabilitation work, for example, or through the reorganization of the use of spaces. In the field of reconstruction, that is to say, in essentially unstable environments, similar problems arise. To give just one example, it was widely reported in the media that fishermen in eastern Sri Lanka preferred to receive new boats rather than new houses, in order to rebuild their lives more rapidly after the tsunami.

Second question: how to organize?

If the answer to the first question calls for building, it becomes necessary to address a further set of questions, which are better considered at both technical and organizational levels. At the *technical* level, choices relate to what the output of the project should consist of (e.g. of what materials and what components it should be built). In terms of *organization* (properly considered in parallel), decisions relate to what processes to set in motion, how tasks are to be performed, to whom they will be entrusted and when, i.e. in what sequence they are to be carried out.

As is well known, any construction project has many participants, ranging from professional offices to enterprises and craftsmen, selected from the building industry, that is to say, from a relatively restricted community in any country or region.[3] The building industry is, in management jargon, a "multi-industry," reflecting the fact that it is composed of a number of different categories of participants, each with its technical competencies and each with its own set of behavioral rules and customs. It exists within a given *national* context (all buildings exist in a national/regional-specific location, even if some participants may be multinational). This national context is, in turn, inscribed in the contemporary *global* environment (political, economic and cultural-media) (Figure 5.3).

The selected project participants constitute what is loosely called "the project team."[3] A relatively limited number of professional and business firms are *chosen* from the range of available professions and trade specialties, shown in black in Figure 5.3 (white circles designate other professionals and businesses probably involved in other projects). They are chosen, but the question immediately arises: by whom and acting on what authority?

The members of the team come together through selection procedures (explained in detail later in this chapter) to design and build the required project. In management jargon, this group of team members is called a "temporary multi-organization." It is *temporary* because it only lasts for the duration of any one project, separating at the end; indeed, its members probably do not all work together on any later project. It is a *multi-organization* because of its necessarily multidisciplinary composition, with each participant bringing his or her specific skills to fit in with the requirements of the briefing, designing and constructing process.

The traditional organization of the building project team operates within certain management patterns; Masterman describes three major types of arrangements:

- *separated and cooperative* – in which project initiation (by the building's owner) and design are separated from production and construction, requiring nonetheless a high level of cooperation between the two blocks of participants;

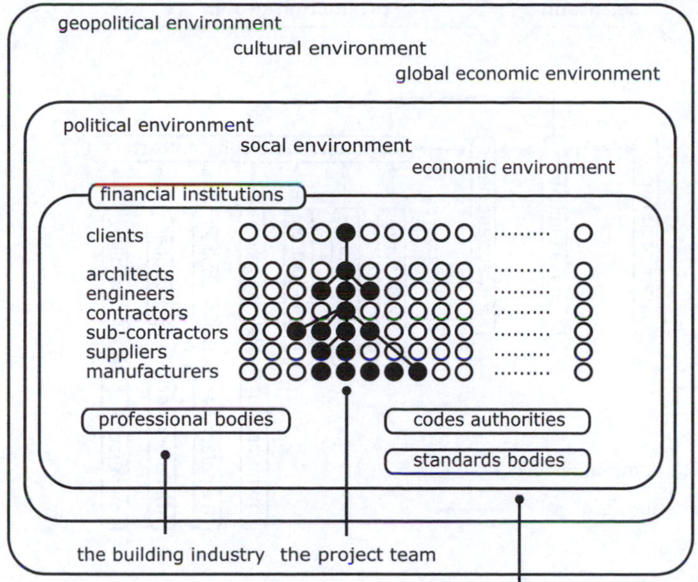

Figure 5.3 The building industry and its principal participants, within their respective environments. In traditional construction contexts, where shared know-how is available nationally or regionally, the global environment has little recognized impact on the project team; in reconstruction projects, the contrary is the case and the impacts of global influences are all-pervading and difficult to cope with.

- *integrated* – in which the owner entrusts all design and construction activities to a single entity, which may even assume responsibility for financing the project during its construction;
- *management-related* – in which the owner turns to a management professional who is appointed to take charge of and *manage* design and construction activities carried out by a number of distinct professional offices and construction enterprises.[7]

In traditional, relatively stable environments, one or other of these organization types is usually successful (projects do get built, and cost and time over-runs fall into a pattern that has come to be commonly accepted, for better or for worse). Each participant in a traditional building project team relies on his or her own accumulated know-how, reassured by the knowledge that the other participants have their share of relevant know-how too (Figure 5.4).

Indeed, Mohsini and Davidson showed that a shared recognition of the boundaries between each participant's intervention, coupled with unbiased and rapid access to information about the project, is a major determinant

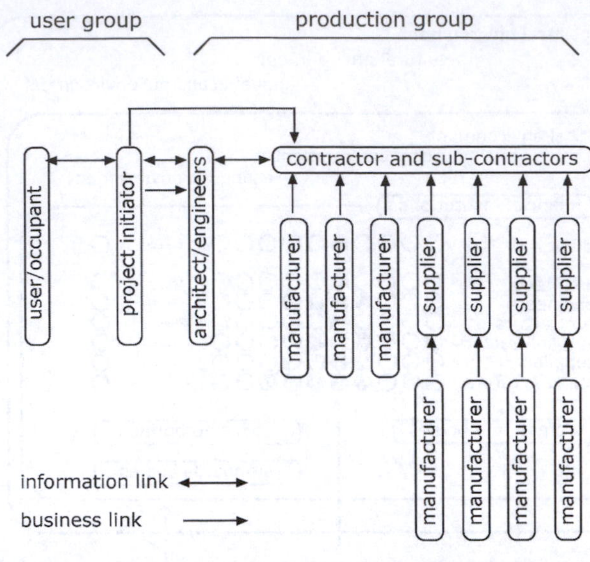

Figure 5.4 Organigram of the formal relationships in the traditional building team. The composition of the "user group" and the "production group" is easy to predict in traditional construction; for reconstruction projects, that is not the case and the make-up of these two groups and their interrelationships has to be carefully designed.

of project success.[9] The United Nations Economic Commission for Europe also expressed the same concern – in terms of the importance of the skills that are required for carrying out work *and for interpreting instructions*, be they explicit (in the form of specifications, drawings, standards, etc.) or tacit (acquired through apprenticeship and practice).[14]

In the unstable context of reconstruction after natural disasters, the traditional approaches to project organization may be entirely unsuitable and/or unworkable; likely participants are many and varied in origin and in motivation, and they have to be selected and organized according to some upfront plan, which may or may not exist (see Figure 4.3 in Chapter 4). Meeting the specific demands for an innovative organizational design follows from the special circumstances and global context of each post-disaster reconstruction project; this organizational design is explained later in this chapter.

Third question: how to initiate a project?

If the answer to the first question calls for building – housing and related infrastructures, for example – and a building project (or a program of projects) is to be launched, and the second question of organizing the building team has been addressed, at least in principle, then it is necessary to move forward into the realm of operational, i.e. contractually binding, decisions, following a logical sequence.

In stable environments, the upfront steps usually take a relatively long period of time, during which various levels of feasibility studies are performed. *Technical* feasibility studies aim at selecting an appropriate level of technical innovation and assessing its predictable impacts on the project's outcome (remembering that the level of innovation may often be virtually nil). *Economic* feasibility studies, conducted in parallel, explore the "profitability" of the proposed project, where profitability may be visible on a bottom line or may translate into social non-measurable benefits felt to outweigh the predicted costs. These feasibility studies are often done out of the limelight, by members of some owner-related inner circle or clique.

Once the feasibility studies have shown the value (assessed in monetary or non-monetary terms) of proceeding with the project, it may be announced publicly and impact studies may be called for. Then the project moves into the realm of procurement, that is to say, of making decisions about how to acquire – i.e. purchase – the services of the necessary project participants who are expected to work in the project. Procuring their services ensures bringing to bear their respective skills and resources in an orderly manner.

Thus giving form to the building team follows from the strategic upfront decisions taken by the intending *building owner* as he or she makes what are considered – in the given context – to be the best possible *procurement* decisions. These procurement decisions determine the roles of all subsequent participants and effectively delimit the interfaces between their activities.[8,9] In a traditional and stable context, the procurement decisions will spread the responsibilities and the risks between the participants according to their skills and robustness, acting singly or in groups; they will take effect as soon as the intended project moves from initial ideas and apply through to completed construction.

This process, flowing as it does from the procurement decisions, includes a set of partially sequential and partly iterative steps, as shown in Table 5.1, whichever approach to project arrangement is chosen from the three classes mentioned above.

The same set of participants does not usually carry out all these tasks. Indeed, the design phases (steps 1 though 4) may be carried out by an architect or by engineers or both (possibly engaged by the building owner in parallel or sequentially) or be split into smaller tasks, starting with separate specialists, e.g. in functional programming (tasks 1 and 2) or performance analysis (task 3). The construction may be entrusted to a general contractor who also assumes responsibility for subcontracting the numerous specialized tasks to trade firms, or it may be transferred directly by the owner to as many specialist trade enterprises – possibly coordinated and managed by a manager acting as agent on the owner's behalf.

In general, the more the process is split up between different participants, the more distinct contracts will be required, defining the scope of the work

Table 5.1 Necessary steps in the process of initiating, designing and producing a building (steps 1, 2 and 3 are sequential, steps 3 and 4 are iterative, then after completing step 4, steps 5 and 6 are sequential)

1	Identifying who the building will be used by (including social and cultural specificities, particularly regarding privacy);
2	Recognizing what users' activities will take place, and when (i.e. in any specific sequence); this is often called the functional programming;
3	Describing the conditions that are required for these activities to take place adequately (taking account of conditions created by the activities such as noise or odors); this takes the form of a more or less formalized performance specification or a specification of requirements;
4	Proposing a design and checking it against the requirements; it is only reasonable to move on to step 5 after making sure that the design meets the specified requirements;
5	Communicating the design to those who will be entrusted with carrying out the construction work;
6	Constructing and supervising the work, including progressively paying for it.

demanded of each and spelling out how the various interventions fit together to form as smooth-flowing a process as possible. As might be suspected, the more contracts there are, the more risk there is for bottlenecks and for litigation, particularly at the interfaces between the various packages of work, since the outputs of one phase are almost always the inputs for the following phases.

To counter the effects of multiple contracts, the "integrated" approach (the second category proposed by Masterman,[7] referred to above), as its name implies, proposes that the building owner entrust all tasks of analysis, design and construction to a single entity, which may also be responsible for interim or long-term financing (the "design-build" or "turnkey" approaches, and the various forms of "build-own-operate" contracts, respectively).

However, the integrated approach presupposes, from the outset, a particularly careful definition of what is required – expressed in terms of the intended occupants and their expectations – without which there can be no recourse in the eventuality of unsatisfactory design and production.

Other options can be observed, lying between the extremes of fragmenting the responsibilities between many participants and integrating the responsibilities into the hands of one major player. If, for some reason, fragmentation is felt to be desirable (for example, where work must be spread within a given community or region or where there is no set of firms large enough to take on the whole project), a centralizing management control is called for (the third category proposed by Masterman[7]).

In other words, there is a continuum of approaches that are available. In general, when there is some degree of integration, it puts more power into the hands of the participant at its centre. This power can be used to exercise control over those whose activities are integrated and to influence – for better or for worse – the other "outside" participants. The traditional organization, with its unwritten rules concerning (i) the frontiers between roles and (ii) the symmetrical access to information, can then no longer be assumed to apply.

In all cases, the distinct motivations of the participants have to be recognized, particularly regarding remuneration. Are they to be paid on a fee basis (usual for professional services) or through a purchasing agreement (usual for construction work)? Or is, for example, some form of "sweat equity" or exchange of services to be applied to some or all of them?

Organizing for reconstruction – also a design problem

Sources of complexity

Initiating and organizing a reconstruction project is a particular instance of the decisions that have been described, but in circumstances that render them more difficult to plan for and to implement.

As has been explained, in all construction projects there are many participants whose roles have to be defined (through organizational design) and whose responsibilities, obligations and remuneration have to be agreed upon in advance (through strategic procurement). This is a challenge even in stable conditions, let alone in reconstruction, where it is possible to rely on relevant past experience neither for the choice of the participants nor for the organization of their respective roles.

In reconstruction, the fact that no pertinent earlier experience is available follows from the unique circumstances that characterize each disaster (location, gravity, time, socio-political context, etc.). It is also probable that potential participants possess many more differences even than in traditional construction: for example, they may come from different countries with different technical, cultural and economic values; they may be non-profit or for-profit; and they may be driven by priorities imported from elsewhere or from another context. In addition, the whole question of the relationship between quality and cost has to be debated from scratch (on cost: how can the available resources be fairly shared, within expected donor-driven time constraints; on quality: how much improvement on pre-disaster standards is reasonable to call for in the name of sustainable development). To further complicate matters, there is no clear project initiator (the equivalent of the traditional building owner).

This is indeed a "wicked problem." The design of an organization for reconstruction presents more options and fewer certainties than for construction in stable circumstances; it is not even clear who should hold an overall responsibility for it.

Who does what and when?

Figure 5.4 shows the formal relationships between participants in the building team. The participants are loosely categorized as the *user group* and the *production group*. In traditional contexts:

- In the *user group*, the project initiator or building owner (who may or may not be a user of the future facility) assumes responsibility for organizing the project on his or her behalf and on that of the users (the users may be individually known in advance or they may be unidentified people from a socio-economic category identified by market research); the building owner has a general responsibility for steering the use-related tasks (tasks 1 and 2, Table 5.1) and is also responsible for setting up the production group, either in detail or in principle (by establishing the strategies that govern its organization and functioning, that is to say, the way the production *processes* will be controlled).
- The *producer group* includes the designers (usually architects/engineers) responsible for determining the nature of the *product*, which should respond to the building owner's requirements (i.e. for tasks 3, 4 and 5 in Table 5.1), and the building contractor and sub-contractors responsible for task 6 (Table 5.1), that is to say, for the actual production of the required buildings. Suppliers and manufacturers support these production activities.

In the reconstruction context, composition of these groups can adopt many forms, as shown in Table 5.2, and it is precisely because of the spread of options that the organizational design assumes so much importance. As will be shown later, the *responsibility* for the organizational design is also variable and depends on business customs and on the cultural and legal systems that survive the disaster in the receiving country. In all cases, however, fair, rapid and transparent arrangements define (i) the roles of each participant within what is to become a team effort and (ii) the sharing of available resources (funds, materials, labor, equipment, etc.).

After identifying the participants from the lists of Table 5.2, the following points must also be taken into consideration:

- The ensuing organizational design has to reflect hierarchies of relationships that must be respected in a given locality, particularly regarding the project initiators; for example, the country's Prime Minister's office may have to be given a key role, or the local religious dignitaries may need to be consulted.
- The relationships that have to be planned for probably fall into distinct categories such as: "authorize," "inform," "give/request prior clearance," "delegate to ...," "carry out," "verify."

- Not all of the participants will be involved with a given project for all of its duration; for example, an off-shore building firm may be best equipped to carry out infrastructure repairs at the start of a project, whereas the house building is best entrusted subsequently to local craftsmen.

Obviously some of the combinations of the participants in Table 5.2 are unlikely; however, the upfront organizational design has to sort out the realistic

Table 5.2 List of likely participants in a post-disaster reconstruction project (compare with Figures 5.2 and 5.3)

User group	*Production group*
The users	*The designers*
Known survivors	Local architects and/or engineers
Unknown survivors of known social categories	External architects and/or engineers (e.g. from donor countries)
Community representatives or leaders	Local technicians
The project initiators	Local craftsmen
Surviving community groups	*Building contractors and sub-contractors*
Religious groups or leaders	Local building enterprises
Local NGOs	"Off shore" building firms
External NGOs (e.g. from donor countries)	Local craftsmen
Local governments at national or regional levels	Self-help laborers
Political entities	Construction manager
Project managers	*Manufacturers and suppliers*
Controlling bodies	Local producers and local resources
Local professional bodies	Local distributors
International professional bodies	National or regional producers
Local codes authorities	International producers
Local standards bodies	Logistics and transport enterprises
International standards bodies (e.g. ILO, ISO)	Customs and shipping agents and brokers
International funding sources (e.g. World Bank)	

from the improbable arrangements and arrive at the most "satisficing," i.e. plausible, combinations.[12] Then the contractual arrangements have to be drawn up through the processes of procurement, discussed later in this chapter.

The question raised earlier about *who* among the potential project initiators should be responsible for the design of an organization for reconstruction remains to be addressed. A priori it is often not clear who should hold an overall responsibility for a given reconstruction project, and indeed it often seems that several entities are attempting simultaneously to assume a lead or coordinator role. To a great extent, the choice depends on the relative power (and policies) of the national government and/or regional or local authorities, on the medium- to long-term upfront presence of one or several NGOs in the affected region prior to the disaster, and on the degree to which post-disaster reconstruction has been planned for – if at all.

The level of chaos that prevails in the post-disaster situation depends, among other things, on the existence of any upfront planning that may have taken place and its fit with the actual circumstances of the disaster. The protagonists in the reconstruction effort, such as NGOs, as they strive to make some sort of orderly space within which they can start to fulfill their mission, actually have to work within a context that is largely defined by any precautionary measures that may or may not have been taken before the disaster, as shown in Figure 4.3 of Chapter 4.

From the point of view of a participating NGO, the organizational design activities (shown in Figure 5.5) start with a reference to its specific mandate and brief, particularly to detect any hidden agenda (e.g. to favor a particular religious group or members of a social class or community). Subsequent steps permit establishing a list of participants, including identifying particular socio-cultural requirements. In these steps, it is also prudent to identify "competitor" service providers (such as other NGOs or local public and community services). Finally, the nature of relationships with the retained partners has to be defined: hierarchical relationships of buyer–supplier, partnerships between equals, mandatory consultations, etc.

Once these organizational features have been established appropriately and woven into a network of relations (for this, the importance of recognizing the local preferences and local customs cannot be overemphasized), it is possible to proceed with the actual procurement, that is to say, to move on to translating the design of the organization into operational procedures, contracts, etc.

Procurement

As a participating NGO moves through the organizational design phases (shown in Figure 5.5), identifying professional, charitable and business enterprises with which it will work, its decisions depend on the degree of local or regional upfront planning, which helps to reduce the prevailing chaos but also imposes procedures and protocols that have to be respected.

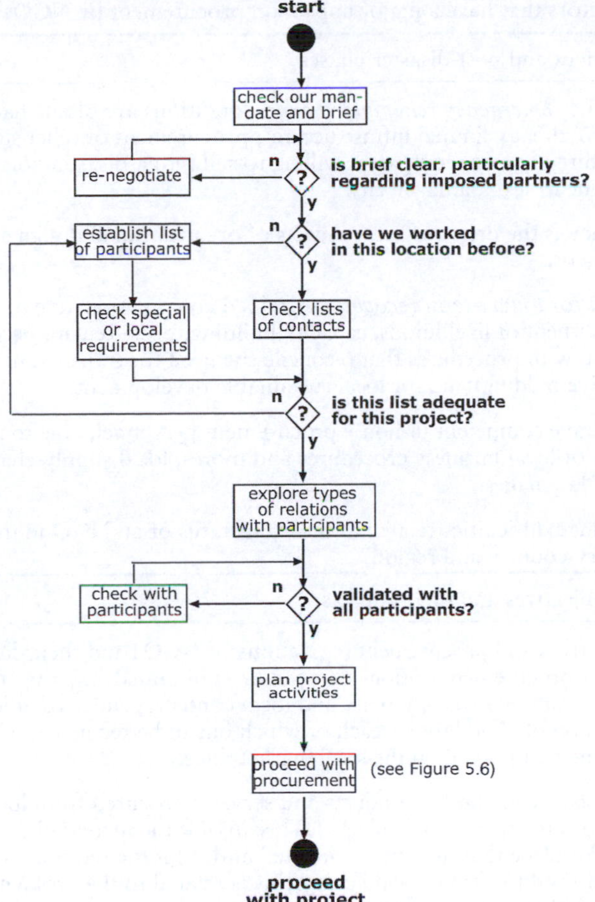

Figure 5.5 Steps in designing an organization for reconstruction, from an NGO's position.

Once the organizational design decisions have been made – and making the best possible decisions falls into the domain of wicked problems mentioned at the beginning of this chapter – it is possible to proceed with procuring the needed services and supplies. Table 5.3 provides some recommendations regarding these decisions and their potential consequences. Figure 5.6 illustrates the sequence of decisions to be made.

Procurement decisions have to reflect apparently conflicting requirements:

- being legally binding and allowing for accounting transparency for the parent NGOs and their funding agencies;
- being compatible with the local business regulations regarding purchasing in the public sector;

Table 5.3 Factors that have a major impact on procurement by NGOs

1	Procurement and post-disaster phases:
1.1	*Provision of emergency relief and shelter*: conditions are often chaotic, with damage to already limited infrastructures; procurement of relief supplies and logistics directly from companies willing to sell into a disaster zone, probably from the nearest undamaged city. Expediency is the driver of most aspects of organizational design and procurement.
1.2	*Provision for longer-term recovery*: sustained construction activities, reestablishment of livelihoods, capacity building, procurement becoming systematic with procedures that reconcile the need for transparency (e.g. competitive bidding) and for local sustainable development. Need to have competent in-house procurement personnel, able to face the problems of local business procedures and mores, local supply-chain capacity and local languages. Need to face difficulties related to the legal status of an NGO in the beneficiary country and region.
2	NGOs' objectives and their impacts:
2.1	The objectives and procurement regulations of NGOs and their donors may affect procurement options that can be entertained, e.g. the need to support community sustainability and local content, gender equality, and the exclusion of child labor – each of which has to be reconciled with the perceptions that prevail on the local marketplace.
2.2	The increased demand for products and services procured from local sources is likely to raise prices, particularly (a) because of the increased demand on a marketplace that may be fragmented and (b) if the required quality specifications differ from local norms; this is related to the problem of finding suppliers with whom procurement contracts can be entered into.
3	Envisaging the suppliers' point of view:
3.1	Making sure the procurement objectives are properly understood by potential suppliers.
3.2	Ascertaining that what is about to be purchased is available from (or through) the suppliers being solicited, particularly regarding dimensions, quantity and quality.
3.3	Using clear bidding procedures, which do not change in the course of a project and which are understood by the firms being asked to bid; coping with suppliers who do not make written bids or provide performance bonds and who never give credit.
4	Making payments:
4.1	Adapting payment procedures to fit with local customs; for example, dealing with suppliers who work on the basis of cash-and-carry.

(*continued*)

Table 5.3 (continued)

4.2	Recognizing the risks perceived by the suppliers in selling to an NGO that is new to the locality.
4.3	Assessing the risks associated with the lowest price and the likelihood of non-performance.

Source: adapted from Ardie (2008).[1]

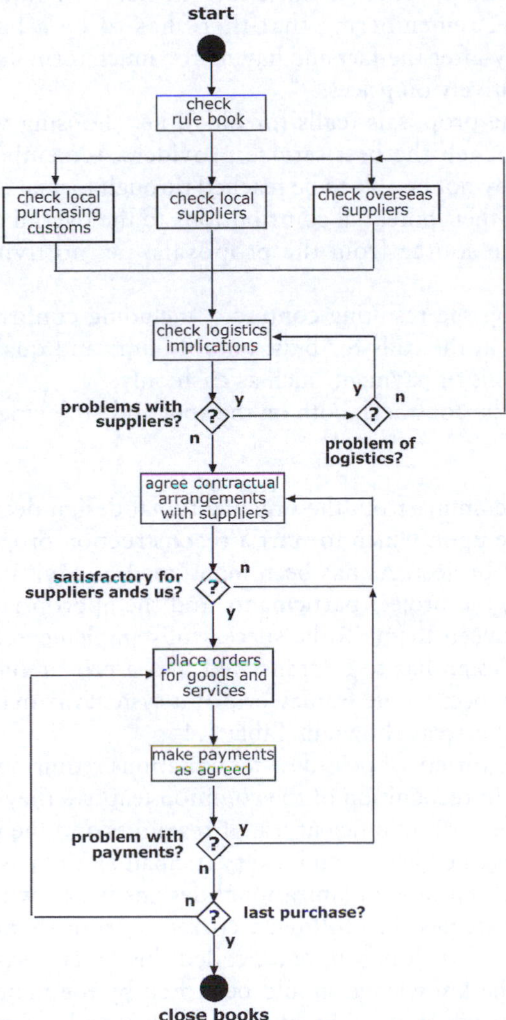

Figure 5.6 Sequence of procurement decisions, following upon completion of the organizational design.

- fitting with the local routines – where a handshake may amply confirm normal trust.

There are six aspects of managing procurement that have to be adapted to these requirements, particularly the local procedures:

- procurement planning, i.e. allocating upcoming expenditure between local and off-shore sources, notably in the NGO's home country;
- planning the approach to solicitation, i.e. how much formality is appropriate, remembering that there has to be a balance between transparency-after-the-fact and having too much formality, which would impact negatively on prices;
- soliciting the proposals (calls for bids), i.e. choosing what is the best method to reach the best service providers, remembering that local resources may not be able to be reached through formal channels, despite the value of their potential contributions to the overall effort;
- selecting the source from the proposals, i.e. notifying the selected enterprises;
- administering the resulting contracts, including confirming the conditions stated in the calls for bids, notably time and quality constraints, and conditions of payment, such as cash only;
- closing out the contracts, both on the spot and archiving for subsequent audits.[10]

Procurement, stemming from the organizational design decisions, provides an infrastructure upon which to start a reconstruction program of projects or an individual project. As has been mentioned, organizational design allows identifying the project participants and the appropriate relationships to be set up between them. To be successfully implemented, however, the organizational design has to be translated into a procurement plan, which in turn has to respect to the framework of a systematic management plan, which includes the areas shown in Table 5.4.

Because of the variety of post-disaster situations requiring reconstruction efforts, but also in recognition of the common features they share (the need for speed, the need for an efficient use of resources and the need to balance the contributions of external and local participants), there is scope for sharing knowledge about how organizational designs which worked and about procurement strategies that followed correctly from them. Some sort of repository is required. Johnson, *et al.* called this "meta-procurement" and suggested that the knowledge should be stored by the major international funding agencies, which would make it (together with supporting learning materials) available to qualified recipients of grants.[5]

Conclusions

On the subject of "repair mechanisms" to be called into action to manage and control the spread and severity of damage induced by disasters, Jessica Flack writes: "… disaster-relief systems could establish back-up relationships among relief agencies to ensure that bottlenecks do not hinder the distribution of emergency resources."[4]

The organizational design that this approach suggests concerns not only the individual reconstruction projects and their teams but also the programmed reconstruction effort in its totality. To do so is not easy, primarily because of the probable absence of a single coordinating authority. Consequently, the best source of efficiency is for the lead entity of each project team to organize its links to other participants – through effective networking within the local technical and social environment – as systematically as possible.

In traditional building under stable conditions, organizing for and obtaining a building (housing, community facilities, public buildings, etc.) is a

Table 5.4 Issues in project management

- Integration management: establishing how the project fits into broader strategic considerations of the participant organizations (e.g. the beneficiaries, the NGOs, the public authorities);
- Scope management: determining what is properly part of the project and what is or has to be excluded (including preparing an analysis of requirements);
- Time management: anticipating the duration and sequences of activities in order to be able to start quickly and finish within the anticipated limits;
- Cost management: preparing a budget and following it as contracts are let and activities monitored;
- Quality management: defining the appropriate levels of quality to be designed for and implemented, bearing in mind the need for sustainable community development within the limits of the available resources;
- Human resource management: planning for and managing the complex links between the various participants in the project, in full recognition of local and regional cultural characteristics;
- Communications management: identifying what information is to be supplied to whom, at what steps in the project and in what form, particularly to motivate key participants such as the beneficiaries and their community leaders;
- Risk management: finding a way to identify unexpected events and developing means to minimize their negative consequences;
- Procurement management (as described on pages 109 and 110).

Source: adapted from Project Management Institute, 2004.[10]

complicated process, requiring careful planning and management in order to coordinate the efforts of the many participants. Indeed, determining what is to be produced is of itself a wicked problem, admitting no single optimum approach. In reconstruction, deciding what is to be produced and who is to participate is difficult, since conditions are not stable and the participants are further differentiated by culture, socio-economic conditions, language and politics.

As a result, the reconstruction context has to be examined afresh in terms of the "who does what, why, and when" questions:

- *who*: the many potential participants in the reconstruction effort have to be identified and their ability to contribute assessed in a way that is not deformed by preconceptions about their competencies;
- *what*: breaking down the multitude of tasks into work packages that correspond to the identified competencies;
- *why*: to reconstruct for sustainable development, of course, but recognizing (and reconciling) the secondary motivations (the "hidden agendas") of the participating agencies;
- *when*: recognizing that time is critical as reconstruction moves from the provision of emergency shelter to permanent housing.

The issue therefore is: how can these four questions be answered in practical terms? Project participants must move from problem identification to organized and efficient production through a systems approach. Organizational design, accompanied by appropriate procurement of services and goods, is the starting point. Upfront planning is the ideal.

Postscript

A comparison between panels A and B of Figure 5.1 reveals the differences between how the formal and the informal sectors function under normal conditions. As shown by Lizarralde in Chapter 2, the *informal* sector provides simple and evolving housing for many more families than the formal sector does, particularly for the poorest sectors of society. It operates in a generally decentralized way; after an initially coordinated effort, e.g. during land invasion, where the coordination is in the hands of a community leader, every family fends for itself, building onto its first core shelter as and when it has resources available.

In a post-disaster context (compare panels A and B of Figure 5.2), the same principles apply. The formal sector focuses its efforts on the building sector, reached through its "procurement gateway," accepting the ensuing delays. The informal sector bypasses this source of bottlenecks; instead, each family has to rely only on a combination of its resources and its inherent resilience. The sheer numbers of people "compensate for" the apparent lack of recognizable forms of organization.

The challenge facing stakeholders in post-disaster reconstruction is to find ways of bridging between the two sectors – formal and informal – in order to benefit from the logic of the supposedly planned operations of the formal sector and from the "strength in numbers" that characterizes the informal sector. This is a wicked problem, the resolution of which calls for flexible organizational designs.

6 Stakeholder participation in post-disaster reconstruction programmes – New Orleans' Lakeview

A case study

Isabelle Maret and James Amdal

The reconstruction effort involves many stakeholders concerned with rebuilding the many aspects of their daily lives; the official processes take inordinate amounts of time and suffer from inherent problems of coordination. Local initiatives, often due to a single person's efforts, can lead to citizen involvement and thence to successful community restoration. A detailed case study in post-Katrina New Orleans illustrates the strength of the bottom-up-model approach.

As explained in Chapter 5, the success of rebuilding after disasters depends primarily on the organization and coordination of a variety of different efforts and programs at all levels of government and society. Extremes of response vary from heightened bureaucratic processes to direct civilian intervention; however, in all cases, cities need to find the right mix to maximize efficiency to affect a timely recovery. The case of post-Katrina New Orleans exemplifies this critical issue in response to a devastating event.

Three years after this massive disaster, the costliest in America's history, there is still no overarching structure to coordinate the multiple recovery strategies in place or pending. Responses originate from individual citizens, neighborhood associations and the City's Office of Recovery and Development Administration, as well as from numerous non-profit organizations mobilized for particular projects or programs. The rebuilding of the city after the disaster involves the integration of many types of stakeholders but within a well-organized structure that, to date, is lacking in New Orleans.

In this chapter, we demonstrate that three years after the storm, the reconstruction of New Orleans' communities is wildly diverse and remains sadly uncoordinated. We emphasize the importance that a diverse set of stakeholder organizations have in the recovery, but we question their coordination. We have chosen one area of the city to illustrate our point: Lakeview. Using this particular subset of seven distinct neighborhoods that comprise Planning District 5, we show the current challenges faced by specific stakeholder groups in the coordination of their recovery efforts. Hence the various efforts occurring in Lakeview help to explain the importance of the timely intervention of engaged citizens in a successful recovery.

Current status: New Orleans three years after Katrina

Hurricane Katrina made landfall at Buras-Triumph, Louisiana, 62 miles southeast of New Orleans, on the morning of August 29 as a category-3 hurricane (200 kilometer per hour winds). Katrina was the most destructive and costliest natural disaster ($75 billion) in the history of the United States, affecting the entire central gulf coast (Florida, Alabama, Mississippi, and Louisiana.) Storm waters submerged roughly 80 per cent of the city of New Orleans (Figure 6.1). Along the Mississippi gulf coast the storm surge was estimated to be 10 meters high in selected areas. The resultant devastation was of almost biblical proportions for an entire region of the United States. Less than one month later, Hurricane Rita devastated large parts of the west/central gulf coast region, making landfall on September 23 at the Texas/Louisiana border, with 190 kilometer per hour winds. The storm caused major coastal erosion, massive evacuations, and localized flooding. In New Orleans, this second storm surge topped 2.5 meters and breached some provisionally repaired levees.

The damages from these two storms were unprecedented for the US: over 1464 lives were lost and many people were still missing in 2008; the total loss has been estimated to be in excess of $100 billion; 200,000 homes were destroyed;[5] some parishes suffered 100 per cent devastation; over 250 square kilometers of wetlands were lost; and 320 million trees were killed or severely damaged in Louisiana and Mississippi alone, making these storms the worst

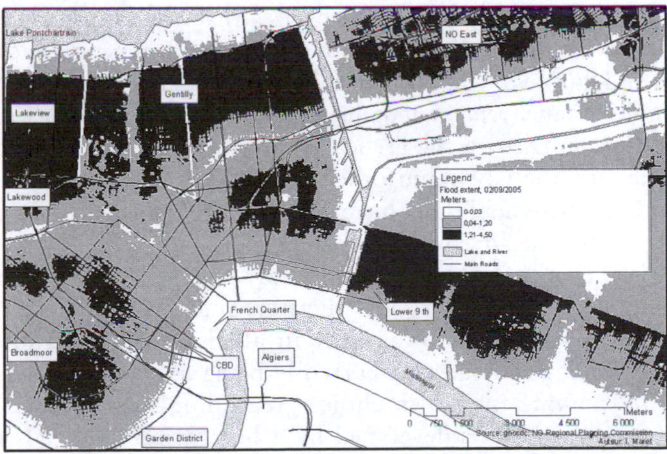

Figure 6.1 Flooded neighborhoods in New Orleans.[3]

ecological disaster in the nation's history.[7] Moreover, 1.3 million citizens were evacuated in the greater New Orleans region; 81,000 businesses were impacted, with over 18,000 that were destroyed remaining closed.[4] Currently over 150,000 displaced residents have yet to return. Due to the storm and its after-effects (business interruption or closure, depopulation, negative tourism impacts), New Orleans' city government lost 50 per cent of its employees (planners, engineers, inspectors, clerical support) just at a time when they were most needed.

The damage to utilities and support infrastructure was extensive and its extent was largely unknown; the impact on health, education, and criminal justice systems was overwhelming; 95 per cent of City-owned properties were damaged; the Army Corps of Engineers took 53 days to "dewater" the city; $14 billion was the residential damage estimate; the City's annual revenue loss was approximately $168 million. Taken *in toto*, New Orleans sustained 57 per cent of Louisiana's cumulative loss. Katrina and Rita represented a deadly assault to New Orleans and the central gulf coast, and they remain devastated to this day.[1]

Three years after having been swamped by Hurricanes Katrina and Rita, New Orleans is far from fully recovered. The numbers speak for themselves: in 2008, the city of New Orleans is housing 67 per cent of its former residents; the current residential population is roughly 308,000 out of a population of over 450,000. Still, this number hides a major aspect of the recovery: the nature of its diversity and its disparate state from neighborhood to neighborhood.

New Orleans' neighborhoods are recovering at different rates. Individual neighborhoods are using diverse redevelopment strategies to recover, with mixed results. Some neighborhoods remain almost unchanged. Due to their natural elevation and historic architectural treatment (raised main floor in Creole cottages, shotgun derivatives – narrow-fronted deep houses with rooms lining up in a row – or grand houses that were typical throughout the older parts of the city), the mainly middle- and upper-class owners of residences and businesses that were not badly flooded during the storms had the capacity to finance repairs of damage caused by wind, fire, or vandalism. Hence the Garden District, the French Quarter, Algiers and the entire West Bank of the city, the CBD, and other traditional neighborhoods located adjacent to the Mississippi River have demonstrated normality since the city was officially reopened in early October 2005.

In 2008, other parts of the city are deeply engaged in various recovery efforts: demolition, gutting, reconstruction, and rebuilding activities are occurring at varying levels of activity in all the "wet" neighborhoods. Different rebuilding strategies are currently being used, showing that many residents are making their own choices regarding recovery, irrespective of overall planning efforts developed by a host of professionals hired by both the public and private sectors or by the City. This is largely due to the mayor's decision in November 2005 to let the recovery be "market-driven."

In many neighborhoods, residents are making the choice to rebuild the same house they had before the storm with little or no modification. New codes and building standards have been adopted, but there remains no effective enforcement of their requirements. Thus, in some areas, the structures are being rebuilt unchanged.

Other citizens are changing the underlying urban landscape of their community. In Gentilly, for instance, hazard-mitigation techniques are being employed: houses are being rebuilt with a mandated raised elevation (minimum 1 meter elevation of the main floor). In parts of Gentilly, the emerging urban landscape (Figure 6.2) demonstrates the strong will of the people regarding their rebuilding choices: they choose the elevation, building height, exterior material, style, etc. of their homes.

A new emphasis has also emerged with the post-disaster rebuilding of New Orleans communities: the adoption of green architecture/sustainable reconstruction. A sub-area of the Lower Ninth Ward, Holy Cross, has chosen to utilize sustainability and green development concepts as an overarching strategy for redevelopment. However, this ward regrettably represents an island of sustainable recovery in a largely devastated area.

Individual communities differ in their degree of progress and the overall redevelopment strategies they are employing. They are using different redevelopment models, different processes, and different strategies. However, one challenge faced by almost all of the neighborhoods is the need to quickly provide temporary housing while rebuilding permanent structures.

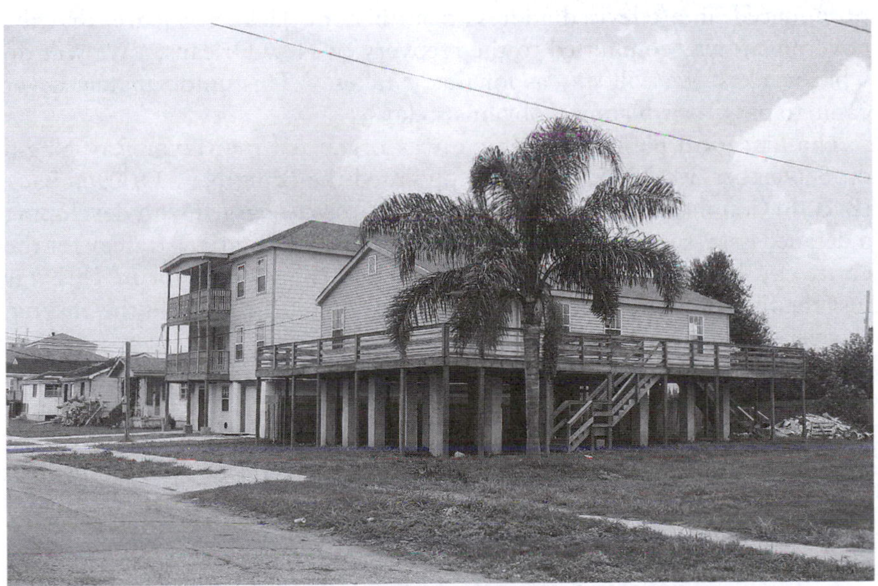

Figure 6.2 Post-Katrina housing style in Gentilly.

The government's solution has been to provide small trailers that appear throughout the city. Attempts at creating temporary clusters of trailers in a semi-permanent setting (traditional trailer parks) have been rigorously opposed throughout the city, therefore most trailers co-exist on individual residential lots where reconstruction of permanent housing (rehabbed or new) is occurring. On-site Federal Emergency Management Agency (FEMA) trailers occur throughout the city, but in some neighborhoods more than others. Currently in Lakeview, few trailers have been located.

A chronology of recovery planning

As soon as the winds subsided and the flood-protection failures became evident, the vast extent of the devastation became obvious to both government representatives (local, state, and federal) and the citizens of New Orleans. It also became obvious to the world via live TV broadcasts and related news media. Residents, civic leaders, and national and international experts debated various options for both short-term and long-term recovery. No American city had been faced with destruction on such a grand scale before, so no organizational model actually existed to guide the process. Consequently, during the first few weeks after the event, overarching questions included: "When can we return home?", "What are we going to do?", and "Where are we going to live?"

There were no clear-cut answers to these and umpteen other questions posed on a daily or even an hourly basis. The first public statement from President George W. Bush was given on September 15, 2005, when he pronounced, in a televised address from historic Jackson Square, that the government was committed to the recovery of New Orleans: "We will do what it takes. We will stay as long as it takes."[2] This unfortunately never came to pass, as is blatantly obvious today.

The first local planning initiative was organized by Mayor Ray Nagin on September 30, 2005, when he appointed the Bring New Orleans Back (BNOB) Commission. This blue-ribbon group was charged with developing a detailed issue-specific recovery plan and an implementation strategy for the entire city. It was given 90 days to complete and deliver the plan. This was just the first of many unrealistic timeframes established during the ensuing recovery process.

The BNOB Commission had 17 members, including attorneys, academics, respected developers, church leaders, and community activists. They were organized into various committees to address a multitude of issues: land use, infrastructure (flood protection, public transit, criminal justice), culture, education, health and human services, economic development, and government effectiveness. Each of these committees had numerous subcommittees that addressed more specific aspects of recovery, such as historic preservation. As the BNOB Commission were deliberating on their respective focus areas, many citizens could not or had not yet returned to the city, let alone to their neighborhood or their homes. It is important to note that the BNOB Commission was developed at a time when the population that had returned to New Orleans was very small and not terribly representative. This ultimately created unique problems for all involved in this process.

The Louisiana Recovery Authority. Further complicating matters were actions being taken at the state level. As the cumulative impact of both Katrina and Rita had severely impacted 19 parishes across the entire southern coast of Louisiana, Governor Kathleen Blanco on October 17, 2005, signed an executive order creating the Louisiana Recovery Authority (LRA). This 33-member entity was charged with the development and implementation of both short- and long-term recovery and redevelopment strategies for all hurricane-affected parishes. The LRA also became the body responsible for the disbursement of all federal funds allocated by Congress. For the City of New Orleans, the LRA became yet another level of authority to deal with, but one with vast powers, particularly financial. The LRA also stipulated that before any funds controlled by it were distributed to an affected parish, a comprehensive parish-wide recovery plan had to be developed and submitted to it for review. Funding would ultimately be provided based upon the planned projects and processes. This requirement became a major issue for New Orleans, as it was the only affected parish whose city limits and parish boundaries are the same.

One of the LRA's first actions was to co-sponsor the Louisiana Recovery and Rebuilding Conference, in partnership with the American Planning Association, the American Institute of Architects, the American Society of Civil Engineers, and the National Trust for Historic Preservation. This event, attended by some 650 citizens of the state (by invitation only), was held in New Orleans during the second week of November 2005. Local, national, and international speakers made a wide array of technical presentations regarding disaster recovery and flood-protection systems used in foreign countries (e.g. the Netherlands), and presentations on related topics were delivered by nationally recognized experts in historic preservation, civil engineering, computer modeling, etc. At its conclusion, probably more questions existed than answers, but the people of the state were getting mobilized and educated. One striking fact discovered during the meetings, partially facilitated by America Speaks, a Washington-based not-for-profit organization, using high-tech polling technology, was that 72 per cent of the attendees had at least three generations of family still residing within the state. This "rootedness" became a major determinant for decision-making as the planning processes progressed both locally and statewide.

Shortly after this most important meeting, other city-sponsored initiatives were also underway. At the request of the BNOB Land Use Subcommittee, the Urban Land Institute (ULI), a Washington-based not-for-profit organization representing the development industry, deployed a multidisciplinary team to New Orleans to conduct an on-site investigation and analysis of the state of New Orleans. Approximately 50 ULI members from both the public and private sectors spent one week studying all aspects of the situation there. On November 18, 2005, they made preliminary (and very controversial) recommendations on the city's overall recovery.

At a well-attended public meeting, the team presented their findings and recommendations. They suggested shrinking the city's footprint to match a reduced residential base and approaching redevelopment in a phased manner.[8] They warned of the "Jack-o'-Lantern" effect (where the pattern of rebuilding will be erratic in areas of uncontrolled redevelopment). They stressed the need to strategically plan for a potentially slow repopulation and suggested the conversion of heavily damaged neighborhoods into open space/retention ponds/nature reserves. They also called for the formation of a powerful development authority to oversee and direct key recovery efforts. None of their recommendations, although based on sound professional judgment, were seriously considered by either elected officials or the general public. In fact, they were firmly and adamantly rejected.

On November 28, 2005, the mayor declared his intention to "rebuild all of New Orleans" by adopting a market-driven approach to redevelopment/repopulation. In keeping with this concept, the City of New Orleans' Department of Safety and Permits continued to issue building permits city-wide, applying great latitude in certifying a structure's degree of damage. Negotiated assessments were made on a structure-by-structure basis with the overall intent of reducing the estimate to below 50 per cent so structures could be renovated and their owners would not be forced to rebuild from scratch.

On January 11, 2006, recommendations and an overview of the BNOB Commission's plan were presented by the mayor, Land Use chair Joseph Canizaro, and Canizaro's handpicked planning consultant, John Beckman, a principal of Wallace Roberts and Todd, a Philadelphia-based firm with years of experience in dealing with various aspects of New Orleans' growth and development. Specific recommendations of the BNOB Commission included the following: areas with little or no flooding would be open for redevelopment/repopulation immediately; a four-month building-permit moratorium would be imposed on flooded neighborhoods; an extensive light-rail transit system would form the city's organizing framework; and a powerful development authority, the Crescent City Recovery Corporation, with broad and vast powers, would be created to oversee the city's redevelopment. In addition, all 13 planning districts, including 73 separate neighborhoods, would be required to prepare individual development plans within four months. This imposed yet another impossible scope of work and deadline. Integral to the BNOB Commission's plan was a mandate that each neighborhood demonstrate their viability – i.e. prove to the City that their residents and businesses would come back. The BNOB Commission and the City Administration also assumed that FEMA would provide the funds necessary to secure the technical assistance needed to develop the neighborhood recovery plans while also proving their viability. After many meetings between FEMA and the BNOB Commission, it was ultimately deemed unlawful for FEMA to fund these activities.

The Lambert Plans. In response to FEMA's decision not to contribute funds to the BNOB neighborhood-planning activities, the New Orleans City Council, using unspent resources of the Community Development Block Grant (CDBG), hired a consortium of local and national planners, led by Paul Lambert, a Miami-based real estate and housing consultant under contract to the City, and Sheila Danzey (of SHEDO LLC), a local real estate and development consultant, to prepare individual recovery plans (46 in all) for each of the "wet" neighborhoods. "Dry" neighborhoods could not utilize CDBG funds for purposes of recovery planning; therefore, the Lambert Plans, from the outset, could not become the city-wide recovery plan as required by the LRA. However, the professionals engaged in the process provided an important and timely service for the neighborhoods in which they worked. Key members of the Lambert Team that were based in Miami (Bermello Ajamil and Partners, Inc. served as principal planner and project manager for the total project) had been intimately involved in multi-year recovery activities in the aftermath of Hurricane Andrew in Miami-Dade County, so they were uniquely qualified for this post-Katrina assignment. These professionals, working in tandem with their local partners, developed neighborhood-specific rebuilding plans that truly represented the projects and programs deemed important by the residents involved in the process.

Projects were illustrated, mapped, and ranked in order of importance and timeliness, and an order-of-magnitude cost estimate was developed for each specific plan element. This process began in April of 2006, and the Neighborhood Rebuilding Plan was adopted by the City Council by unanimous vote on November 2, 2006. When presented, the full report was 1200 pages in length and truly represented the will of the people within the "wet" neighborhoods; there were also several additional reports for neighborhoods that had chosen to develop independent plans. The total estimated cost for projects and programs included in the Lambert Plans was $4.4 billion.

Qualifying neighborhoods were clustered into designated planning districts (based on previous work done by the City Planning Commission). The University of New Orleans (UNO), at the direction of Chancellor Ryan, a resident of Lakeview, partnered with both District 5 (Lakeview) and District 6 (Gentilly) to assist in their overall recovery efforts, starting in March 2006, prior to the Lambert Team being assigned the contract for recovery planning. Given UNO's close proximity to both District 5 and District 6, the objective was to involve university personnel, along with the affected district residents, business owners, and institutions (churches, schools, police and fire departments), in creating a vision for their neighborhood with specific expertise provided pro bono by UNO faculty and staff, many of whom lived in one or the other district. In both instances, UNO eventually partnered with the district's Recovery Steering Committee as well as the Lambert Team to develop the adopted Neighborhood Rebuilding Plan.

The Unified New Orleans Plan (UNOP). While the Lambert Plans were still under development, an independent group of architects/planners, citizen/neighborhood activists, local and national foundation leaders, and political officials (elected and appointed) determined that a more inclusive process was needed – one that encompassed all 13 planning districts (both "wet" and "dry") to satisfy the requirements established by the LRA for eventual project funding. The scope of UNOP also required the consultant team to address city-wide infrastructure issues and stress hazard mitigation in their overall planning approach.

Financially supported by a consortium that included the Rockefeller Foundation, the State of Louisiana, the Greater New Orleans Foundation, and the Bush-Clinton Katrina Fund, UNOP was managed by an independent not-for-profit organization: the New Orleans Community Support Organization. UNOP was also overseen by a nine-member advisory board, which was composed of both elected and appointed representatives including Albert Petrie, Jr. a recognized Lakeview community leader who served as the City Council District A representative.

These organizations selected and oversaw 16 separate consultant teams that were tasked to prepare recovery plans for all planning districts as well as a city-wide recovery plan that addressed issues such as infrastructure systems, public services, and facilities. During this six-month process, all existing plans developed by the BNOB Commission and the Lambert/SHEDO consultant team were reassessed, refined, and amended for the "wet" neighborhoods that had been previously adopted. New plans, developed from scratch, were prepared for the "dry" neighborhoods. It should be noted that although "wet" neighborhoods incurred varying degrees of physical damage, the "dry" neighborhoods were and to some extent continued for several years to be devastated by economic and demographic impacts. The total estimated cost for UNOP was $14 billion. For District 5 and Lakeview in particular, the UNOP process basically reinforced the findings of the Lambert Plans with minor additions and revisions.

Since a major criticism of both the BNOB and Lambert Plans was their lack of true citizen representation/participation, America Speaks used all-day community congresses to educate, inform, and poll participants (in excess of 1200 New Orleans citizens participated in simultaneous meetings conducted in New Orleans, Baton Rouge, Atlanta, Houston, Dallas, and Memphis), and these meetings were all broadcast electronically and in real-time. This technique, employed during three different congresses, convinced the LRA that the UNOP process was indeed democratic and truly representative.

An unintended consequence of the UNOP process was "planning fatigue": a malady experienced primarily by those citizens who had actively participated in either or both the BNOB and Lambert Plans and then were called upon again to participate in the UNOP process. Citizens felt required to participate in all sorts of meetings, public hearings, topical presentations and issue-specific briefings (e.g. lake area zoning revisions) in order to be fully informed on proposed processes and projects for their neighborhoods. They felt compelled to attend every meeting called by either their neighborhood leaders or the consultants. After enduring this regime week after week (even months), the "citizen-driven planning process" took its toll. The citizens of District 5 were just one of many groups afflicted by this phenomenon.

Dr. Ed Blakely's One New Orleans Plan. On January 8, 2007, Mayor Nagin announced his selection of renowned academician and developer Dr. Ed Blakely as "Recovery Czar" for the City of New Orleans. His official title became the Director of the Office of Recovery Management. For many citizens of the city, the mayor's decision was too little too late. Although everyone recognized the need for a point-person within the city's administration for all matters relating to recovery, Dr. Blakely's arrival was initially greeted with both anticipation and sarcasm. He did create a small but dynamic core of senior staff, but their numbers were a bare minimum.

One of their first challenges was to understand the evolution of the various plans (including UNOP, which was still being developed) and forge a workable and doable plan. The result was the "One New Orleans Plan" (ONOP), which incorporated five key concepts: 1) healing and consultation; 2) physical and emotional security; 3) twenty-first-century infrastructure reconfiguration; 4) economic diversification; 5) developing a safe, secure, and environmentally sustainable settlement pattern. In addition, the plan had to be realistic in scope and budget. By mid-2007, it was also quite apparent that the funds required to implement the Lambert Plans ($4.4 billion) or UNOP ($14 billion) were unlikely to materialize. Consequently Dr. Blakely's approach was to downsize the total effort and approach implementation in increments. He and his staff identified 17 target recovery areas (TRAs) where initial efforts and funds would be focused. The total budget for ONOP was $1.1 billion, with 40 per cent to be spent in the TRAs and the remaining to be spent on city-wide improvements (primarily infrastructure projects). The TRAs did reflect elements of previous recovery plans but at a significantly reduced scale and cost. In 2008, efforts to realize ONOP are ongoing.

Current rebuilding challenges

Resiliency is increasingly present in the literature on rebuilding in post-disaster environments.[6,10,11] The term involves the capacity to restore not only buildings but also social systems.[9] The case of New Orleans helps us to understand its different forms and timeframes. Time and coordination remain very important factors in reinforcing resiliency while achieving a successful and viable recovery. Moreover, different levels of resiliency, involving different types of stakeholders, can be distinguished after a disaster.

Short-term resiliency in New Orleans first involved rebuilding the primary infrastructure systems and city services. The daily lives of residents depend on complex technologies that provide safe drinking water, adequate and reliable drainage and sewage, a 24/7 communication network supported by an adequate infrastructure, flood protection (levee/floodwall reconstruction), debris removal, sanitation services, mail delivery, and the provision of public safety (police and firemen) – i.e. the mundane and normally taken-for-granted city services provided for all citizens in a fully functioning city. These systems are essential for the survival of the population and have to be rebuilt quickly and efficiently post-disaster.

In the case of New Orleans, this phase of recovery has been relatively quick, given the scale of the destruction; however, even in 2008, the city still faces many challenges. For instance, many parts of the drainage systems are not back to their 2005 condition, due to the extensive damage caused by the weight of the floodwater that pooled in some neighborhoods for more than 40 days. The same statement can be applied to roads, bridges, the sewage system, etc. Many basic services still need varying, and in some cases yet to be determined, repair or reconstruction. The flood-protection system has been improved incrementally, as this involves not only the rebuilding of the physical infrastructure (floodwalls and levees) but also the restoration of the natural protection of the city (wetlands).

The stakeholders involved in this phase and in these projects are often far removed from the decision-makers who function at various governmental levels, and they represent discrete agencies or entities representing city, state and federal interests. In Lakeview, for example, floodwall breaks from the 17th Street Canal have been rebuilt by the US Army Corps of Engineers (USACOE); however, additional reinforcements and enhancements still need to be completed. Temporary pumping stations have been constructed by USACOE at the Lake Pontchartrain outfall canal (a recommendation made in the original BNOB Infrastructure Committee report); a permanent pumping station is scheduled for completion by 2010 in roughly the same location.

What can be termed mid-term recovery (5–10 years) will be measured by two indicators: the strength of the economy and the number of permanent residents. The citizens' return is dependent on at least two variables: the availability of housing and the perception of normalcy (functioning city services and support systems). Of particular importance to repopulation is the availability of affordable housing (currently in short supply). In turn, the lack of affordable housing has a dramatic impact on the overall economy. Workers need housing they can afford, and businesses need workers if they are to function and hopefully grow. This forms a closed loop with many major and minor implications. Some segments of the tourism industry have been slow to recover, as many restaurants and hotels have had to adjust to a shortage of employees. The low-wage population is still struggling to come back, as many low-income neighborhoods have not been rebuilt, and, as mentioned, affordable housing is still in short supply.

Economic recovery can be demonstrated both quantitatively and qualitatively. One measure can be the resumption of normal or near-normal operations. Immediately post-Katrina, the Port of New Orleans showed an aggressive resolve to reopen when they serviced their first vessel a few weeks after Hurricane Katrina hit New Orleans. Granted, this was the exception and not the rule; however, the Port has continued to operate as a fully functioning leader in the maritime industry since the arrival of that first ship in mid-September 2005. In 2008, other sectors of the local economy are still struggling (tourism, the hospitality industry, specialty retail). For many sectors of the economy, survival is still the operative mode.

Rebuilding initiatives such as the Road Home Program (administered by the state's LRA) have become synonymous with bureaucratic nightmares: endless paperwork, redundancy at all levels, and poor management and performance. According to some community activists, these state-run programs have actually slowed the rebuilding process. Hence, more than three years after the disaster, New Orleans' economic and repopulation recovery is far from complete. As just one example, in 2004, the total visitor count for the city was estimated to be 10.1 million; in 2008, the total will be roughly 7.6 million. Another indicator is public transit ridership: pre-Katrina daily ridership averaged 135,000; current ridership averages 31,000 per day.

Long-term resiliency requires the rebuilding of the informal social and cultural networks present pre-storm, as these serve to preserve and enhance neighborhood identity and uniqueness. This type of recovery is more difficult to assess, as it is not based on specific measurements. It encompasses formal institutions: churches that serve their respective congregations or build new ones; functioning neighborhood or parochial schools; operative and accessible health-care systems; and adequate police and fire protection with sufficient support facilities (police and fire stations repaired or reconstructed and fully operational). It also encompasses the informal institutions unique to New Orleans culture: an interconnected network of bars, restaurants, lounges, clubs, etc. that have always played a major role in the life of the city.

Lakeview

Lakeview was one of the most devastated areas of the city. Its western boundary was the infamous 17th Street drainage canal, the location of one of the most serious floodwall failures. Its northern boundary was the Lake Pontchartrain shoreline, where the storm surge overtopped the earthen levees; portions of Lakeview were covered with over 4.5 meters of water, and flooding of 2.5 to 3.5 meters was not unusual. It is estimated that only 42 per cent of the residents have returned to the neighborhood.

Lakeview was one of the city's most desirable residential areas. It included early-twentieth-century suburban neighborhoods (Parkview, a historic district adjacent to Bayou St. John and City Park, one of New Orleans' finest urban amenities), post-Second World War tract housing (primarily built slab on grade), and genteel upper-income lakefront estates located in progressive "new town" developments adjacent to Lake Pontchartrain. Taken *in toto*, Lakeview contained a unique mix of building types that illustrated various phases of both historic and contemporary urban development.

One of Lakeview's claims to fame was its central locale, situated midway between the central business district and Lake Pontchartrain. It was located next to City Park and the lakefront's multiple amenities. It retained historic remnants of the pre-jazz West End entertainment district, with a collection of legendary seafood restaurants, a small but functioning commercial fishing fleet, a municipal yacht harbour, and the New Canal Lighthouse. Verdantly landscaped sunken gardens were planted within its central roadway median. Its main street, Harrison Avenue, was populated by churches, parochial and public schools, and a public library, as well as shops and restaurants catering to the local trade. Tony Angelo's, a restaurant frequented only by locals, for which signage wasn't necessary, was a well-known culinary landmark. It was a healthy, happy neighborhood that served as "home" to families for multiple generations.

For Lakeview's residents, this close-knit neighborhood was a diverse collection of both formal and informal networks. After Katrina, in response to the often-asked question "What do you want for your neighborhood?" the standard and most common response was "I want it to be just like it was on August 28, 2005." Whether this remains feasible is still an unanswered question.

All of the ills first described by the ULI team in November 2005 can be seen in 2008: haphazard development patterns reflecting the "Jack-o'-Lantern" effect (occurring in some areas more than others), strained city services, and depopulation or erratic repopulation.

However, much progress has been and continues to be made. Recovery is extremely varied, even by block or individual street. Some residences have been completely renovated or rebuilt, while others haven't been touched since the storm, presenting an eerie sight to the unknowing. On a number of lots, "McMansions" (super-sized houses) have sprouted (like overgrown weeds). On other blocks in particular neighborhoods (such as Lakewood South), most houses are repaired.

In yet others, however, there is little evidence of any progress. House demolitions are rare in 2008, as are house guttings, although these activities still take place on occasion. The roads, never anything to write home about pre-storm, remain miserable to this day, particularly the side streets. Potholes of enormous dimensions lurk around many street corners. City parks remain overgrown and lack adequate maintenance. The library remains shuttered. The public elementary school site is now vacant, awaiting a new complex of buildings. However, most of the churches and their schools are fully functioning, drawing their faithful congregations back home. Starbucks (a well-known chain of coffee shops) has moved into the neighborhood, but several banks are still operating out of temporary trailers while new replacements are being designed and constructed. Most of the lakefront properties have been rehabbed. The lakefront parks and levees are being repaired and reconstructed. Most utility systems are fully functional.

A key recovery factor

Pre-storm, Lakeview had multiple neighborhood associations and special-purpose organizations that were extremely well organized and politically connected. They had real personal bonds (both formal and informal) that were established over the years pre-Katrina, and these bonds were used post-storm to form the basic recovery organization and social network used so effectively by area residents to confront their post-Katrina reality. Perhaps most important to their collective recovery has been the institutional framework created by these individual neighborhood organizations: specifically, the Lakeview Civic Improvement Association (LCIA). The new Lakeview is more connected both formally and informally; residents now know that they cannot rely on the government to solve their problems, but they can and do rely on themselves and on their community organizations and leaders to resolve both short-term and long-term issues, projects, and programs.

Stakeholders in Lakeview

If a disaster-mitigation plan had been in place before the storms, the city's recovery would have been quicker, more coordinated, and probably reinforced by more initiatives with the private sector or other non-traditional partners. Unfortunately, no such plan existed, so post-disaster planning/recovery efforts remained unorganized and in some cases redundant. Many plans have been developed over the period 2005 to 2008 by a multitude of well-meaning and dedicated professionals: planners, architects, social scientists, engineers, geographers, community organizers, advocacy interests, etc. However, the cumulative impact remains spotty, at best. Throughout this often-times frenetic period, a constant presence has been the *citizen activists*: individuals from all areas of the city, representing all races, incomes, and ages, who have remained actively engaged in this arduous series of processes and dialogues, which continue unabated to this day.

As in any other disaster, a multitude of stakeholders are involved and playing specific roles, and as time passes, their mix and focus changes. In the case of New Orleans, the first wave of returnees was mostly made up of residents from non-flooded areas as well as FEMA employees, state-agency officials/staff, public safety and security personnel, the National Guard, essential city staff, port employees, demolition contractors, a smattering of contractors and laborers, and a massive number of volunteers (initially deployed for debris removal and house gutting). It should be remembered that for the first several weeks access to the city was restricted to essential personnel, who gained access using specially issued clearance passes. Most city services were non-existent at this point. As time went on, the mix changed. Residents were allowed back into parts of the city in a phased manner, with non-flooded areas being given first priority. As conditions improved, more areas of the city were opened and occupied.

Throughout this long and involved process, what has remained constant is the struggle to build an integrated strategy among many differing stakeholders, each having their own individual priorities and needs. The variety of stakeholders is still growing, but they all share one quality: they remain committed citizens (either New Orleans residents or out-of-town volunteers) representing many diverse interests (faith-based organizations, community activists, environmentalists, etc.). However, one overarching question remains as we watch this recovery saga unfold: who is doing what, with what impact, and is it integrated into a larger context? Unfortunately, the answer given by many remains "Who knows?" Stakeholders have formed the opinion that they "can't afford to miss meetings or not participate," fearing their interests won't be represented in the final product or included in the ever-changing decision-making process.

Each of the recovery plans and their respective authors has strived to develop a coherent rebuilding blueprint or redevelopment strategy with varying degrees of success. All have employed unique processes that have involved differing professionals (both local and national) and lay participants (primarily concerned citizens and neighborhood activists). During the development of each of these planning processes, unique challenges have occurred. However, one overarching hurdle for consultants has been to engage the affected citizens in a meaningful manner while overcoming their inherent scepticism.

A complex rebuilding process

One of the first challenges for the communities in Lakeview was to reorganize and re-establish their civic networks and prove their viability. Lakeview was fortunate to have an active set of neighborhood associations in place and operational pre-storm. Pre-eminent was the LCIA. It had been the largest civic association in Louisiana for over 60 years. Post-storm, being one of the city's oldest and most active civic organizations, the LCIA (both its membership and its leaders) formed a cohesive and powerful force for the area's survival and recovery. They were instrumental in organizing themselves and others in the difficult tasks to be faced in the months and years to come.

During the initial post-Katrina period, the citizens of Lakeview and of many other areas of the city had many questions that could not be answered: For example, what level of pollution existed in their heavily flooded community? Was the soil contaminated? Who could provide answers? But the answers were insufficient, incomplete, and hard to obtain.

By October 2005, residents were getting more and more frustrated about the lack of information being provided by the authorities at all levels of government. Many realized that "their government" either didn't know the answers or wouldn't tell them. They therefore decided, almost by default, to take things into their own hands. They held their first general meeting at the Heritage Plaza. Hundreds of citizens showed up to vent their frustration, ask questions, and attempt to understand what they might be facing in the immediate future. As the elected officials had no plan to propose and few answers to provide, people were understandably upset. Fortunately, key community stakeholders who held important civic positions in the community (within both the public and private sectors) had knowledge of the actual infrastructure-rebuilding process. Some of these spokespeople were able to share important information, as they were acting as contractors for federal agencies involved in various activities of the recovery process (e.g. debris removal), and they gave both concrete information and hope to the residents.

The USACOE, the federal agency responsible for repairs to the levees and floodwalls, had been developing a new strategy for the 17th Street Canal and other elements of the area's flood-protection system. However, they were not communicating their plans in an effective manner. At this critical juncture, it was important for Lakeview's citizens to know as much as possible so they could make an informed decision about whether to return and whether they would ultimately be safe in their neighborhood in the event of future storms.

While individual neighborhood organizations were reorganizing themselves, the citizens who could come back were returning at a slow pace, with many being forced to live in temporary housing (such as trailers provided by FEMA).

At the suggestion of BNOB leaders, LCIA leaders mobilized to re-establish their respective neighborhood organizations and to establish a communication network (normal communication systems did not function at this time, so cell phones and the internet became the foundations for all communication).

The decision to organize the city into distinct geographic districts was in direct response to a decision made by the City to organize overall planning activities on the basis of specific geographic areas, using the somewhat arbitrary planning districts developed before 2000 as part of the City Planning Commission's initial Master Plan organization.

Members of the District 5 Recovery Steering Committee (RSC) included the presidents of the seven affected neighborhoods within District 5 and other uniquely qualified residents of the affected areas with particular skills (public relations, finance, engineering, project management, etc.). The RSC members organized themselves into a very complex network of 72 issue-oriented committees and subcommittees. This was already established and operational before the UNO began its partnership with the RSC. At the first joint meeting, held during the second week of March 2006, UNO faculty and staff were assigned particular responsibilities and points of contact with the RSC leadership.

Weekly RSC briefings and committee meetings were held so that individuals, as well as the overall group, were kept informed of the neighborhood's status. Formal committee and subcommittee reports were also required. This reporting tool was later used to great advantage by the infrastructure committee to establish and maintain direct communication links with key City department heads and staff members: e.g. the City Planning Commission, the Sewerage and Water Board, and the Department of Public Works.

Pre-storm, the general area had a crime-prevention district committee organized by representative block captains. Post-storm, the District 5 RSC used a similar structure to organize their efforts, the block captains being the spokespeople for the needs and desires of their respective areas. Although the BNOB Commission did not provide productive rebuilding guidance, it forced the community to re-energize their informal social network and revitalize their neighborhood organizations, in order to organize and guide their collective efforts to save their community. It was clear that citizen activism was essential.

District 5 (the greater Lakeview area) includes seven distinct neighborhoods as well as City Park. The neighborhoods' relation to the local authorities at that point was: "Lead us or get out of our way." They decided to carefully organize and coordinate their efforts to demonstrate a united front, while presenting one comprehensive recovery plan.

One of the most organized and effective committees was the infrastructure committee. This committee was essential from the outset, as the neighborhood was initially lacking all forms of functioning infrastructure: utilities, sanitation services, communications (including telephone and cable TV), street lighting, drainage and sewage systems, mail delivery, fire and police protection, etc. The first concern was to determine the state of the infrastructure so that Lakeview could be rebuilt as a community based on fact, not on fiction or guesswork. Therefore, accurate and timely information on all aspects of the infrastructure systems was vital.

Meanwhile, resident-generated surveys showed incremental improvements (number of permits issued by type, number of demolitions underway, status of streetlights, etc.), which were shared with the rest of the residents through the efforts of the communications committee. Each committee, regardless of its specific focus, had timelines and benchmarks, which were essential to delivering tangible and useable products to both the RSC and the city.

A vision for the future

Soon after UNO partnered with the District 5 RSC to assist them in the development of a recovery plan while simultaneously proving their viability, the Lambert/SHEDO Team was designated by the City Council as technical support to assist distressed neighborhoods in developing their individual recovery plans, as mandated by the mayor. Using professional consultant firms from Florida (who had extensive experience with recovery planning) and other national and local architecture and planning firms, this professional consortium undertook a massive public planning and educational effort, requiring exhaustive community outreach and engagement. For District

5, this required developing consensus on six separate neighborhood plans (Parkview and City Park were combined into one recovery plan). Each plan identified specific projects that were reviewed and approved or rejected by citizen participants in numerous public hearings in each of the seven distinct neighborhoods. The projects and programs were also ranked according to their degree of importance and need (immediate, mid-range, and long-range). Upon completion and adoption, the New Orleans Rebuilding Plan (the Lambert Plan) was estimated to cost $4 billion.

There were underlying assumptions made by the Lambert Team from the outset. They included: 1) the federal government would provide a secure flood-protection system capable of withstanding a one in one-hundred-year storm; 2) the City would adopt and enforce new building code standards to improve wind resistance; 3) the City's basic street grid and urban structure was sound and should be maintained/enhanced; 4) an operable hurricane evacuation program would exist.

One significant accomplishment of the Lambert Plan's consultants was to work in close consultation with FEMA to establish an adjusted base flood elevation (ABFE) for all structures that were to be either substantially renovated or rebuilt at a 1 meter elevation (ABFE was measured from the crown of the street fronting the property). This established a minimum elevation for the first floor of all residences; many newly constructed homes have been raised to higher elevations (2.5 meters or higher). This has presented (and continues to present) a unique challenge for architects and owners (see Figure 6.3).

Difficulties

One major problem city-wide is that City government has not been enforcing rules currently "on the books." This situation exists due to either a manpower shortage or a lack of focus within several city departments. The need for a new zoning ordinance specific to District 5 became painfully obvious to many citizens as they struggled to rehabilitate their homes. After working for months with representatives of the City Planning Commission, District A Councilwoman Midura and a special committee of the District 5 RSC spearheaded a new zoning ordinance for the lake area, which was adopted on October 18, 2007. It is currently included in the *Comprehensive Zoning Ordinance* (CZO) as Chapter 28. However, at this time, the City Planning Commission, working in close coordination with their consultants led by the Goody-Clancy firm of Boston, Massachusetts, is in the process of developing a new city-wide master plan, which, based upon a recent vote, will have "the force of law." It is expected that the entire process, including a rewrite of the CZO, will be completed by the end of 2009.

Blight is also a major challenge. To address this problem, the Lakeview Blight Committee has been created. It has identified roughly 1700 homes in various stages of "blight" or neglect within their specific area. Batches of 200 notices are sent out weekly to the property owners in question, so

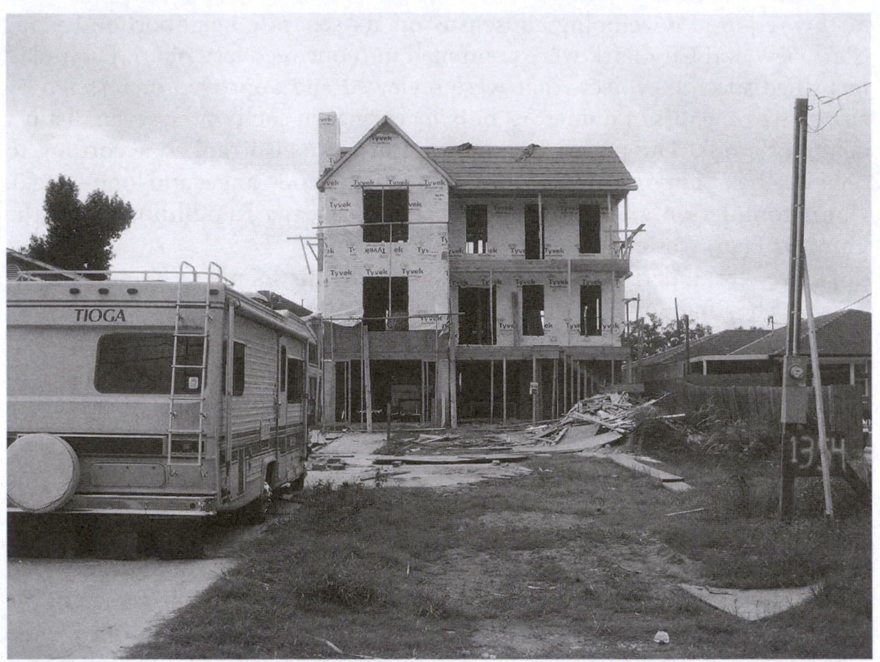

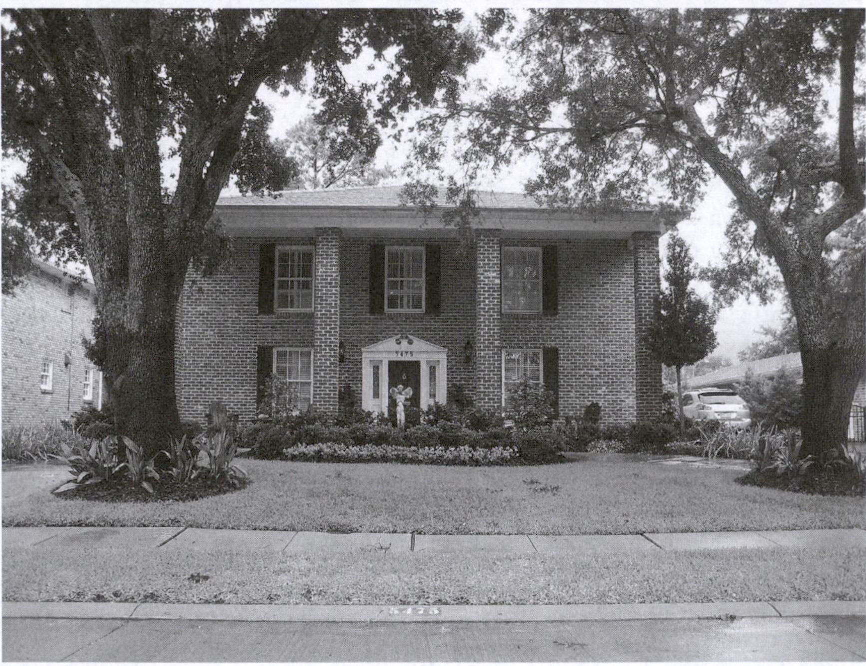

Figure 6.3 Rebuilding houses in Lakeview: a unique challenge for architects and owners.

that the volunteer staff can keep up with the paperwork, man the phones, and monitor the legal process. The "blight fight" is working in Lakeview because the area has a dedicated base of residents who remain active and persistent. The committee now works closely with the tax assessor's office, which maintains cell phone contact information and property addresses for tax purposes. Therefore the committee can now reach citizens who have not even gutted their house or mowed their lots post-Katrina. Unfortunately, the committee and legal council have to resort to lawsuits (citations for benign neglect) to get the lots mowed or the houses gutted.

Lack of funding is another major challenge. Major projects funded by the public sector have been scarce. More prevalent have been projects undertaken by the private sector. These have included numerous reconstructions of commercial structures at strategic locations within District 5. City Park has recently begun a series of projects to reinforce its primary civic function: a major urban open space serving as the location of many regional assets, including the New Orleans Museum of Art, the Bestoff Sculpture Garden, the Pavilion of the Two Sisters, the botanical garden, and Storyland (a kids' mini-park), as well as major recreational facilities.

The area's main street, Harrison Avenue, now has reopened businesses and vibrant churches, with their affiliated parochial schools. This is successful largely thanks to the infusion of private investment, not public funds. Other institutional anchors are back and thriving. The public library, currently operating out of a donated trailer with funds provided by the Bill and Melinda Gates Foundation, is a new addition to the street. A new permanent library is scheduled for completion in 2018, when it will be the second largest library in the city. Starbucks has opened, as have several mainstay restaurants, banks, a new pharmacy, and assorted specialty retailers.

To date in 2008, as far as public involvement is concerned, the main results are a multitude of plans, with a litany of projects identified and illustrated, but with little or no money available to implement them. Significant funds, from various public and private sources, are just beginning to arrive in New Orleans.

The residents of Lakeview feel more connected since the storm. They have faced their common adversity together, and in doing so, they have built and maintained strong linkages and relationships. The citizens of Lakeview and District 5 have revealed the importance of working incrementally (step by step) in an organized manner. They have shown that ordinary people can accomplish superhuman achievements. The fact that this community had a powerful organization in place prior to Katrina was essential: the citizens knew who could assume leadership, organize, and ultimately act for the betterment of the entire area and its respective citizens.

One citizen can make a difference in a profound manner: the Beacon of Hope

Two neighborhoods within District 5, Lakewood North and Lakewood South, were the nexus for a particular not-for-profit organization that sprang from the efforts and example of one woman and her trials and tribulations in rebuilding her house. Recognizing from the very beginning that recovery would be a painful process, Denise Thornton, a typical yet very focused community activist, demonstrated by doing and in the process created a non-profit structure that has been replicated as a model of community recovery: the Beacon of Hope.

This highly motivated, dedicated, and organized resident decided to rebuild her house months after Katrina tore through this neighborhood and in doing so helped her community come back. Her first issue was to repair her home – to show her neighbors that it was feasible. In doing so, she began to learn all the ins and outs of home reconstruction: what forms and permits are required, what contractors can be trusted, what financial tools are available, what volunteers are available to gut houses or mow the grass, etc.

Then she needed a mechanism to "spread the word." The idea was to share her personal experience and use it as a tool for rebuilding her neighborhood. Information and access to resources (tools, computers, printers, forms, email lists, personal recommendations on reliable resources, etc.) formed her recovery model. Her router helped residents get connected as well, via the internet, so they could identify additional resources and contractors. During reconstruction, she started a database, based at her house, for the multitude of issues that her returning neighbors would need as they faced the many trials and tribulations of recovery, house by house and neighbor by neighbor.

She informed the 12 families who were already rebuilding their houses that she was going to open her house, even if it was not finished, on May 20, 2006, the primary election day for the mayor's race, to show what progress could be made. The goal was to show how she was able to restore her own house and welcome returning residents or potential residents back home. A map of the neighborhood and open houses was available to people. The event included food, music, and a tour of the gutted homes and houses for sale (opened by the listing realtors). JRS Rentals donated 20-foot by 20-foot tents, which were used to host any representative associated with home repair or reconstruction, including mold remediation, electrical contracting, and utilities (Energy, Sewage and Water Board, etc.).

In February 2006, neighbors and other types of stakeholder, such as the St. Paul Episcopal Church and Lakeview Christian Center, committed to helping reorganize the neighborhood. The Lakeview Christian Center was the first local, organized group to volunteer on a regular basis. This group has continued its ministry through volunteer service and is still very active today. One of the most important needs at the beginning was to clean the debris, exterior and interior, so as to give some sense of normality and order. The first volunteer groups came to help clean the devastated lots and gut houses. Simultaneously, the Beacon of Hope (mentioned above) was created, thanks to grants that helped to buy the essentials for neighborhood and individual recovery. Gardening tools lent to neighbors so that they could keep their lots clean, computers, printers, a website, and publicity were all used to organize and aid the community. The Beacon of Hope thus became the center of activity and information for these neighborhoods.

The initial outreach event was successful, as many evacuees showed up and signed a mailing list to receive information on the progress of recovery and revival. They looked at the 12 houses in progress and became convinced over time that recovery was possible and achievable. When people needed equipment, advice, or just a place to share their challenges and anxieties, the Beacon was open to help them and send them back stronger and more educated to face their difficulties. This resource center served as an independent recovery node within the wider District 5 community. This small-scale bottom-up initiative had and still has a strong administrative structure that has been codified for other Beacons to follow as they establish their own individual nodes in other neighborhoods. Figure 6.4 shows some of the stakeholders of the Lakewood Beacon of Hope.

This type of bottom-up organization is an excellent recovery model to "rally the troops." Lakewood in 2008 is more than 80 per cent rebuilt. Maps are updated with the status of houses, and the ongoing recovery is communicated to the citizens as well as to the City. Communication and accurate information have been and continue to be key, and this structure has made it possible not only to show the progress but also to reach out to evacuees. Members of the organization have contacted former residents who have done little or nothing to their property to urge them into action.

Other Beacons are being opened in neighborhoods such as Gentilly or Ninth Ward, where this type of grassroots organization is most needed. The organizing team of the Lakewood Beacon also went to Iowa after the 2008 spring flood to share their experience in Cedar Rapids. They provided the civic leaders in Cedar Rapids with both the Beacon volunteer manual and the Beacon administration manual. This non-profit organization is a model of a small-scale resident-driven initiative to help communities regroup and rebuild their long-term resilience after a disaster. The challenge is now to learn, replicate, and link the process to the larger plan developed by the City.

Conclusion

Many stakeholders have been working for the last three years toward the same goal within the same city: recovery and the return to normalcy for the citizens of New Orleans.

One of the main challenges seems to be the issue of coordination and timing. The process to date has been never-ending for those who have actively participated in it. It also has been quite challenging, involving both top-down strategies and bottom-up "happenings." Hence, in this context, communities are managing to come back, each in its own way and sometimes in spite of the government. There still needs to be a greater effort to integrate the public visions, as expressed in the various planning processes, with both public and private investments.

The Lakeview community provided some "knock out" lessons that can usefully be learned: change the mindset regarding risk and learn from the arduous Katrina experience; organize at the grassroots level; stay focused; recover incrementally; and remember that information in a post-disaster environment is like "gold in the dust." Furthermore, do not wait for the government; do what you can, independent of them, and lead, do not follow. The role of the local community is to support the rebuilding effort; it is not supposed to take the main leadership position, but it has to be respected, as the success of the recovery depends on its input and support. Recovery also has to be guided and grounded in reality.

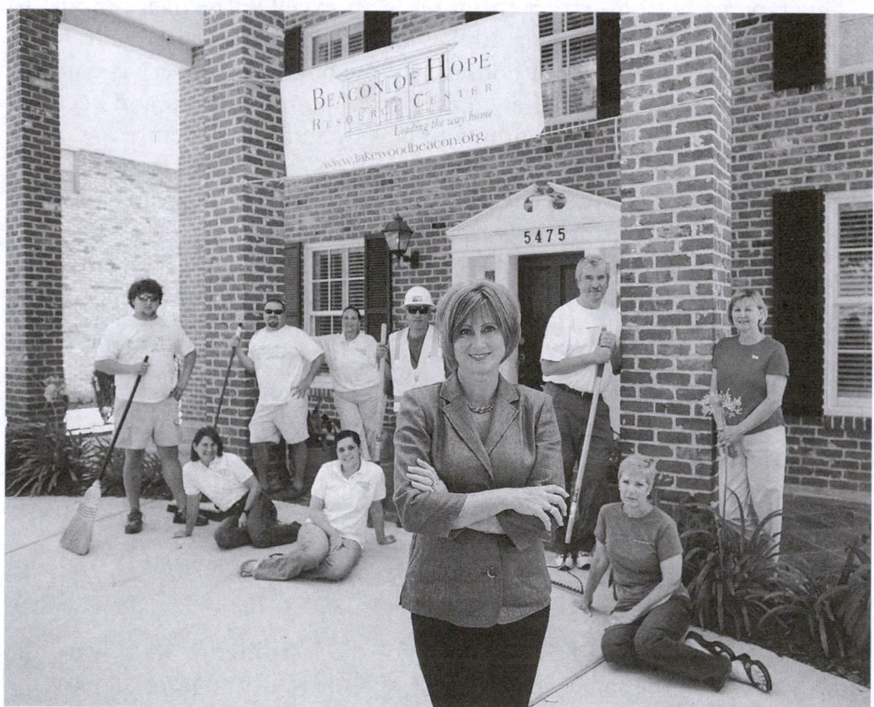

Figure 6.4 The stakeholders of the Lakewood Beacon of Hope.
Source: R. Romaguera.

7 Surviving the second tsunami

Land rights in the face of buffer zones, land grabs and development

Graeme Bristol

> The developers have tried before to chase people away. Now the tsunami has done the job for them.
>
> A Thai senator commenting on the aftermath of the tsunami.[1]

Government institutions, corporations and individuals will make use of the opportunities afforded by disaster. The confusion, tragedy and loss offer the opportunity for them to implement plans for development. This second wave of what Naomi Klein calls 'disaster capitalism' dashes any hope of communities returning to their normal lives. Post-tsunami development plans along the coasts of the most heavily affected countries of Sri Lanka, India, Indonesia and Thailand clearly show a pattern to this second wave. In much the same way that communities must plan for disaster, they must also be prepared for the aftershocks of development that follow.

Introduction

Daeng had never intended to be a community leader. Personal tragedy brought that task to her, along with grief and outrage.

It began in December 2002, when soldiers appeared in Laem Pom, a community of some 50 families just to the south of the larger fishing village of Baan Nam Khem. They informed the residents that this land was no longer theirs. For many years this whole area had been the site of a thriving tin mine, but by the middle of the 1970s the tin had been extracted, and the company left their workers to their own devices. While some left, many stayed and rebuilt the economy of the Laem Pom and Baan Nam Khem around fishing. By the late 1990s the economy was successful enough that the population of Baan Nam Khem had reached about 5000.

The armed soldiers informed the residents of Laem Pom that the land had been sold by the previous owner to the Far East Company. They were there to survey the land and to put up a barbed-wire fence around it. If this was a legitimate claim, though, Daeng thought, why did they need armed soldiers? How did this state-owned land become private property? If either the selling company or the buying company had a legal deed, surely they would simply go to the courts to resolve the dispute in their favour. There would be no need to intimidate the residents with these soldiers. She started to fight back by organizing her neighbours and collecting documents to prove the fact that they had been living there for more than 25 years. However, after two court appearances and the murder of one of her allies, there was still no resolution to the land dispute by December of 2004.

On the morning of the tsunami, Daeng had headed out early to one of the resorts about ten kilometres south of her home at Laem Pom beach. There was a prospect of becoming one of the suppliers of fish to the resort, and this additional source of income could be an important boost to the family income.[12] She was still at the resort, waiting for the purchasing manager, when the first wave struck. That she survived at all was really a matter of luck, if one could call it that.

It took her nearly two hours to get back to the road into Baan Nam Khem, the fishing village about 500 metres north of Laem Pom. As she came down the hill into the town, she could see there was little left but rubble. If Baan Nam Khem was so thoroughly destroyed, there was no chance that the unprotected hamlet of Laem Pom would have been spared. When she finally arrived, there was nothing left but broken bodies of her family, friends and neighbours, many of them cut and tangled in the razor-wire fencing the soldiers had erected. After a few hours of finding bodies, she could stand it no longer and headed back up to the main road. She found her husband alive and sitting in the back of a truck. They went back to the hospital together.

The next morning she continued her search for her children. When she reached the area where her house used to be, she was stopped by men standing by the barbed-wire fence. 'I begged them in tears to let me in so I could find my daughter and my relatives. They said the tsunami could not kill me, but they could.'[7]

She didn't find the badly decomposed body of her daughter for another ten days. 'Had I found her earlier, my daughter wouldn't have been in this condition,' she says, her voice full of rage. 'Look! Look at what they did to my little girl. Look at her!' ... 'I can no longer stand their inhumanity; I can't bear the injustice.'[7]

Two months later, when I first met her in Laem Pom, she was living in a tent, but she was on her land. About 300 metres away from her and the shore, there was an encampment of armed men. They were clearly waiting for all the prying eyes of the foreigners to simply go away. Part of what kept them from acting against Daeng was the fact that a small BBC crew had set up a tent next to hers. These crew members were witnesses but they would not be there forever.

The plight of the residents of Laem Pom is by no means unique. It is, pointedly, typical. There are patterns to development, and these patterns are made more obvious and urgent through the 'opportunities' afforded by disaster. I want to look a little more closely at some of these patterns and how they were enacted in policy responses at the international level. From there, based on work done in the recovery process with architecture students and with UN-HABITAT, I will look more closely at the responses in Thailand. Finally, I would like to raise a few points about preparations communities can make to resist the cruelty of the few.

The international response

What is this pattern represented by the experience of the Laem Pom community? What emerges from that experience is well described as 'disaster capitalism' by Naomi Klein in her book *The Shock Doctrine*.[11] Her observations about the response governments and the private sector have to the typical circumstances surrounding a disaster provide a valuable context for understanding the decisions made in the aftermath of the tsunami. With that in mind, I want to review seven different issues/responses arising from the tsunami disaster and briefly indicate the responses to them in Sri Lanka, India and Indonesia.

The shock doctrine

Klein recognized that in natural disasters such as the tsunami and Hurricane Katrina or in man-made disasters such as the war in Iraq, the acts visited upon the Laem Pom community and so many others like it were actually a strategy and not an anomaly.

The shock doctrine is a product of Milton Friedman and the neo-liberal philosophy of economics that took hold at the University of Chicago Department of Economics in the 1950s. Klein's contention is based on the writing of Friedman and his disciples, on policies put into place in a number of countries in the name of this approach to economics, and on the premise that these policies are politically unpopular. These policies cover three areas of concern: deregulation, privatization and dramatic reduction in the funding for social programmes. Klein gives substantial evidence that they are deeply unpopular. In order to implement such politically unpalatable policies, there is a need for what Friedman called 'economic shock treatment'.[11] Although shock treatment refers to the 'speed, suddenness and scope of the economic shifts', these shifts are most readily performed in the midst of crisis. As Friedman put it:

> … only a crisis – actual or perceived – produces real change. When that crisis occurs, the actions that are taken depend on the ideas that are lying around. That, I believe, is our basic function: to develop alternatives to existing policies, to keep them alive and available until the politically impossible becomes politically inevitable. (page 6)[11]

These crises can be created or they can be natural disasters. They can be economic free-fall or hurricanes. The key to the production of 'real change' is that these ideas are, in fact, lying around as alternatives. In other words, it takes planning in order to be prepared to use crisis as an opportunity for turning the politically impossible into the politically inevitable.

In addition to the implementation of these unpopular economic policies, the other aspect of these 'shock treatments' is memory loss. Klein uses the CIA electroshock therapy experiments at McGill University in the 1950s as a metaphor for the larger societal shock treatments. Dr. Ewen Cameron, the doctor who conducted these experiments, stated that the 'massive loss of all recollections brought on by intensive ECT wasn't an unfortunate side effect; it was the essential point of the treatment.' In the first real opportunity to test the strategy of economic shock treatments – the Pinochet coup in Chile in 1973 – the erasure of memory was also a key component in the spread of uncertainty and terror. People simply disappeared along with their histories.

I raise these points because the implementation of a number of the tsunami recovery policies involved similar strategies.

Policy responses

The object of any recovery process is the return to normalcy, which is to say 'whatever existed before the disaster'.[5] There is, of course, the urge to improve on 'whatever existed before'. In many instances, this is absolutely necessary. We do not want to rebuild schools that will again collapse in earthquakes. We want to build new housing that can perform better under the forces of storm surges or a tsunami. Or, to take this idea of improvement further, we rebuild the housing so it never faces the threat of the tsunami. If we move people off these beaches or away from that floodplain or out of the delta area or the fault line, everybody will be safe from that kind of disaster. This urge to improve on the safety of survivors might work but for the fact that that would mean finding other land for these people, uprooting communities from their history and culture and removing them from their sources of employment.

More often, the urge to improve on whatever existed before the disaster is related more to the sense of opportunity arising from the slate having been wiped clean. While the protection and safety of citizens is presented as the rationale for the policy decision to move people away from the danger zone, the underlying motivation has much more to do with the opportunity to take advantage of the shock of disaster and the temporary relocation of traditional landholders by claiming ownership of the land for development purposes. In this case, the beach has been wiped clean of traditional landholders and all their housing, docks, boats and storage. With survivors located in relief camps, this provides an opportunity to use the now unoccupied land more effectively for a 'higher economic purpose'. As Klein points out, this is not the aberrant behaviour of a few greedy people; this is standard operating procedure for 'disaster capitalism'. It is out of this conflict that the issue of land rights is raised.

The resolution of the conflict over land and the right to it is a central issue for the recovery process. Without access to land, the recovery of both housing and employment become problematic, if not impossible. Agencies funding the recovery process will not begin building until outstanding land disputes are resolved.

How are these disputes manifested in practice? I see eight different conditions and/or responses to conditions that affect the access to land after the tsunami.

1 *Buffer zones (the land-use planning response)*. Buffer zones are often set up between conflicting parties – at abortion clinics in the United States, for example, or demilitarized zones between states in conflict. They also apply to protective zones between different activities, such as those between forest reserves and industrial development, where mangrove forests act as a buffer zone between the sea and human habitation, or those between hazardous activities and protected areas, such as zones where pesticides can be used and those where they cannot.

   After the tsunami, the common and very understandable approach was to treat the sea as the hazardous area and then to set up a buffer zone between any habitation and that danger. However, access and proximity to the sea is critical for two key activities – fishing and tourism. With the former, this is focused on traditional fishing communities rather than commercial fishing. With the latter, the focus is on commercial tourism rather than community-based tourism. Where the livelihoods of traditional fishing communities were at stake, the need for buffer zones was critical. Where commercial interests were at stake, the exceptions to the buffer zones were essential.

   Initially, the buffer zones in Indonesia were set at an extravagant two kilometres.[21] UPLINK (Urban Poor Linkage) and other Indonesian NGOs successfully fought this policy, and the two-kilometre setback was rescinded.[1] In Sri Lanka, the Task Force to Rebuild the Nation (TAFREN), formed the week after the tsunami, decreed a buffer zone of 100 metres in the south and 200 metres in the north and east.[6] Given that the extent of inundation of the tsunami was as much as 400 metres,[24] there was a well-founded justification for local communities within these proposed buffer zones to believe that the purpose of these buffer zones was not their protection but simply to remove them from these commercially valuable zones.

2 *Land disputes (the legal response)*. In many instances, opportunities were taken to pursue legal claims that had existed before the tsunami or to fabricate legal claims. These actions were taken by both private developers and public authorities. Where the creation of buffer zones used land-use planning as a policy tool, land disputes used the courts. With the reliance on records, the courts provide a natural advantage to those who can produce records of ownership, of sale, or even of identity.

Traditional landholders are seldom able to do so. Where they did have any such records of continuous possession of the land, in many instances these records were swept away in the tsunami (see 6, below), which left them much more vulnerable to other claims to the land, whether legal or fabricated.

Public authorities such as ministries of forests, parks, fisheries or harbours would often use the tragic removal of people from the land as a means, finally and more easily, to enforce the existing laws against habitation in specific protected areas of land, such as mangrove forests and national parks.

Another form of dispute concerns inheritance. This was particularly the case under Syariah Courts in Indonesia, and it was a central issue of women's rights to land. The most common land disputes involved complex inheritance issues. '[T]he sheer number of deaths means land-related inheritance cases still constitute the predominant form of land-related conflict after the tsunami.'[9]

3 *Threats of violence (land grabs)*. The story that introduced this chapter indicates the nature of land grabs at their most personal and threatening. There are other levels, both less personal and less violent, but the results are the same. One example is the occupation of land while the former landholders are absent and living in a relief camp. While the former landholders are away, the invading land grabber – often a corporation – will erect barbed-wire fencing around the land and post armed guards around it to ensure that the former residents cannot return to occupy it.

Another form of threat of violence is the military. As with any disaster, the national military forces are called upon to assist in rescue operations, clean-up, the building of relief camps and, often, the rebuilding of housing and infrastructure. In the conflict areas of Indonesia and Sri Lanka, the presence of the military is itself seen as a threat. The Indonesian military (TNI) had imposed martial law between 1989 and 1998. It was reimposed in 2003–2004. The day before the tsunami struck, the TNI had killed 18 guerrillas in Aceh. More than 3000 had been killed since the imposition of martial law in May of 2003.[17] Before the tsunami hit, the civilian population was terrorized by the TNI and was justifiably fearful and suspicious of any of their actions. The military, on the other side, viewed all Acehnese as likely members of the Free Aceh Movement (GAM). These attitudes had a significant effect on the relief efforts and reduced the flow of aid because it was seen as 'forming new supply lines for rebels in the hills'.[17] Under such circumstances, for many Acehnese, returning quickly to their land to reclaim it became a larger nightmare.

4 *Development (higher economic return)*. A statement made by the Tourist Board of Sri Lanka typifies the development response to the tsunami: 'In a cruel twist of fate, nature has presented Sri Lanka with a unique opportunity, and out of this great tragedy will come a world class tourism destination.'[19] Land, in other words, is viewed as being cleared of people

and therefore of any title or right of use they may have had over the land they occupied before the tsunami. That view only applied to traditional landholders, mainly fishing communities. It certainly did not apply to the land occupied by existing tourist resorts.

Klein pointed out that in Arugam Bay on the east coast there had been disputes between hotel owners and the traditional fishing community. The hotel owners wanted exclusive use of the beach and to be rid of the sight of the traditional houses on the beach and the smell of drying fish. The tsunami came and swept all that away. The hotel owners then only had to keep the survivors from returning. In addition to the buffer zone, the national government prepared the 'Arugam Bay Resource Development Plan'. This plan called for transforming the town, though most of it was largely undamaged, into a 'boutique tourism destination'. This $80 million redevelopment was to be financed out of the aid money raised in the name of the tsunami victims.[11] This was all part of a broader tourism plan developed two years before the tsunami with the support of the World Bank, the US Agency for International Development (USAID) and the Asian Development Bank. While the regional population had resisted these plans prior to the tsunami, the shock of the disaster gave the national government the opportunity to pass legislation that paved the way for privatization of public services, of land and of development. TAFREN was put in charge of the implementation of this plan. 'Somehow, in only ten days, and without leaving the capital, the business leaders on the task force were able to draft a complete national reconstruction blueprint, from housing to highways.'[11]

At Kaipanikuppam in the Indian state of Tamil Nadu, 'real estate agents have been buying up land and selling it on to tourism developers for ten years.' Their jobs have been made easier by the tsunami. Fishing catches have reduced dramatically, in part as a consequence of the tsunami, and this has left local fishing communities in ever-increasing poverty. This has increased the already great pressure on the community to capitulate and sell to the developers. In addition, '[t]he village is now hemmed in on all sides by land that no longer belongs to them, but urgently needs space to rebuild homes destroyed in the tsunami.'[22]

Such opportunistic development, largely focused on tourism, was the post-disaster norm. In the competition for land between traditional fishing communities and international hotel chains and their supporting agencies and governments, there was little doubt about who had the power to demand the ownership to land, despite any prior claims to the right to the land.

5 *Land has disappeared or become unusable*. Particularly in Banda Aceh, closest to the epicentre of the earthquake that precipitated the tsunami, the loss of land to the sea was substantial. The land has been rendered inaccessible by being under the sea or rendered unusable by salinization of agricultural land or of well water. Under such circumstances, national

governments would often provide either replacement land or compensation for the land lost. However, this restitution was also dependent on the validity of the claim to ownership. In turn, that depended on the claimant's records. Without those records, the process of restitution was slowed down or stopped.

6 *Records have been destroyed*. This applies in some cases to the loss of government records, but more often it is that case that personal records are lost. After the tsunami, as many as 70 per cent of the survivors lost their documents.[10] These records relate to identity and to the ownership or occupation of land. When people are unable to prove identity and citizenship, access to services can be curtailed or even denied. Where these documents relate to land, both personal records (where there are any) and government records may well have been destroyed.

7 *Conflict*. Both Banda Aceh and Sri Lanka were conflict areas prior to the tsunami. The disaster provided opportunities for revenge or for resolution. The former fits well into the pattern of the shock therapy of disaster capitalism described by Klein, and it is the opportunity to take advantage of weakness. The latter takes advantage of solidarity in the face of disaster and finds common ground from which to resolve outstanding conflicts.

In Banda Aceh, the conflict between GAM and the national government had been going on since 1976. The military practised what 'President Suharto described in 1989 as a kind of public "shock therapy" designed to restore public order.'[16] This involved the rounding up and torturing of civilians. Mutilated bodies would be left by the roadside for the shock value. The worst years of the conflict were in the 1990s and then in 2003–2004.[20] In large part because of the overwhelming media, NGO and agency attention to the area because of the disaster, the two sides were pushed into dispute resolution. A Memorandum of Understanding was signed between the two parties on 15 August 2005. With such a resolution, it became much more feasible to move forward with land claims and adjustments.

In Sri Lanka, '[e]ven the government's first anniversary report on tsunami clearly indicates that there have been aid inequities and more aid was distributed more quickly to the south than to the north and east.'[18] This uneven and discriminatory distribution of funds, housing and infrastructure came at the worst possible time. Negotiations in the peace process had been stalemated since 2003, but there was a process, however fragile. Such obviously discriminatory behaviour on the part of the government became a clear indication of bad faith in these negotiations. Renewed attacks began in August of 2005 with the assassination of the Foreign Minister.[15] This further worsened the situation for those trying to return to their land and rebuild their houses.[3] Not only were the buffer zones creating displacement, but the renewed conflict was as well. Access to land was dramatically reduced.

8 *Discrimination*. In general, the recovery process favoured those who had land before the tsunami. Although there were, as discussed, many ways for that land to be taken away from them, they did have something. On the other hand, renters and undocumented workers had few, if any, options. In all affected states this was a problem.

In Sri Lanka, renters who formerly lived within the area designated as a buffer zone were to receive no housing relief at all.[3] In Aceh, 25,000 households were left landless, and another 15,000 households had been renters or squatters before the tsunami.[14] Oxfam noted that with the inflation of land costs, the regulations passed by the national government in June of 2006 would never be adequate to allow for the resettlement of this 70,000-strong population to leave the relief camps. While Oxfam applauded the recognition by the government of the neglect of this population, they said that with land costs rising by 40 per cent in 2005 the meagre restitution for renters of $2,800 USD and for squatters of $1,150 would confine them in these relief camps for the foreseeable future.[14]

The Thai response

In Thailand, as in all the other affected countries, land was most critical to the recovery process. Survivors along the Andaman coast of Thailand were faced with all of the above issues. Those who stayed the longest in the relief camps were those for whom the access to land was unresolved – often renters but not always. Most communities were involved in some form of land dispute or related issues as described above. The land disputes raised broader issues about rights, minorities, cultural traditions and employment, and they raised an opportunity to address some of these issues.

Rights: In many of the coastal areas, people had been living on the land for generations and doing so without any legal title. Like most traditional cultures and communities, they were there before the concept of the commodification of land had taken hold – before there was a ministry of forests or parks or tourism. Does their right to be where they are – held prior to any notion of property rights – take precedence over any subsequent legal constructs? This is a question that arises in courts of law regularly in Canada and Australia with regard to the land claims of indigenous populations. Even in those countries not faced with the immediate threat of natural disaster, the issue remains contentious.

In Tap Tawan, one member of the community stood up and said that she couldn't understand these people who come from the city with a piece of paper. They knew nothing of this land and how this community and their ancestors had lived on it. How could they own the land without knowing anything about it? How could a piece of paper be more important than this relationship she and the rest of the community had to this land? It was not understandable. Her right to be there, then, arose out of a relationship between a specific community and a specific piece of land.

In Laem Pom, a few kilometres north of Tap Tawan, Khun Daeng asked a similar question. In her case, though, not only was this the place of her parents, grandparents and beyond, it was also the place from which five members of her family were swept away. She was not going to abandon her loved ones because someone with a piece of paper and the power of some distant authority had laid claim. The right she claimed came from history and sacrifice. Is that a valid right?

Minorities: Whether they were the Moken (semi-nomadic sea-based culture), Moklen (land-based), Muslim communities, fisherfolk or Burmese immigrants, these people were most often without the identity papers necessary to receive government services. Without papers they were often rendered invisible to aid.

Traditions: Many traditions of a community and a culture are directly connected to the land on which they live. For example:

> Unlike their Buddhist neighbors (who cremate their dead), the Moklen bury their dead, and have a tradition of planting a coconut seedling in the burial place. In the past, when many Moklen people lived on remote islands, the coconut was an important ingredient in their survival – when there was nothing else to eat or drink, the coconut offered flesh, juice and some basic nutrition. The Moklen also use coconut trees to measure the passing of years. As a coconut tree grows, each year's growth produces a ring, so you can count the rings to determine how old a coconut tree is. This has made it possible for many Moklen communities to prove how long they had stayed on their land, by showing the trees they had planted themselves 40, 50, 60 or even 80 years ago.[4]

This connection to, and understanding of, a place was also in evidence with the Moken people of Surin Island in terms of their understanding and use of the local flora as materials for their boats, houses, food and medicine and in terms of the placement of their homes in relation to the sea.[8] All of this important information is developed in anthropological research that is often the key to establishing tenure and to the appropriate design of housing and communities.

Buffer zones: This idea of creating buffer zones was presented at a landowners' meeting held with government officials at the Andaburi Resort in Kaolak in March of 2005. While it was favourably received by some hotel owners who wanted to use this as a form of control over beachfront vendors, it never got off the ground as a serious policy in the way it did in Sri Lanka and Indonesia.

Employment: For communities dependent on the sea for their livelihoods, any kind of buffer zone would be a terrible blow to the recovery process. In many cases, even moving 50 metres away from the shore can make a hard life that much harder. Professor Narumon pointed out one of the requirements of the Moken people in village planning:

> [A] beach area with suitable degree of slope – if there is too little slope, if the beach is rather flat, then it will be difficult to bring boats in and out at low tide. One will have to wait until high tide before taking boats in or out.[13]

It is clear from her observations that there is an important relationship here – one that is clearly understood by the people using the land and the sea for their survival. It is a relationship that is most often disregarded entirely by those who view land as a commodity, for whom this relationship is an abstraction, not a daily struggle to get a boat in and out of the water. The people making decisions that fishermen can be relocated up to two kilometres away from the sea have failed to move beyond the abstractions of land and ownership into the much more critical area of livelihood. These traditional landholders need a form of advocacy that does not resort entirely to deeds, titles and courts.

How did the people of Thailand and their government resolve these issues of land rights? In addressing that question I want to look at one government body (the Land Sub-Commission) and a number of different communities (Laem Pom, Ko Mook, Ko Kho Khao, and Tungwa).

The Land Sub-Commission

In Thailand, the Land Sub-Commission was a successful response to these land problems after the tsunami. The Land Commission was started in 1992 under General Chawalit Yongjaiyut. There were encroachments on army-held land, and at that time General Surin Pikulthong drafted procedures to solve the land problems on army land. The process accomplished its task and, while the Land Commission did not meet again, it was never disbanded. Twelve years later, when similar disputes arose over land after the tsunami, this commission was revived and headed by the deputy prime minister, who formed a special sub-commission for the resolution of disputes related to the tsunami. General Surin was called upon to chair this sub-commission.

Of all the 412 affected communities, 56 had land disputes that could not be solved at the local level. The first stage in addressing these land problems was the collection of information. Because it was already engaged in many of these communities, and in many cases had been even before the tsunami, a national agency, the Community Organizations Development Institute (CODI), was the key organization in collecting the necessary data for the Land Sub-Commission to be able to assess the problem and derive some amicable solution. Of these 56 outstanding problems, 53 of them – including those at Koh Mook and Tungwa outlined below – were resolved so that the communities were able to stay on the land. All of those 53 involved disputes with government departments. The remaining three were disputes between private developers and traditional landholders.

In the resolution of these disputes, the Land Sub-Commission had a number of criteria by which it judged the validity of the claims of communities resisting the state's demands that they not be allowed to move back to where they had been before:

Date of occupation: As indicated above with the Moklen people tracing their time of occupancy to the rings of the coconut trees, it was important for the community to be able to trace back to the period of time when the people moved onto that land. In most cases they occupied the land before any regulations had been created for the use of the land – such as the law to reserve land for national parks, national marine or forest conservation areas and so on. Those that were there before these laws and regulations existed could stay. The Baan Ta Seh community, for example, was there 165 years before it was announced by the Forestry Department that the mangrove forest would be protected. Not all 53 communities, though, could stay exactly where they had been. The Tungwa community moved a short distance closer to the main road. Other communities, for whom it had been determined that they had moved there after a law was in place, could stay but they would likely be required to pay a nominal rent on the land (5 baht/rai/year), by which a landlord/tenant arrangement was established.

Safety and environmental condition: Where there were specific environmental or safety problems, such as steep slopes, the community would be given land nearby.

Maintaining traditions: This applied to a number of Moklen communities as well as to fishing communities where an order to move away from the coast would directly affect their livelihood. Another aspect of this criterion was the opportunity for the development of tourism for the community.

Quality of life: As above, the Land Sub-Commission did not want to create conditions where villagers would have to carry 50 kilograms of their fishing equipment great distances from their houses to the shore. On a daily basis, such hardship creates very definite quality of life issues.

Fifty-three of the 56 disputes were settled with relevant government departments using these criteria. The three outstanding disputes all involved the private sector – in Laem Pom, Tap Tawan and Baan Nairai. Here the Land Sub-Commission had far less negotiating power. In all three of these disputes between the private sector and the traditional landholders, the Sub-Commission suggested land-sharing as a possibility but this was rejected by the private-sector claimants holding the disputed title to the properties. An investigation was then ordered into the claims themselves to see who issued the titles and when as well as the legality of the claims. Eighteen months later, these three claims were still unresolved, but the communities were still on the land[2] and remain there in 2008. Considering the extent of the problem, though, the fact that 95 per cent of the land disputes were quickly resolved was one of the most impressive responses on the part of the government to a problem that could have stopped the recovery in its tracks for many communities.

It is useful to look more closely at some of these land issues by outlining the circumstances that created the potential for dispute. There are three specific communities that faced problems with government departments, individuals, provincial governments and potential development. One is a Muslim community on the island of Ko Mook. A second is on another island, Ko Kho Khao. The third is a Moklen community at Tungwa.

Ko Mook

Prior to the tsunami there had been an ongoing dispute over the use of this Forestry Department land. The community on Ko Mook, of course, was not the only one facing problems with land use. After the tsunami there were many such disputes, enough to give rise to the special Land Sub-Commission that was set up to resolve them. Until the dispute on this piece of land was settled, no building was going to occur.

The dispute was further complicated by a separate claim from a local resident. While the Land Commission had resolved the dispute with the Forestry Department in favour of the community, the project was not going to move forward without a resolution to this other claim. Initially it appeared that it should have been a dispute between this individual claimant and the Forestry Department, both of which were laying claim to the same piece of land – a dispute that would be resolved by the courts. However, it was also clear that the residents planning to build on this land had to live with this claimant. He was not only a member of the community but also related to the local authority that was responsible for issuing permits. They had to resolve this by further negotiation rather than resorting to any heavy-handed approach from the outside. The issue, then, was not about the law but about the way the community continues to live together after all the outsiders have gone home.

A signing ceremony was planned for early March 2006, in which the land would be handed over from the Forestry Department to the community. About a week before this event, it appeared that the other claimant had put up concrete fence posts along the edge of this property, indicating that he still considered it his land and that the dispute was not resolved. On the day of the ceremony, after the officials and the residents had signed the document, a number of them went out from under the tent and removed each of these loosely placed concrete posts before they came back and placed the ceremonial footing and first post into the ground. The dispute had been settled amicably and it was then possible to begin construction of the new housing.

It is important to note that this land was handed over to the community as a whole. What this meant was that there were no individual lots to be sold. The land itself belongs now to the whole community. At the ceremony, members of the community and representatives of the Chumchonthai Foundation (CTF – a Thai national NGO), CODI, the United Nations Development Programme (UNDP) and the Save Andaman Network (SAN – a

Thai umbrella NGO formed immediately after the tsunami) all signed the Memorandum of Cooperation that committed the community to rehabilitating the mangrove forest in which they were about to build their houses.[23]

Ko Kho Khao

On the north-western corner of the island there is an old airstrip ready for future development. The Tourism Authority of Thailand had already proposed that this airstrip be rebuilt and upgraded to improve access by air.

There is an existing road going east from the airstrip to the location of a future bridge to the mainland. When the bridge is built, that land along the existing road to the future airport is going to be up for grabs to the highest bidder – that is, unless the community makes some plans for other forms of development that support the community and the island environment.

As part of the recovery process, UNDP, in conjunction with UN-HABITAT, organized a capacity-building programme with the local authorities and the communities of Ko Kho Khao. Over a period of 18 months they went through a participatory process of identifying recovery projects in the community. With the prospect of this future development and the possibility of the loss of land to developers, the community needed to use the planning experience they gained through the UN-HABITAT programme to consider the implications of this future development on the Ko Kho Khao communities and on the ecosystem itself. As the UN project ended in October of 2006, the communities had not yet initiated any planning process to prepare plans for appropriate development. It is likely, under such circumstances, that they will lose this land even before the bridge is built.

Tungwa

The original Ban Tungwa village occupied 26 rai (4.16 hectares) of land. That land, and the land to which they relocated, a few hundred metres from the shore, is all public land. The land on which they rebuilt is right on the highway, so it has a greater market value because of its high commercial exposure and because of rapidly increasing development along the highway prior to the tsunami.

Immediately after the disaster, while the community was still in the Kuek-Kak relief centre, the district administration and the provincial governor took their absence as an opportunity to seize the land for development purposes. They put up a signboard announcing that a hospital was to be built on the site with funds donated by the German Embassy in Bangkok. Further investigation by the community and supporting NGOs uncovered the fact that the hospital project was a fabrication invented in order to seize the land for the 'public good'.

Like many other communities up and down the coast, the people of Tungwa found that, in order to prevent its being taken over, they had to get back on the land and start building as soon as possible. This was a technique utilized effectively by the Human Development Foundation in a number of other communities along the coast. Using techniques they had perfected years ago during the 'development' fires in the Klong Toei slum by the port in Bangkok, they got simple structures up as quickly as possible so that the villagers were back in occupation of the land instead of waiting at a relief centre. If they had waited, the land would have been lost for them by the time they tried to return. If they had a presence on the site, they had at least a negotiating position.

When the Tungwa community began negotiating, with help from the Land Sub-Committee, the idea of land-sharing came up, whereby the people would keep part of the land for redeveloping their housing and give part to the Province for 'public use'. This compromise solution was seen as a way of avoiding a protracted legal battle and allowing the villagers to rebuild their community and for the Province to carry on with its development plans right away. Initially, the Governor of Phang Nga wanted at least half the land, but finally, after some very tough haggling and many tense meetings, it was agreed that the villagers would keep 16 rai (2.56 hectares) and give 10 rai (1.6 hectares) to the Province. The village people were not too happy about having to give up any of their land like this, and a supporting national NGO, the CTF, had to argue that this compromise was going to be their most effective way forward.

The compromise resulted in a five-year communal lease on this land. The obvious unanswered question is: why a five-year lease? It has been asked by every visitor to the site, and it continues to be asked by everyone in the community itself. They are concerned, of course, about their tenure status on the land. They have invested their labour and their lives. The community, volunteers from around the world, UNDP and many other organizations have put their time and money into this recovery effort at Tungwa. Would the provincial authorities actually have all of this torn down and removed in 2010? That seems highly unlikely, particularly considering the international exposure that this community now has. What, then, does a five-year lease achieve but to increase the community's apprehension about their future? Many people will be watching what happens in 2010.

Conclusions

In October of 2005, UN-HABITAT organized an international workshop in conjunction with World Habitat Day. About 100 people attended from the region and from international agencies. One of the site visits made over the two-day workshop was to Laem Pom. There, at the beach, people gathered around the community leader, Khun Daeng, as construction of new Laem Pom houses continued in the background. In the six months since I first met her sitting on a makeshift bench outside a tent that was her home, she had faced the grief of the loss of most of her family and had taken up the mantle of community leadership and faced down the threats of the henchmen of the nai-toon (money baron). She was addressing UN representatives and NGOs from India, Sri Lanka and Indonesia. Although the henchmen were no longer in sight, she knew that this did not mean she and her community were safe from claims. The assembled workshop participants wanted to know what she needed for her safety and for the recovery of her community.

She said that the Laem Pom community had help from the Law Centre at Thammasat University in dealing with the legalities and research on the land claims. They had also involved the National Human Rights Commission of Thailand. However, they needed more. Along with the help from these organizations, there were, for Daeng, four important elements to restoring and maintaining a secure community:

- access to information;
- access to skills;
- access to resources;
- and, she said, 'We need a plan.' She knew that plans would be a tool of negotiation for this community. They needed an alternative to the plans that were already being made by the nai-toon and by different government agencies, including the Tourism Authority of Thailand.

It is with the recognition of the need for local planning that the resistance to the effects of disaster capitalism can be most effective. Communities can prepare for disasters such as earthquakes, floods, cyclones or tsunamis. National governments can develop disaster-preparedness plans (for example, after the tsunami, warning systems were initiated and evacuation plans were developed). However, what communities must also do is be ready for the second tsunami, the 'aftershocks' that follow. For that, it is clear that if they do not have a plan, there will be developers and agencies ready with their own plans.

8 Who governs reconstruction? Changes and continuity in policies, practices and outcomes

Jennifer Duyne Barenstein

Post-disaster policy-making processes, practices and outcomes depend on a number of contextual factors, such as the capacity of local communities to articulate their needs and demands; the relation between state governments, national civil-society organizations and international agencies; previous disaster experiences; the balance between public and private actors; and the amount and source of funding for reconstruction.

Guiding principles for post-disaster reconstruction – between theory and practice

For over twenty years international agencies have stated that disasters are an opportunity to 'build back better' and to enhance community resilience. This underlying principle was already implicit in the United Nations Disaster Relief Organization (UNDRO) guidelines for shelter after disaster,[32] was reiterated by Sphere,[28] for example, and became the reconstruction slogan after the Indian Ocean tsunami and the Pakistan earthquake of 2004.[7,33]

Numerous manuals, international policy frameworks and guidelines indicate a growing consensus regarding the importance of community participation, of linking reconstruction to long-term development and livelihood restoration, of encouraging local building technologies, of avoiding relocation, of paying attention to local contexts, of gender-sensitive planning, of cooperation with local governments, of capacity building, of cultural sensitivity and so forth.

In spite of all these generally accepted principles, reconstruction practices and outcomes continue to differ distressingly from policy declarations. This has led several authors to argue that post-disaster reconstruction is one of the less successful areas of international cooperation.[4,5,8] There is no evidence that the reason for discrepancies between intentions and outcomes is caused by policy deficiencies, yet international agencies keep responding to these discrepancies through investing heavily in refining their policy instruments. The recent mega operation to revise the 1982 UNDRO guidelines[22] and the World Bank's ongoing effort to produce a housing reconstruction handbook[26] are just two examples of international agencies' profound trust that they will be able to influence reconstruction practices on the ground through better guidelines and manuals.

In this chapter I argue that large international NGOs, in particular, in spite of their vast experience and their discourses emphasizing equity, sustainability and participation, are often unable or unwilling to follow their guiding principles on the ground. Through a review of reconstruction policy-making processes, practices and outcomes in the Indian states of Maharashtra, Gujarat and Tamil Nadu, which were affected by severe disasters between 1993 and 2006 (Table 8.1), I will show that local stakeholders, including state governments, civil society organizations and local communities, have more influence on reconstruction approaches and outcomes than international actors do. However, whether local actors' role in shaping reconstruction leads to equitable and sustainable reconstruction depends on a number of factors, such as previous disaster and post-disaster recovery experience, the relation between the state and civil society, and local power structures. Variations related to these factors, in combination with the availability of

Table 8.1 Three disasters in India at a glance

Affected states	*Maharashtra*	*Gujarat*	*Tamil Nadu, Andhra Pradesh, Kerala, Andaman and Nicobar Islands*
Type of disaster	Earthquake	Earthquake	Tsunami
Date of the disaster	30 September 1993	26 January 2001	26 December 2004
Number of deaths	7928	19,727	12,405
Number of injuries	16,000	167,000	6,913
Affected districts	Total 13; over 50% of human losses and damage in Latur and Osmanabad districts	21 out of 25; over 85% of human losses and damage in Kutch district	Over 80% of human losses and damage in Tamil Nadu's Nagapattinam district
Number of affected villages	2500	7633	1089
Number of fully damaged villages	52	450	NA
Estimated number of fully damaged houses	27,000	344,000	157,400

Sources: Government of Maharashtra 2005; Gujarat State Disaster Management Authority 2005; Asian Development Bank, United Nations Development Program and World Bank 2005.

external financial resources, explain the differences in reconstruction outcomes between the three states. In certain cases it became apparent that the reconstruction practices of most international NGOs continue to be primarily dictated by the pressure to spend money and to present quick results to their constituencies, a state of affairs that leads them to ignore local favourable conditions and challenges and to deviate dramatically from international guiding principles.

This chapter is based on a review of policy documents and literature and on field research in numerous villages in Tamil Nadu and Gujarat between 2004 and 2008. The three interlinked research projects were funded by the Swiss Agency for Development Cooperation and the Swiss National Science Foundation. They involved several junior and senior Indian researchers as well as five Swiss graduate students who conducted, under my supervision, several months of anthropological village studies in Gujarat and Tamil Nadu for their master theses.[6,17,21,29,30,31]

Reconstruction policies and practices in India

India is a federal state characterized by a clear division of roles and responsibilities between the central government and state governments. In the wake of a disaster, the central government has an overall policy-development and supportive role and a key role in mobilizing financial resources. The basic responsibility for rescue, relief and rehabilitation lies with the state government, which enjoys relative autonomy in organizing relief operations, long-term disaster preparedness and rehabilitation measures. At the district level, the district collector prepares district-level action plans, directs, supervises and monitors relief measures and reconstruction and also assumes a major role in regulating and coordinating NGOs.[13]

In spite of India being characterized by strong governance, recent disasters have shown that while government institutions are very effective in managing rescue and relief operations, no state appears to be prepared for reconstruction through clearly defined pre-disaster policies. Accordingly, reconstruction policies are generally only designed following specific disasters.

Whereas recent examples indicate that national civil-society organizations have a tangible influence on state governments' reconstruction policies, there is little evidence that these are being influenced by international principles such as UNDRO's guidelines for shelter after disaster.[32] This does not necessarily mean that the latter's reconstruction policies contradict or impede the adoption of good practices, but simply that at least in India they appear to have a rather marginal role in defining reconstruction at the local level. To a large extent, reconstruction is determined by negotiations between the state government and national civil-society organizations.

The case of Maharashtra

Maharashtra's historical Marathwada region, located about 500 kilometres east of Mumbai, was hit by a massive earthquake of the magnitude of 6.4 on the Richter scale on 30 September 1993. The earthquake killed nearly 9000 people, and there were over 16,000 reported injuries. It affected over 2500 villages, of which 1191 are located in the districts of Latur and Osmanabad. Fifty-two villages, consisting of a total of 27,000 houses, were completely destroyed.[14]

Maharashtra's reconstruction policy

The earthquake caught government and communities totally unprepared, for the region was not believed to be seismically active.[23] Yet, only a few days after the quake, the Government of Maharashtra announced that all devastated villages would be rebuilt on safer sites. Resettlement was thus emphasized from the very beginning. By December 1993, the government had developed the Maharashtra Emergency Earthquake Rehabilitation Programme (MEERP), a comprehensive rehabilitation plan, which was the first of its kind in India. The plan was conceived and executed with the help of a soft loan from the World Bank and was also supported by the United Nations Development Programme (UNDP), several bilateral donor agencies and NGOs.

MEERP proposed a comprehensive approach towards resettlement and rehabilitation, emphasizing the construction of permanent houses in relocation sites.[14] The quake-affected villages were divided into three damage categories: relocation and full reconstruction of about 28,000 houses was suggested for the fifty-two most heavily damaged 'category A' villages; reconstruction *in situ* through financial assistance was suggested for 'category B' villages; and repair and seismic retrofitting of about 190,000 damaged houses was suggested for 'category C' villages. The new houses to be provided were again divided into three categories: landless and marginal landholders (owning up to one hectare of land) would be given houses with a carpet area of 250 square feet; households owning between one and seven hectares of land would get houses of 400 square feet; and large farmers (owning more than seven hectares of land) would get houses of 750 square feet. This policy implied that wealthier people would benefit significantly more than poor households, regardless of their own endowments and individual requirements.

As already mentioned, the Maharashtra's reconstruction programme strongly emphasized relocation. There is a growing consensus among development agencies and social scientists that resettlement is a painful and socio-economically risky process that people generally are not undergoing voluntarily. In Maharashtra, however, villagers did not oppose resettlement. Moreover, the twenty-two less severely damaged 'category B' villages refused housing assistance *in situ*, demanding to be relocated instead. According to

Vatsa, these earthquake victims had lost faith in their traditional building capacity and thus preferred to move to modern and seismically safe villages.[35] Jigyasu maintains that people's preference for relocation and modern houses was influenced by the negative attitude towards traditional housing of the junior engineers who surveyed the earthquake-damaged villages, as well as by the fact that people were forced to make decisions about their future too soon after the quake, at a time when they were still deeply traumatized.[18] Another reason why the villagers from the less severely affected villages opted for relocation may be related to the fact that international NGOs were more interested in building new villages in relocated sites than in supporting communities to rebuild their own houses by themselves. By offering modern 'ready-made' houses to people who, according to the government policy, were entitled to a financial compensation of only 62,000 Rs to rebuild their houses *in situ*, NGOs created an artificial demand for relocation. Maharashtra reconstruction policy thus led to massive resettlements and to the replacement of traditional, compact settlements of stone masonry houses by grid-patterned endless rows of concrete houses occupying up to ten times more land than the original villages.[19]

The role of NGOs

Most NGOs involved in reconstruction after the earthquake in Maharashtra came from outside the state. Several Indian NGOs challenged the government's top-down reconstruction approach, which was based on resettling people in urban-like settlements and which failed to take into account vernacular housing designs and spatial arrangements. This led to some amendments in the policy, in that a participatory planning element was added to the reconstruction process. This policy change in turn caused some national NGOs to assume an enabling role, that is, to conduct meetings with the communities aimed at involving the latter in village planning. As a result, some of the houses and villages that were built at later stages incorporated some vernacular features. Nevertheless, they were built with industrial materials by outside contractors. The participatory process thus remained limited to a certain amount of consultation at the stage of design but did not allow local masons and artisans to participate in construction.[25]

In contrast to national NGOs active in policy advocacy and in promoting participatory planning within the framework of the state government's reconstruction programme, some twenty-five large, internationally funded NGOs and private corporations preferred to 'adopt' entire villages for reconstruction work within the government's notion of public–private partnership. By promising 'modern' houses and villages in relocated sites, they were also able to persuade less severely affected communities to relocate. No agency involved in reconstruction in Maharashtra relied upon local technologies by promoting the use of locally available materials such as stone and by involving the local building industry. Community participation, if such participation took place at all, was limited to a few village meetings aimed at communities approving the housing designs and settlement layouts. The fact that reinforced concrete was the only building technology that was considered implied that local masons and artisans were completely marginalized from reconstruction.[24]

Reconstruction outcomes

The earthquake-affected Marathwada region was revisited by Salazar and Jigyasu in 2001. Both found that the outcome of the reconstruction programme that the Government of Maharashtra had followed was highly problematic and led to an increased vulnerability of local communities.

The quality of construction of the houses was generally found to be poor. Salazar attributes quality problems to the inappropriateness of concrete in extremely hot temperatures, which made the process of curing difficult to control. In addition, water shortages led to severe shortcuts, with curing taking place for only a few days instead of the required three weeks. This caused severe cracking and water infiltrations, leading to a rapid decay of the houses. Local communities did not have the capital and the skills to repair and maintain these buildings, with the result that they are now gradually being abandoned. Salazar estimated that at the time of his last research in Latur in 2001, only 50 per cent of the houses were inhabited.[26] In some cases people started building new houses near the dilapidated agency-built houses using salvaged materials, corrugated metal sheets, stones and bamboo. These materials were also used to make extensions, such as additional rooms, to NGO-supplied core units, external kitchens and compound walls.

Resettlement proved to be unsustainable. Due to the villagers' inability to pursue their livelihoods and to adjust their lifestyles to the urban-like settlements and house designs, many people abandoned the relocated villages and moved back to their old villages. There they started to rebuild their old houses following their traditional building technologies, without employing any earthquake-resistant features. Not only was the opportunity to improve resilience through enhancing local building capacity missed, the fact that reconstruction relied on imported industrial building materials led to a tremendous waste of financial and material resources, a built environment with a high environmental impact and the loss of valuable agricultural land.

The case of Maharashtra confirms the serious drawbacks and risks of post-disaster resettlement and contractor-driven reconstruction, which, although they were acknowledged internationally and well documented, the actors involved in reconstruction failed to fully understand.

The case of Gujarat

The disaster in Gujarat (also presented by Jigyasu in Chapter 3) was about thirty times larger than the Maharashtra quake, and it was the worst that

India had experienced in the last fifty years. The earthquake affected twenty-one of Gujarat's twenty-five districts and 7633 out of 18,356 villages. It completely flattened 450 villages. It destroyed 344,000 houses, and 888,000 reported damages. Over 90 per cent of the deaths and an estimated 85 per cent of the asset losses occurred in Kutch, one of the state's poorest and most vulnerable districts.[34,37]

Gujarat's reconstruction policy

Less than two weeks after the earthquake, the state government established the Gujarat State Disaster Management Authority (GSDMA), which announced its rehabilitation policy only a few days later. The Gujarat Emergency Earthquake Reconstruction Programme (GEERP), to be funded by the World Bank, proposed relocation of the most-affected villages, assistance for the *in-situ* reconstruction of severely affected villages, assistance for repair and *in-situ* reconstruction in less-damaged areas and assistance for the construction of modern buildings in urban areas.

The proposed policy was almost identical to the one followed by the Government of Maharashtra after the earthquake of 1993. However, whereas in Maharashtra there appeared to be a relatively high societal consensus over the proposed reconstruction policy, this was not the case in Gujarat, where it met with stiff public resistance. The Maharashtra experience was still fresh in the memory of professionals and civil-society organizations, and it had a considerable impact on public awareness. Civil-society organizations had more experience and were thus better prepared to influence reconstruction policies. Prominent public figures, including the former district collector of Latur district, warned the Government of Gujarat against repeating the same mistakes.

A systematic public consultation carried out in 468 villages by the NGO network Kutch Navnirman Abhiyan (known and hereafter referred to as Abhiyan) revealed that over 90 per cent of the villagers refused the idea of relocation. When it became clear that relocation was not only opposed by professionals, civil-society organizations and the concerned villagers, but that it was also unacceptable to the World Bank, the government abandoned its relocation plans. The Government of Gujarat thus adopted an 'owner-driven' reconstruction approach, as opposed to the 'contractor-driven' approach that was followed in Maharashtra.[16] Its reconstruction policy consisted in offering financial assistance (40,000–90,000 Rs, depending on the damage and the type of house), technical assistance and subsidized construction materials to all those who preferred to undertake reconstruction on their own and who rejected relocation and full-scale 'adoption' by an external agency (Figure 8.1). Given that option, 72 per cent of people opted for financial compensation and to reconstruct their houses on their own.[1]

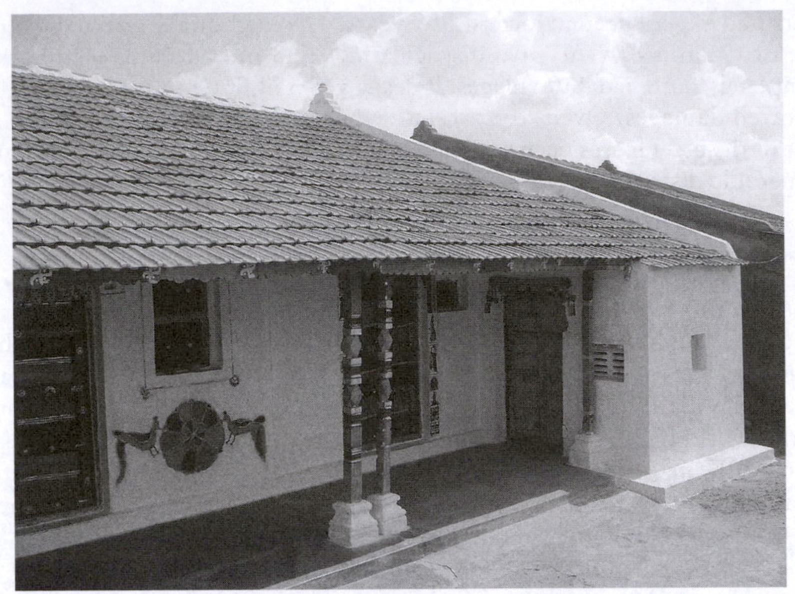

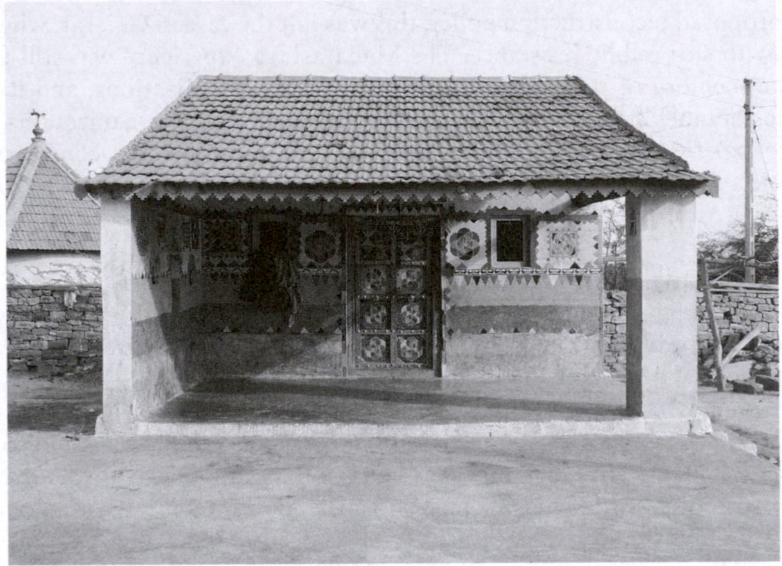

Figure 8.1 Self-built houses in Gujarat.

The role of NGOs

In order to analyze the role of civil society and NGOs after the 2001 earthquake in Gujarat, it is necessary to make a clear distinction between local and international actors. Gujarat was the home state of Mahatma Gandhi, whose teaching inspired many of its vibrant local NGOs and civil-society organizations. In particular, Abhiyan, which was founded in response to the devastating cyclone of May 1998 with the aim of enhancing communities' disaster preparedness, had a pivotal role in policy-making. It facilitated a dialogue between the government and communities through a massive information and consultation campaign. This allowed people to express their opposition to relocation and contractor-driven reconstruction. During reconstruction Abhiyan and several other local NGOs focused on supporting the government in creating an enabling environment.

Owner-driven reconstruction does not necessarily lead to a sustainable built environment and resilient communities. The application of local knowledge and building technologies may be constrained, for example, by inadequate building capacity, lack of information and building codes and guidelines. Abhiyan ensured that people would be informed about their entitlements and options through information campaigns and rural information centres. Abhiyan collaborated with the government in organizing training campaigns for masons and homeowners. It trained retired masons in advocacy for safety and posted them in villages to supervise reconstruction at community level. Furthermore, Abhiyan set up demonstration camps to inform people about different technological options, including low-cost, eco-friendly, earth-based building technologies. The use of alternative building materials was regulated through guidelines that were endorsed by the government.[16]

Most local NGOs supported self-help construction programmes through additional construction materials, training and technical assistance to communities that opted for financial compensation. However, as argued by Jigyasu in Chapter 3 of this book, in some cases NGOs' concept of 'enablement' was rather patronizing and led them, instead of building upon local practices and traditions, to persuade communities to adopt their house designs and building technologies. Most international NGOs, in contrast, proved to be less comfortable with owner-driven reconstruction and went ahead with the same village adoption and contractor-driven approach they had followed eight years earlier in Maharashtra. Several international NGOs and private corporations persuaded villagers to relocate and built exactly the same Maharashtra-type grid-patterned settlements with large, medium and small houses for different landholding categories of people. In fact, though the government changed its own policy, it still offered communities the option of entering an agreement with NGOs to rebuild their houses. This led numerous villages to renounce the financial compensation offered by the government and to opt for agency-built houses.

Reconstruction outcomes

In 2004, three years after the earthquake, we conducted research with the aim of assessing citizens' perspectives on different reconstruction approaches. By that time reconstruction in rural areas had been completed, and in most cases people had moved to their new houses at least one year previously. As shown in Table 8.2, for the purpose of the study we made a distinction between five reconstruction approaches that were pursued by different agencies after the earthquake of 2001. The outcome of these different approaches and citizens' perspectives were evaluated qualitatively through observation, focus groups and semi-structured interviews with stratified samples of men and women, and they were evaluated quantitatively through a survey covering 434 households, which represents 5 per cent of the households in sixteen villages.[10]

Our multi-sited research in Gujarat showed that owner-driven reconstruction, supported by the government and also by some local NGOs, was the fastest and, according to local citizens, the most satisfactory approach. In villages where people benefited from this type of support, everyone felt that their housing situation was significantly better than before the earthquake. With regard to size, location, quality of materials and quality of construction,

Table 8.2 Satisfaction with different reconstruction approaches in % (N = 434)

	Owner-driven reconstruction	*Owner-driven with NGO top-up*	*Participatory reconstruction*	*Contractor-driven* in situ	*Contractor-driven with relocation*
Financial support per housing unit (in Rs)	40,000–90,000	40,000 + 25,000	47,000	85,000	124,000 (average)
Overall satisfaction with quality of housing	93.3	100	90.8	71.6	22.8
Satisfaction with...					
House location	99	95	96	95	64.5
House size	90	95	85	89	51
Quality of materials	94	95	93	64	38.5
Construction quality	95	95	93	69	3.5
Average	94.50	95.00	91.75	79.25	39.37

Source: Joshi and Barenstein 2005.

95 per cent of the households were fully satisfied. This approach proved to be an effective way of mitigating some of the risks of owner-driven reconstruction as pursued by the government, namely the risk of the special needs of the most vulnerable people being neglected.

The government's owner-driven approach without any additional NGO support was almost equally popular, with 93.3 per cent of households reporting satisfaction with their post-earthquake housing situation. Ironically, satisfaction was highest among those who obtained the minimum compensation of 40,000 Rs, which was given to rebuild dwellings classified as 'fully damaged huts'. Before the earthquake, their housing situation was generally poor, so even the minimum compensation allowed for an improvement. People's positive judgement about the quality of their new houses was confirmed by our detailed observations, which indicated that the quality of construction was generally good and that the houses were seismically safe. High construction quality was also found by the National Council for Cement and Building Material (NCCBM), which was appointed by the GSDMA as a third party quality audit. By December 2002 the NCCBM had inspected nearly 100,000 houses and found a rate of conformity with the governmental building codes of over 95 per cent.[1] Citizens' clear preference for owner-driven reconstruction was also confirmed by a survey carried out by Abhiyan, which found that only 39 per cent of the people who obtained a house from an NGO would opt for this solution in the case of a future calamity. On the other hand, 91 per cent of the people who opted for financial compensation would again choose the same option.[1]

Our research also covered three villages that benefited from what we defined as a participatory housing reconstruction approach. The approach gave people an active role in the construction of their houses and a say in choosing the materials and determining the design and location of the house. The case refers to one of the few agencies that relied on local building skills by promoting improved stone masonry. This resulted in houses that did not differ significantly from those reconstructed by the people themselves, under the owner-driven approach. The overall satisfaction with the participatory housing approach averaged 90.8 per cent. The reason why the houses built under this approach were less appreciated than self-built houses is that they were comparatively small and people believed that with the same amount of money they could have built larger houses themselves.

The level of satisfaction decreased significantly when houses were built by contractors. Only 71.8 per cent of the people who received a house built by a contractor *in situ* were generally satisfied and only 64 per cent expressed satisfaction with the quality of construction materials. The agency replaced local materials such as stone-masonry walls and tiled roofs with flat concrete-roofed houses, which are poorly suited to the local climate. Contractors' profit-oriented approach was also held responsible by many people for the low quality of construction, which manifested itself through the same problems as found in Maharashtra.

The least popular approach that had been pursued in Gujarat was the most expensive, namely contractor-driven reconstruction in a relocated site (Figure 8.2). Only 22.8 per cent of the people who had received a NGO house built under this approach were satisfied, and only 3.5 per cent considered the quality of construction to be adequate. People also complained about

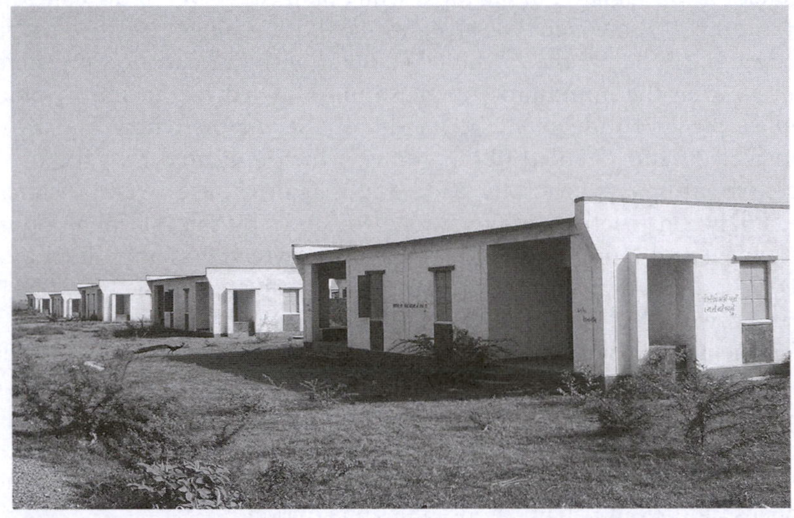

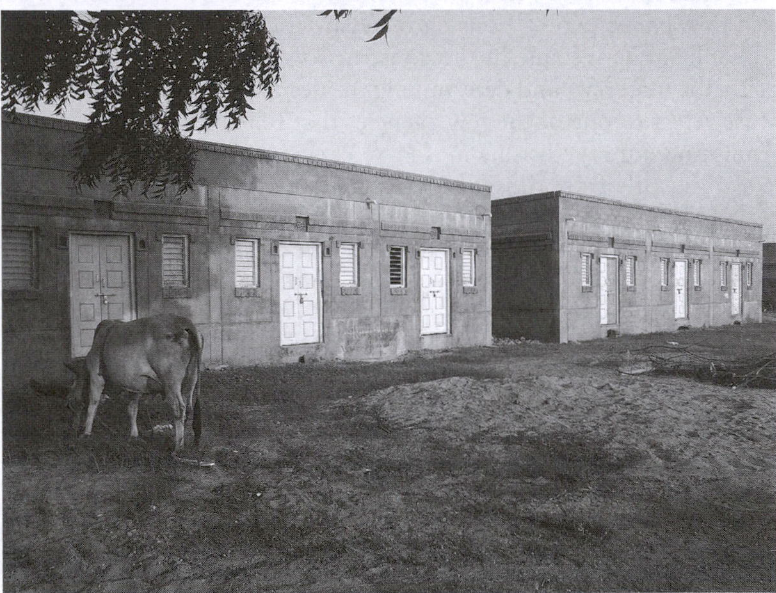

Figure 8.2 Unoccupied contractor-built houses in Gujarat.

the lack of participation, the elite's monopolizing of decision-making and project benefits, discrimination in favour of local elites and the disruption of family networks caused by the relocation. Where people had the option of rebuilding their old houses, they almost always refused to move to the new village. It is ironic that the project that enjoyed the lowest level of appreciation among its beneficiaries was the most expensive one, with housing units costing around three times more than owner-built houses.

Gujarat's reconstruction experience proved that people have the capacity to build houses that are more likely to respond to their needs than are houses provided by external agencies if adequate financial and technical support and other enabling conditions (e.g. good supervision, massive training of local masons and access to subsidized construction materials) are provided. People who managed reconstruction by themselves were able to move back to their houses earlier than those who depended on NGOs. This shows that owner-driven reconstruction was not only the most cost-effective but also the fastest reconstruction strategy.

Citizens' satisfaction is a critical indicator for assessing the degree of success of reconstruction. Yet there are other important issues that need to be considered, such as the reconstructed built environment's resilience and the social and environmental impact of different reconstruction approaches. Also, from these points of view we found several drawbacks of contractor-driven approaches. First of all, it became apparent that self-built houses often made extensive use of recycled and locally available construction materials, which was not the case with contractor-based reconstruction. Most contractors promoted the use of reinforced concrete, a construction material with a large ecological footprint. Another environmental problem related to the use of concrete is the high demand for water for the process of curing, which is particularly problematic in semi-arid zones, where over 85 per cent of the reconstruction took place. In many places the water demand for construction competed with domestic and agricultural requirements, leading to social conflicts. The quality of construction suffered due to the lack of water, as curing was hardly ever done with sufficient care. Another problematic aspect from a socio-economic point of view is that contractors privileged building on new sites, which led to significant losses of agricultural land. Damaged villages were simply abandoned, which is undesirable not only from a psychological point of view but also from an environmental and landscaping one.

Contractors proved to have vested interests in maximizing construction and often managed to create an artificial demand for houses. NGOs that pursued this approach showed no interest in supporting the repair of partially damaged houses, and it is estimated that over 38 per cent of the houses built by NGOs replaced houses that would have been reparable.[1] In Gujarat we found that contractor-driven reconstruction led to a massive increase in the number of houses. Our survey in sixteen villages revealed that the increase in the number of houses was an average of 59 per cent. It was, however, particularly high in contractor-built villages, where the number of houses increased by up to 83 per cent. When relating the village population to the number of houses, we found that an increase of houses of only 5 per cent could possibly be justified in terms of pre-quake shortages. The new houses were not equally distributed among community members, and influential households inevitably succeeded in getting more houses. In the contractor-built sample villages covered by this study, we found that it was not unusual for people belonging to dominant communities to have obtained two or three houses. Some people managed to secure as many as seven houses for themselves. This is one of the factors explaining the low occupancy rate and also the social tensions and conflicts.

From a socio-cultural point of view, it was shown that contractor-driven reconstruction led to several other negative impacts. Houses and settlements built by contractors strongly deviated from the local housing culture and were perceived as incompatible with local livelihoods. This is another factor that explains the low occupancy rate in some villages; many people rejected these houses and ended up building their own. However, as they had officially received housing assistance from an NGO, they were not entitled to financial assistance from the government and did not receive any technical guidance.

To conclude: the case of Gujarat shows that in terms of the overall reconstruction policy and practices there has been a significant improvement since the Maharashtra earthquake. Increased awareness of the risks associated with relocation and with contractor-driven reconstruction has led the government to adopt an owner-driven reconstruction policy. The positive outcome in terms of citizens' satisfaction, cost- and time-effectiveness and the quality of construction proved that owner-driven reconstruction is a viable and appropriate approach for rural India. Whereas local stakeholders had clearly learned a lesson from the reconstruction experience of a previous disaster, this was not the case with large international NGOs, which went ahead with the same approach and committed the same mistakes as in Maharashtra eight years earlier.

The case of Tamil Nadu

On 26 December 2004 a severe earthquake measuring 8.9 on the Richter scale hit northern Sumatra. The quake resulted in one of the most powerful tsunamis of recorded history. In India the tsunami killed over 12,000 people, and approximately 5800 people remain missing.[15] The tsunami lashed over 2260 kilometres of India's coastline, with waves of three to ten metres high penetrating the inland up to three kilometres deep. Nearly 80 per cent of the human and material losses were concentrated in the state of Tamil Nadu. The vast majority of the tsunami victims belong to the coastal fishing communities.

Tamil Nadu's reconstruction policy

Soon after the disaster, the government estimated that over 130,000 new houses were needed for the people made homeless by the tsunami. These figures were not the result of an accurate damage assessment.[3] In fact, the first reconstruction policy issued by the government in January 2005 envisaged permanent relocation of all coastal communities, which implied the need for new houses for all affected people. Another factor that contributed to giving little importance to a housing damage assessment was the assumption that 87 per cent of the coastal people were living in *kachcha* (semi-permanent houses) and that reconstruction would be an opportunity to upgrade these people's housing condition.[3] The Hindi word *kachcha* literally means 'raw' and generally has a negative connotation. Its opposite, *pucca*, means 'ripe' or 'mature' and has positive connotations. The terms *kachcha* and *pucca* are far from neutral, with *kachcha* being associated with poverty and backwardness and *pucca* with progress and modernity. The words *kachcha* and *pucca* are officially used by the Government of India to differentiate between houses built with industrially produced construction materials, on the one hand, and vernacular houses built with locally available construction materials, on the other. Of particular importance for this classification are the roofing materials. All houses with thatched roofs are considered *kachcha*, those with tiled roofs as *semi-kachcha* and only those with concrete flat roofs as *pucca*.

Most tsunami-related reconstruction-project documents follow these categories. Besides the fact that these documents provide no qualitative details about pre-disaster housing culture and building practices, they erroneously translate *kachcha* as 'temporary', as if the majority of the people in Tamil Nadu were living in temporary shelters already prior to the tsunami. Our appraisal in twelve villages in Nagapattinam district revealed that this was not the case.[9] Though housing conditions were not homogeneous, we found that a significant proportion of households had owned comfortable and beautiful houses that were well adapted to the local climatic conditions and were environmentally sustainable (Figures 8.3, 8.4 and 8.5).

The negative attitude towards vernacular housing explains why immediately after the tsunami the Government of Tamil Nadu announced that it would replace all damaged *kachcha* houses with *pucca* houses. It also shows that the government understood post-tsunami reconstruction as an opportunity to upgrade *kachcha* into *pucca* houses, even though the cost of building a *pucca* house is approximately thirty times higher than the cost of a *kachcha* house.[3]

According to the government's initial reconstruction policy – as described in the project document of the World Bank-funded Emergency Tsunami Reconstruction Programme (ETRP) – housing reconstruction was to be either supported through financial assistance from the government or ensured through public–private partnerships. Contrary to the central Government of

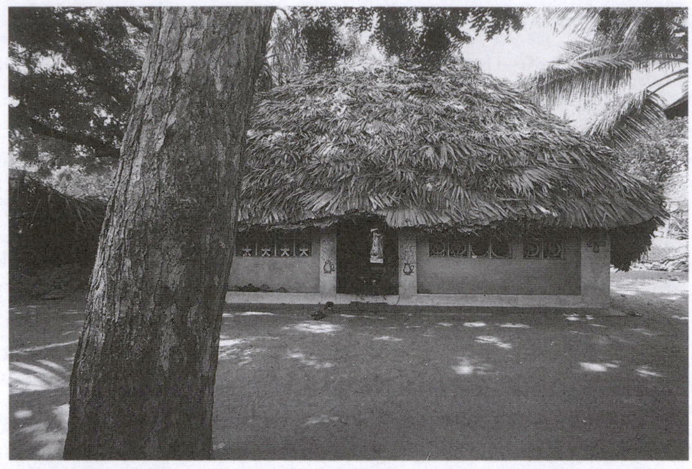

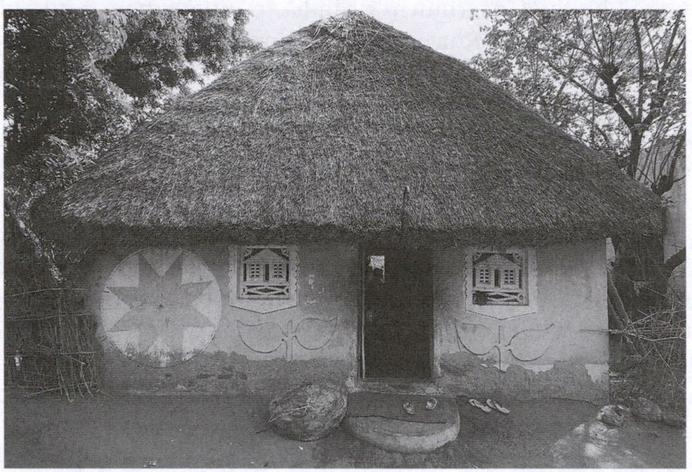

Figure 8.3 Two different types of thatched roofs of vernacular houses in coastal Tamil Nadu.

India, which officially declared that international humanitarian aid was not required for post-tsunami recovery, the Government of Tamil Nadu invited NGOs, voluntary organizations, public- and private-sector enterprises and national and international charity organizations to adopt particular villages for their reconstruction programme. Though the government issued detailed guidelines and building codes, the organizations were free in choosing their own architects and reconstruction approach.[15]

Tamil Nadu's initial policy proposed that new villages should be built at a minimal distance of 500 metres from the coast. This led to immediate tensions on the ground and to stiff public resistance. Fierce opposition and

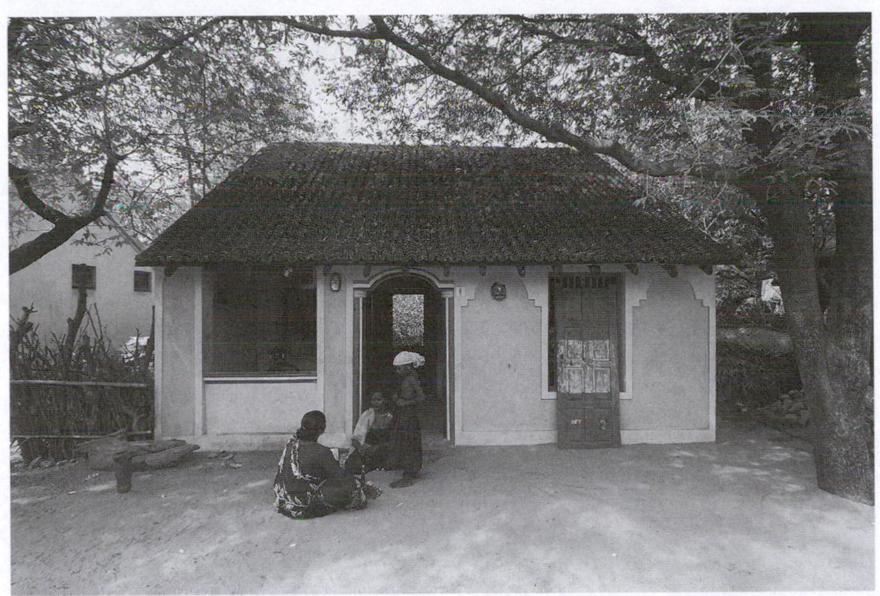

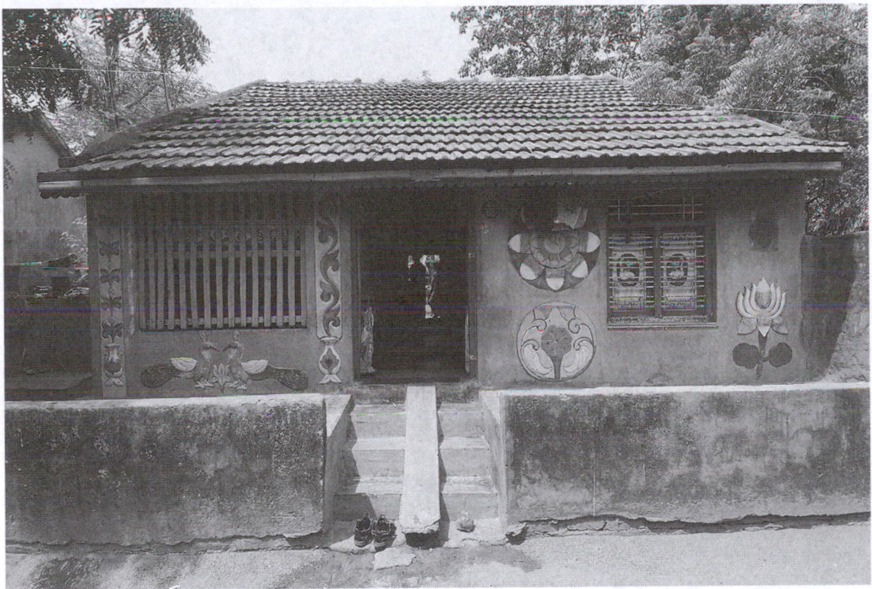

Figure 8.4 Traditional houses with tiled roofs.

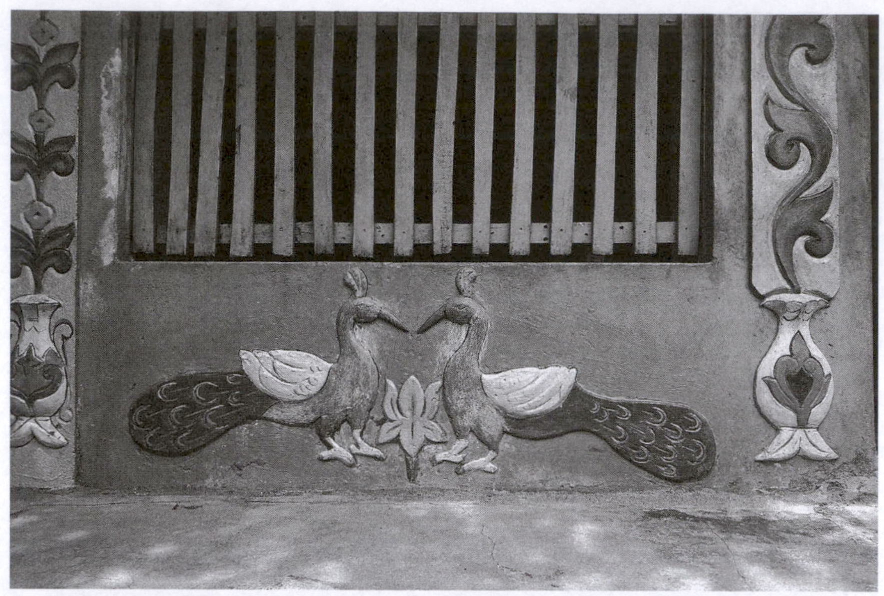

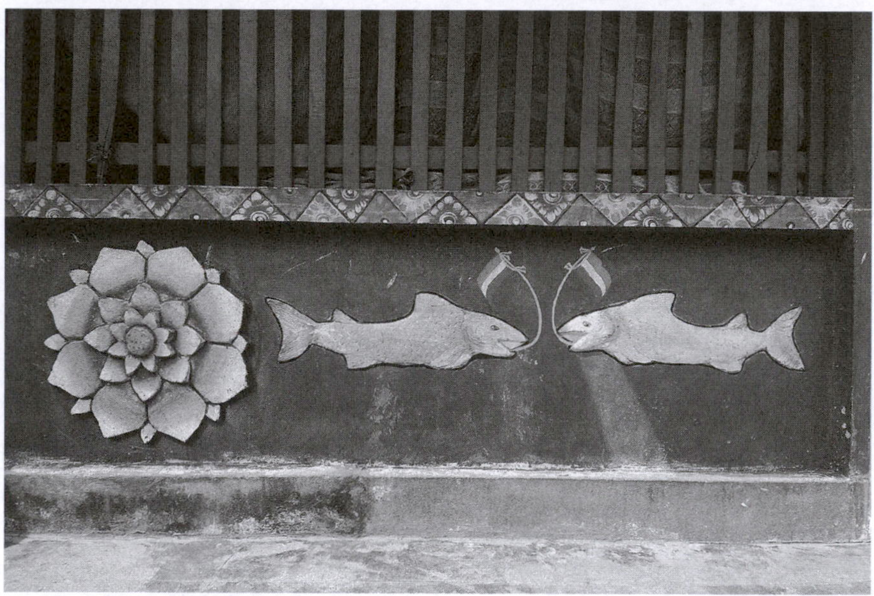

Figure 8.5 Details of vernacular houses in Tamil Nadu.

the difficulties of finding land for relocation led the government to amend its policy. The revised policy retained the essence of the previous one in terms of public–private partnerships but modified the relocation issue. Relocation remained mandatory only for people residing within 200 metres of the high-tide line, and it was optional for those at a distance of between 200 metres and 500 metres. Those beyond 500 metres would be entitled to housing assistance *in situ*. Allowing communities to remain in their original villages would make it necessary to reconsider the number of new houses required, as not all had been damaged by the tsunami. This, however, was never done. The abundance of funds for reconstruction and agencies' vested interest to build as many houses as possible, combined with prejudices towards vernacular housing and the fishing communities' own feeling of being entitled to free houses, led to the continued assumption that the number of required houses was to be based on the number of families living in coastal villages affected by the tsunami.

Tamil Nadu's initial reconstruction policy appeared to have much in common with that of Gujarat. However, whereas in Gujarat communities could choose between financial assistance and agency-driven reconstruction, this was not the case in Tamil Nadu. Once the government realized that there were sufficient non-governmental agencies and funds to ensure housing reconstruction, it withdrew from offering financial assistance for housing and handed over the reconstruction task to NGOs.

The role of NGOs

The Indian Ocean tsunami led to unprecedented global solidarity and massive private donations, and it brought hundreds of volunteers and civil-society organizations to the affected areas. In Tamil Nadu, efforts were concentrated primarily around the small coastal town of Nagapattinam, which accounted for over 50 per cent of the human losses.

One of the first Indian NGOs to come to Nagapattinam was Abhiyan, which aimed at sharing with the local government, with communities and with civil-society organizations its recent experience of post-disaster emergency management and reconstruction. Abhiyan supported the district administration and local organizations in setting up a system to coordinate the massive external aid, and it strongly advocated for an owner-driven approach, also with regard to temporary shelters. Considering that only a small stretch of the coast was affected by the tsunami and that the economy of the interior area was intact, so there was no scarcity of locally available, appropriate building materials, this would have been the most effective and empowering approach towards supporting communities. However, while the district administration appeared to be convinced of this approach, the state's chief minister ultimately ordered the top-down delivery of highly inappropriate shelters to temporarily accommodate those rendered homeless by the tsunami. Abhiyan was equally unsuccessful in influencing the government policy and local agencies' approaches towards permanent reconstruction. In fact, due to the unprecedented scale of private donations, all tsunami-affected villages in Tamil Nadu ended up being adopted for reconstruction by NGOs and private corporations. In December 2005, the government reported that forty-three agencies were in charge of the construction of 17,461 houses in eighty villages.[15] All of these opted for contractor-driven reconstruction, and in most cases, community participation was minimal.

Abhiyan's and other civil-society organizations' failure to contribute to an equitable, sustainable and empowering reconstruction programme for tsunami-affected communities may be explained by a number of factors. First of all, fishing communities, although marginalized, are not particularly poor and thus had previously not been among the NGOs' target groups. Accordingly, there were hardly any local NGOs that had knowledge of, experience with, and the trust of fishing communities. On the other hand, fishing communities enjoyed a good relationship with the state, from which they were used to receiving all sorts of assistance and subsidies prior to the tsunami. Fishing communities are well organized and characterized by powerful informal governance systems. They were thus used to voicing their demands and did not feel the need for being supported in the articulation of their needs by well-meaning NGOs. As did the government, they merely considered NGOs to be contractors from whom they did not expect anything other than houses. At the same time, the tsunami brought to coastal Tamil Nadu many profit-seeking agencies that were little more than disguised contractors waiting for opportunities to get involved in construction through international funding. International NGOs uncritically channelled their reconstruction funds through these agencies, expecting from them little else than the construction of as many houses as possible. With lots of money in their pocket and promises to build as many houses as demanded by local communities without interfering in their internal affairs, it was not too difficult to persuade the *panchayats* (informal leaders) to support top-down contractor-driven reconstruction.

Reconstruction outcomes

This section is based on research conducted in twelve villages in Tamil Nadu's most severely affected Nagapattinam district between October 2005 and March 2008. Our original intention was to start with a first phase of qualitative research, to be followed by a household survey aimed at assessing people's satisfaction with their new housing situation. But this turned out to be a difficult and also pointless enterprise. In fact, Tamil Nadu's reconstruction was entirely contractor-driven. Accordingly, it was not possible to analyze the reconstruction outcome in relation to different approaches. In addition, our qualitative research revealed a number of issues that could not have been captured through household surveys.

We discovered that reconstruction in Tamil Nadu led to the massive demolition of undamaged houses. Preserving as much as possible of the pre-disaster built environment is important from a psychological, socio-cultural, economic and environmental point of view. However, this was recognized neither by the government nor by the agencies involved in reconstruction, and in many cases not even by the community leaders themselves. The promise of getting new houses led several communities to ask for relocation, with the hope of local people ultimately being able to own two houses. However, while agencies were eager to spend their funds on building new houses, finding land for relocation turned out to be very difficult. Agencies thus started pushing for reconstruction *in situ*, which was possible only through demolishing the existing housing stock. In a survey we carried out in summer 2006 in two villages in Nagapattinam district, we found that out of 1500 houses an NGO was planning to build, over 780 were going to replace good-quality, undamaged or reparable houses. Though the communities had found a plot for relocation, its small size provided space only for about forty houses. Those were distributed among the most influential people, who, because they owned the best houses in the old villages, were not prepared to give these up for the sake of getting a new house. Although the key reason for reconstruction *in situ* was the difficulty of finding land for a new village, the NGO in question referred to anti-relocation discourses to legitimize its policy and to the Sphere standards to justify the demolition of undamaged vernacular houses.[12]

But not only vernacular houses were demolished to allow the building of new houses. In fact, some agencies went as far as to demolish houses built by other agencies, promising villagers even better houses. In one village we found that an NGO demolished 110 undamaged concrete houses that had been built by the fishery department a few years earlier within the framework of a social housing scheme and which after the tsunami had already been upgraded by another NGO.

Not all house owners voluntarily surrendered their houses, but they were often forced to do so by their local leaders. Villagers who tried to resist this process were put under tremendous pressure by being excommunicated from their communities. They were thus not allowed to go fishing and they were cut off from services such as water supply and electricity, and the rest of the community was not allowed to interact with them. Such repressive measures are possible in fishing communities, were the *panchayat* are very powerful.[2,30,36]

Reconstruction in Tamil Nadu further led to a severe depletion of the natural habitat. Coastal villages in Tamil Nadu are traditionally immersed within the thick vegetation of a large variety of bushes and trees. This shade-providing vegetation protects people from the scorching heat and is of vital importance in a very hot climate. Trees further supply local communities with important livelihood resources such as fuel, fruits, vegetables and fodder. The importance of paying sufficient attention to the natural habitat during reconstruction has been underlined by international environmental organizations such as the International Union for Conservation of Nature (IUCN) and the World Wide Fund for Nature (WWF).

The Government of Tamil Nadu and a number of NGOs initiated several coastal forestry projects. These, however, were dominated by exogenous species, such as *cajurina*, and the projects did not protect communities' own trees that had not been affected by the tsunami and that had an inestimable value for their livelihoods and wellbeing. In several villages the contractors employed by NGOs for housing reconstruction refused to start any reconstruction work before the ground was completely cleared of pre-tsunami houses, trees and other vegetation. In some villages, people estimated that 800–1200 trees were cut down in the process of building the new village, which consisted of endless rows of concrete houses without any vegetation. Naimi-Gasser found that the absence of trees in post-tsunami villages had severe consequences on coastal communities' livelihoods, social life and health situation and was considered by villagers the most dramatic consequence of contractor-driven reconstruction.[21]

The houses built by contractors in Tamil Nadu are also inadequate from a socio-cultural point of view (Figure 8.6). Fishing communities in Tamil Nadu have a strong housing culture that reflects their specific way of life and religious beliefs. Building a new house in 'normal times' is a social event that involves many specialized castes and therefore consolidates the ties among different coastal communities. Fishers generally venture into the construction of a new house at the occasion of a son's marriage. When the time to build a new house has come, they consult an astrologer, who decides in whose name it should be built and draws the house plan. Among the critical issues are the cardinal orientation of the main entrance, the length of each wall and the number of doors and windows. The astrologer fixes an auspicious date and time to begin the construction. He also performs a ritual on the construction site to protect all people involved in construction from accidents. Further rituals are carried out at different stages of construction and in particular before people begin to actually occupy the new house.

The size and construction materials depend on the house owners' age and socio-economic status. The first house of a newly married couple, if they can afford a separate house from the husband's family, may be a small and entirely thatched house. With increasing age, family size and financial resources, the couple may decide to build a new house with plastered brick walls and a thatched roof. A further improvement that, however, only the better-off households can afford consists in replacing the thatched roof with tiles, and even fewer families have the means or desire to build a flat-roof reinforced-concrete house. Those who have gone for this type of house realize after some time that it is not very comfortable under the local climatic conditions and may end up building a thatched roof on top of their flat roof.

Fishers' houses generally consist of only two to three rooms: a large veranda at the front leads to the main room. If the family can afford it, the house also has a small prayer room. By far the most important room is the

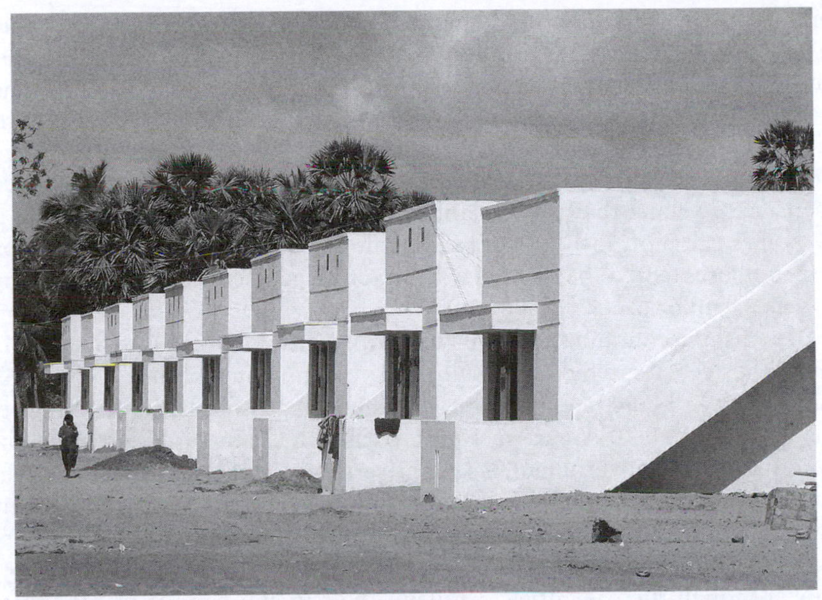

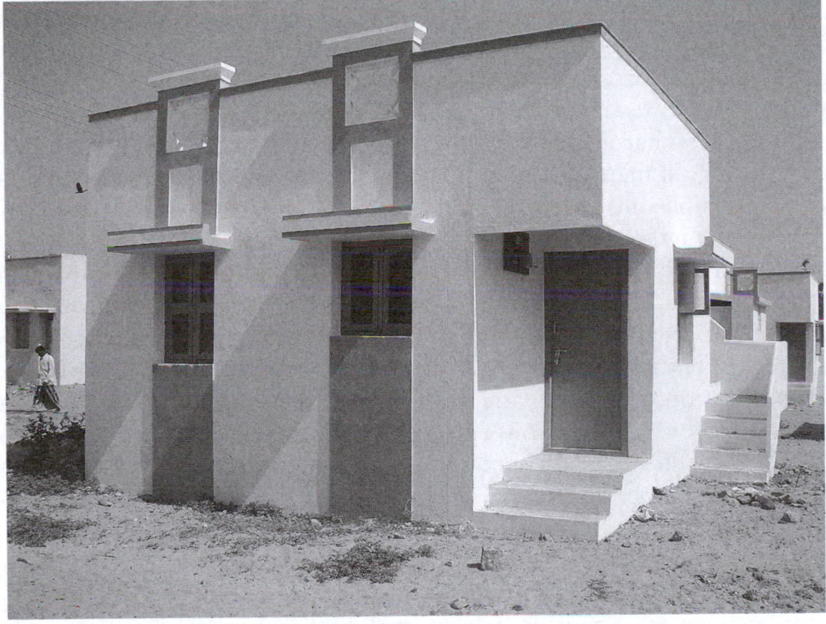

Figure 8.6 Post-tsunami houses in Tamil Nadu.

veranda. During the day this semi-open room is where people spend their leisure time and entertain their guests. At night, when straw mats are rolled out on the floor, the veranda is transformed into a sleeping area. The inner room is mainly used to store the family's belongings and as a sleeping area during the monsoon season. Besides containing a small shrine, the prayer room, too, is used for storage purposes. In most cases the kitchen constitutes a separate dwelling that is invariably located in the south-eastern corner of the homestead plot. Fishers like bright colours. The doors, walls and floors of their houses tend to be painted with beautiful geometric patterns depicting flowers or animals.

These fishing communities' housing culture was not taken into account by any of the agencies, which, following the government guidelines, invariably built one-fits-all-concrete, flat-roof, matchbox-type houses, sometimes even smaller than the 320 square feet (approximately 31 square metres) in size prescribed by the government. As per government regulation, all homestead plots have a size of 235–50 square feet (23–5 square metres), which means that though the houses are far too small for the average family, there is no space for extensions.

Even though the casualties following the tsunami cannot be attributed solely to the vulnerability of the built environment, the government directed much effort towards promoting multi-hazard-resistant concrete houses. In Tamil Nadu, the lack of supervision and the lack of control of the activities of profit-oriented contractors, too, led to poor construction quality. This problem was exacerbated by poor labour skills, poor quality of materials, housing design features that do not match with local building capacities, and insufficient curing. In many cases the consequences of poor construction quality were irreversible, ultimately leading to a higher degree of vulnerability.[11]

Post-tsunami reconstruction led to conflicts, anomy and social disarticulation. Conflicts of interest between those who managed to take advantage of the reconstruction programmes, on the one hand, and those who were negatively affected by them, on the other, split communities that before the tsunami had been living in relative harmony with each other. In some villages the confiscation of private land and the forced demolition of undamaged houses led to overt and serious episodes of violence.[30]

In Tamil Nadu's coastal communities, women traditionally have a central role in the construction of a house. As their husbands are mainly occupied with fishing, the mobilization of local masons and carpenters, the purchase of construction materials and the supervision of the work are often in women's hands. Women had clear and articulated ideas about their housing requirements but were never consulted. In general, participation in decision-making was minimal and only involved interactions with the male-dominated *panchayats*.

By distributing free houses to all young married couples, the reconstruction process also dismantled coastal communities' informal old-age insurance system. In fact, the possession of a house, which the youngest son inherits in exchange for support to his aging parents, has close links to the informal social-security systems. After the tsunami, however, the allocation and distribution of houses were decided by the *panchayats*, who developed their own eligibility criteria. These criteria did not consider whether a person had been rendered homeless by the tsunami, but whether he or she was married. According to the *panchayats'* criteria, widows were not entitled to houses, because they were expected to live with their children. But the new houses were small and clearly designed for nuclear families. The change from being house owners hosting their grown-up children in their own houses to being guests in their children's homes made a big difference to old-aged people's security. There were no solutions for childless people. One village leader explicitly told us that it was not worth giving houses to widows because they would die soon anyhow.

Conclusions: continuity and change in post-disaster reconstruction

This review of India's reconstruction experiences with regard to the 1993 and 2001 earthquakes in Maharashtra and Gujarat respectively and to the 2004 Indian Ocean tsunami in Tamil Nadu shows that policy-making processes, practices and outcomes depend on a number of contextual factors, such as the capacity of local communities to articulate their needs and demands; the relation between state governments, national civil-society organizations and international agencies; previous disaster experiences; the balance between public and private actors; and the amount and source of funding for reconstruction.

All three cases demonstrate that state governments in India have a proactive role in post-disaster reconstruction and the political will to devolve power and responsibilities on the bureaucracy and that they are responsive to communities' and civil-society organizations' demands. These factors greatly contributed to fair participatory and non-politicized approaches towards post-disaster reconstruction processes. In fact, by repeatedly amending their policies, state governments have shown continuity in terms of their willingness to engage in a dialogue with civil-society organizations and communities and to respond to their demands. At the same time, these states' reconstruction approaches and outcomes are, in many respects, remarkably different, which shows that the specific conditions, interests and priorities prevalent in a given context are not homogeneous and may strongly influence reconstruction outcomes. In this concluding section, I will examine similarities and differences between the three cases in relation to a number of key parameters.

Reconstruction in situ *versus relocation*

First of all, it has been noted that in all three cases the state governments initially proposed to relocate affected communities to new villages. Only in

Maharashtra, however, did communities accept this solution. In Gujarat and Tamil Nadu the relocation plan led to fierce opposition and to the governments ultimately amending their policies. This reflects an increased awareness concerning socio-economic and environmental risks and the negative impacts of relocation among communities, governments, civil-society organizations and the World Bank. Several international NGOs and private corporations, however, showed little concern for such risks. Whenever land was available, they urged communities towards accepting resettlement, because building a village on clear ground is less complex than reconstruction *in situ*. Nevertheless, both in Gujarat and Tamil Nadu we noticed that local communities, too, sometimes took advantage of agencies' preference for relocation, as this may offer an opportunity to obtain new houses without having to give up the old ones. This factor, more than the presumed loss of people's faith in their own building capacity and the post-tsunami fear of the sea, may explain why several communities in all three states voluntarily accepted, or even demanded, to be relocated. This kind of unnecessary relocation gives communities the option of returning to their pre-disaster villages in case they do not like what they obtained, but it constitutes a waste of resources that may have serious socio-economic and environmental consequences.

Even though the enhanced awareness of the risks and drawbacks of relocation represents an important step forward, it is important to note that reconstruction *in situ* does not necessarily or inevitably lead to better outcomes. In Gujarat we noted that *in situ* reconstruction generally led to poor outcomes when adequate settlement plans were absent, when reconstruction happened on the basis of the contractor-driven approach, or when exogenous building materials and designs were employed. In Tamil Nadu, in particular, reconstruction *in situ* ended up having severe negative effects on communities' cultural identity and natural habitat, because contractors would refuse to start reconstruction before the ground was completely cleared of houses and vegetation. Reconstruction *in situ* thus often led to the erasure of much of people's history and cultural identity, which had detrimental psycho-social consequences.

Owner-driven versus contractor-driven reconstruction

The potential advantages of owner-driven reconstruction in terms of cost- and time-effectiveness and in empowering citizens to rebuild their houses according to their individual needs and preferences are increasingly being recognized on the international level. A number of international agencies, such as the World Bank, the International Federation of Red Cross Societies (IFRC), the Swiss Agency for Development Cooperation (SDC) and the American Red Cross, have adopted owner-driven reconstruction in Sri Lanka and Indonesia following the Indian Ocean tsunami, as well as in Pakistan after the earthquake of 2005. However, in India – the country where the approach was successfully adopted for the first time on a large scale by the Government of Gujarat – post-tsunami reconstruction was entirely contractor-driven. Tamil Nadu's reconstruction outcome added yet another piece of evidence that contractor-driven reconstruction leads to environmentally and socio-culturally inadequate housing and settlement and to poor construction quality. It was shown that one of the main reasons for the prevalence of this approach was the fact that reconstruction was fully taken over by private organizations that were funded primarily by international agencies.

The observation that many international NGOs continue to support contractor-driven reconstruction is a matter of concern, especially if one considers that the associated processes and outcomes deviate substantively from all international guiding principles and standards. The discrepancies between principles, on the one hand, and the practices on the ground, on the other, point to the need to refine instruments that may enhance accountability towards local governments and communities. In India, state governments have the capacity to develop such instruments. However, governments need to recognize that financial assistance for owner-driven reconstruction is not just the most practical solution for a state agency in managing post-disaster reconstruction but also the most empowering and the most sustainable approach. Once the overall benefits of owner-driven reconstruction and the risks of contractor-driven reconstruction are recognized, governments should ensure that all agencies follow an owner-driven approach. The lack of a regulatory framework has given excessive freedom to private agencies to pursue whatever approach meets their own interests, which all too often leads to contractor-driven reconstruction.

Post-disaster building technologies and practices

India is a country with a well-established environmental housing movement that has its roots in Gandhian ethics and principles. In Maharashtra, however, this movement had but a marginal and inconsistent impact on post-disaster reconstruction. Local civil-society organizations' advocacy for participatory and culturally sensitive reconstruction led to communities being involved, to a certain degree, in settlement planning and housing designs, but it failed to result in reconstruction processes relying on local building skills and technologies. The adoption of industrial building materials led to the exclusion of local masons, so the opportunity to strengthen their building capacity by integrating safety measures within their traditional building technologies was missed. The case of Gujarat exhibits significant progress in building upon local capacity by linking owner-driven reconstruction with the training of local masons. Moreover, official building codes and guidelines aimed at improving the safety of local and alternative building technologies. Nonetheless, several local and most international NGOs did not take advantage of this favourable policy environment and went ahead with promoting exogenous building technologies.

In Tamil Nadu, prejudices towards vernacular housing had dramatic consequences. In spite of the fact that local building technologies could not be blamed for the disaster, reconstruction became a pretext to demolish thousands of undamaged, locally appropriate and beautiful houses. In this regard, therefore, there has been a significant setback that is closely linked to the combination of overfunded private organizations involved in reconstruction, lack of knowledge of, and prejudices towards, local housing culture and building capacity as well as technocratic views of multi-hazard-resistant housing.

In conclusion, this chapter has shown that in spite of increasing knowledge and awareness of what are the best reconstruction practices and a growing consensus on international guiding principles and standards, progress has not been linear. In India, Maharashtra's reconstruction approach was still based on a modernistic and top-down approach towards housing development. In Gujarat, local awareness of the failure of this approach in enhancing people's resilience contributed to the adoption of a more empowering approach a few years later. A regrettable setback was, however, observed in Tamil Nadu, where reconstruction outcomes were disastrous. While it is clear that this was due to a number of factors, it is a special matter of concern that the single most important of these was the unprecedented availability of enormous international private funding for reconstruction.

9 The politics of participation

Involving communities in post-disaster reconstruction

Alicia Sliwinski

There is a common consensus about the importance of community involvement in post-disaster projects. However, there is often less clarity on what type of participation is most advantageous and how a 'community' is defined. A case history in El Salvador illustrates the importance of matching participation to the expectations of the beneficiaries.

Community participation: from development to reconstruction

In post-disaster contexts, humanitarian builders, which can be international and national NGOs as well as state and multilateral organizations, often design projects that aim to involve local populations. This is generally called community participation.

The fact that community participation is regularly adopted in reconstruction is not surprising. Involving disaster victims in the rebuilding of their lives is understood as a sustainable way of doing things. It also follows from the consideration that reconstruction professionals wish to better connect their work to sustainable development goals. And this is not a new question, quite to the contrary, as the important work of Anderson and Woodrow attests.[1] These authors were precisely advocating a stronger participation of disaster victims in reconstruction activities in order to reinforce communities' local capacities and foster their empowerment.

If community participation in post-disaster reconstruction initiatives is often favoured as both an execution methodology and a morally legitimate theoretical framework, this is due to at least three factors: 1) the fact that the particular space-time of reconstruction leads on to that of development and that the aim is to better articulate the two; 2) the fact that many actors, especially NGOs, that operate in reconstruction also operate in the world of development; and 3) the fact that community participation has become a dominant 'paradigm' for the development world[8] – a paradigm that has logically spilled over to influence many post-disaster reconstruction practices.

However, after twenty years of experience in applying participatory methodologies, the outcome is not undisputed, and participation has been the object of various critical writings. Certainly, under the label of participation there exists a whole range of activities that are qualified as 'participatory'. For example, there is an enormous difference between people's participation as a form of free labour and their active involvement at all stages of a given housing project. This is where post-disaster builders must remain vigilant.

This chapter starts with a theoretical overview of the concepts of 'participation' and 'community' according to recent analyses from the development field. Indeed, many of the more critical assessments on the topic of community participation offer sound recommendations for post-disaster builders. A case study from a Salvadorian initiative that followed the two 2001 earthquakes illustrates how people's participation in reconstruction can lead to tensions and conflicts. However, let me emphasize that the aim is not to condemn participation but to highlight some of its shortcomings, as there are real risks in idealizing participatory techniques and reifying the notion of community. No doubt, ignoring them may cause more harm than good.

Community participation: theoretical contours

Although the notion of community participation is now often found in the sphere of reconstruction, it articulates itself to development theories, policies and practices. It is therefore from this perspective that I begin the examination. Regarding participation: most would agree that participation was a much-needed answer to the top-down development approaches, where projects were mainly designed by foreign experts, as Lizarralde explains in Chapter 2. With the introduction of participation, the objective shifted to encouraging the beneficiaries' involvement in the interventions that affected them and over which they had had limited control.[15]

An important figure having a significant impact on the institutional acceptation of participation is Robert Chambers, who, with his book *Rural Development: Putting the Last First*[7] and his subsequent works, developed the well-known participatory rural appraisal (PRA) methodology. Paolo Freire, the Brazilian educator associated with liberation theology, in his 1970s writings clearly influenced the more radical and emancipatory visions of participation understood as a mechanism that fosters the 'conscientization' of poor people and, ultimately, their empowerment.[29] In the following years, many participatory techniques and methods were developed, such as participatory action research, rapid rural appraisal and PRA, of course, all of which became more and more utilized by NGOs. At its beginnings, participation was seen as a means allowing for the social, cultural and political emancipation of people, and participatory instruments reserved a special role for 'local knowledge'. In this sense, participation announced a new approach to development, a salutary alternative to the top-down, modernizing and 'one size fits all' models of the establishment, which would ultimately answer poor peoples' needs.

The 1980s are said to be the 'lost decade' for development. It was also during this period that the soviet bloc dismantled itself, engendering a democratization process through the fall of the Berlin Wall and the opening up of communist countries. Confronted by these profound geopolitical changes, and also considering the multiplication of the number of NGOs on the international scene adopting participatory methodologies, the World Bank also started to incorporate them in its programmes.[39] Participation then became a condition for the financing of projects.

In the 1990s, participation no longer represented a threat, and it acquired its place in the then-dominant institutional practices and discourses. In other words, it became mainstream. Hence the participation of local peoples (called *primary stakeholders* in the language of the World Bank) became understood as the means through which development would better ensure the sustainability of its endeavours. Under the label of 'participatory development', community participation became an official development policy. But, as mentioned, after some two decades of experimentation in a variety of contexts, many would agree that participation has, in turn, become almost a dogma, a belief or an act of faith that has not delivered on its promises and requires a profound and thorough re-examination.[13,48]

Within the scope of this book it is not possible to do justice to the many analyses and reflections that have addressed the notion of community participation; nonetheless, some overarching principles that stand out in the literature are introduced. These considerations are important if community participation is to remain a significant practice and conceptual framework for all actors involved, in the context of development or of reconstruction.

Participation – between the technical and the political

Misgivings about participation, as found in the literature, include the articulation between its 1) technical and 2) political/conceptual dimensions, where the first are criticized for their excessive standardization and the second for missing their objective while being instrumentalized.[15] Initially, participatory development, linked to a leftist ideology and to popular movements, was considered for its potential to transform societies for the better.[34] The incorporation of participatory methodologies in projects was seen as a means leading to a precise end, and ultimately that end was to be the comprehensive empowerment of poor and marginal communities, which, bit by bit, would take over the reins of their own development.[43] However, through participation's ongoing incorporation into the operations of NGOs, a process of normalization ensued to the extent that participation became more akin to a technical instrument ensuring the efficiency and effectiveness of projects, to the detriment of any substantial integration of the different members of a given community.

Confronted by the many forms participation may take in development projects, some authors have elaborated frameworks that better categorize the possible level of participation. The precursory work of Arnstein[2] specifically focussed on the field of housing construction, and that of Choguill[11] offers good examples. For instance, Arnstein developed a *ladder* of participation, reputed to be a rather formalistic tool but holding a definite heuristic value. The author explains how community participation can range from 'manipulation' to 'empowerment' through various other levels of autonomy and control. These analyses have recently been the object of a methodological synthesis, proposing a comparative analysis of various post-disaster reconstruction projects that reveals how the adopted organizational structure affects the degree of participation.[20]

Indeed, it is important to define what kind of participation is really taking place in any given project. It is naive to think that a loosely defined notion of participation can reduce vulnerability, as if by the mere fact of being 'involved' in a housing reconstruction project, beneficiaries will automatically develop a sense of ownership of the project, reinforce their local capacities and resilience and empower their community. Such an assertion would bring with it a few problems, such as:

- the degree of participation (i.e. what is meant by involvement);
- the length of the project;
- the need to identify who effectively participates and how;
- the way participation takes into account intra- and extra-communitarian power dynamics; and
- its concerns with issues of local governance that articulate themselves to the wider ideological, political and economical context.

This leads precisely to the questions of power and empowerment.

The communitarian ideal

No doubt it is on the question of power that a number of important criticisms have been addressed to community participation. In the 1990s, the influence of social theories that analyze the politics of discourse, the question of power and the complex social relations between structure and agency increased. The writings of Foucault,[27,28] Giddens[30] and Bourdieu[4] have definitively influenced the social sciences and the more academic side of researches on development, as the works of Escobar,[24] Ferguson[26] and Long and Long[40] attest. If, overall, their impact on practice and official policies has been rather weak,[13] there is nonetheless a growing unease with the failed promises of community participation that cannot be ignored. It is precisely from this stance that a series of critical analyses examining the failures of participation have emerged. From this literature, we retain three publications: *The Myth of Community*,[32] *Participation: The New Tyranny?*[15] and *Participation: From Tyranny to Transformation*.[34] These writings offer a good understanding and overview of the more recent debates that post-disaster builders cannot afford to not take into account.

As its title indicates, the first work (*The Myth of Community*) concerns the notion of community as a reified entity. The authors' fundamental criticism points to the gendered bias inherent in participatory techniques that are applied in development projects; in other words, to the fact that many practitioners forget or underestimate the gender dynamics in their way of thinking about a given community and in planning their interventions. Too often, community participation actualizes the sole participation or the dominant presence of the male members of a community. In many social contexts in the developing world, men still occupy a dominant position and are those who verbalize the needs of their 'community'. However, this does not mean *ipso facto* that adequate account is taken of women's perspectives – perspectives that may not just concern them but the entire social group. Hence the authors of this work insist on the 'micro-politics of gender relations'. By ignoring women's roles, opinions and needs, and by basically turning a blind eye to the hierarchical relations and processes of social differentiation that characterize a community, participatory methodologies cannot presume to ensure a community's full empowerment.[16,17] Indeed, we shall see in our case study how gender relations did not enhance the emergence of 'a sense of community' within the reconstruction project.

All this comes from the fact that the social sciences have had – and still have – the unfortunate tendency to 'mystify' the concept of community. This idealization dates back to the work of Tönnies[54] on the distinction between the communitarian and the non-communitarian, between the *gemeinschaft* (community) and *gesellschaft* (society), where we (as a Western readership) entertained, vis-à-vis the first term, a nostalgia of enduring social ties based on territoriality, kinship relations and the existence of tradition and custom as a glue that ensures the cohesion and shared identity of a social group generally considered small.[31,55]

In development and reconstruction, we still find this tendency to imagine a community as a homogeneous entity occupying a clearly defined territory. There is often the risk of underestimating the presence of internal tensions and the effects of differentiation processes that articulate themselves in terms of gender relations and also in terms of people's socioeconomic status, their level of education, their religious and political affiliation and other socio-cultural markers. To underrate their importance renders fragmentary, if not just plain prejudicial, any initiative that hopes to empower communities.

An often-quoted text by Etzioni[25] discusses the shortcomings of the community as a unit of analysis and intervention according to five points:

1 the lack of definitional clarity;
2 the normative usage of the concept that reproduced a conservative attitude (as in the idea of the 'weight of tradition');
3 the romanticism associated with it;
4 the lack of attention given to minority groups; and

5 the fact that the communitarian approach can oppress individuals when they find themselves constrained to follow the values and norms of the majority that they do not share entirely.

All communities are dynamic and changing entities composed of various social sub-groups and traversed by tensions and conflicts. These observations are important for post-disaster builders when planners envision new habitats for disaster victims.

Participation and power

The second book retained, *Participation: The New Tyranny?*, prolongs these remarks. From the start, the authors find a harmful potential in participation. Indeed, various contributors to the volume, inspired by the writings of Foucault, show how many aspects of participation reveal an exercise of power when those who intervene in communities neglect the political dimensions and effects of their initiatives. Recall that for Foucault, power is something that circulates in everyday life and that manifests itself on people's bodies (through the notion of biopower) and through techniques and systems of knowledge that frame them. Power is realized in norms, in practices and in the production of knowledge and discourses at all levels of social life.[27,28] So, for instance, all the attention given to 'local knowledge' in projects (which, in reconstruction, may concern the cultural values of modes of spatial occupation as well as local representations of the built environment – as Nese Dikman in Chapter 10 and Rohit Jigyasu in Chapter 3 discuss in this volume) often reveals the extent to which foreign, Eurocentric conceptual frameworks are used in order to generate what is then considered local knowledge.[41]

Time and again, it is the dominant groups who are best able to express their 'needs', which, moreover, will often be formulated according to their perception of what a given initiative may or may not offer them.[42] In a Foucauldian perspective, any model of community participation is ultimately an external system of knowledge production, foreign to the practices of local social groups that are targeted by development experts. Foucault's perspective has the advantage of revealing how discourses and practices said to be participatory can operate a subtle (or not so subtle) exercise of power on the 'communities' that are to be developed or rebuilt.

Of course, there are other analytical approaches that expose problems with participation. For example, the reflection on the relationships between structure and agency[30] may also explain how and why certain local institutions participate, who composes them and why others may choose not to do so, as people may find it more profitable to *not* participate.[13] Many participatory approaches assume that people *should* participate and therefore encourage the creation or the mobilization of committees, preferably democratically elected. But the institution of a new committee does not absolutely guarantee that decisions will better reflect the needs and opinions of the group, nor that internal divisions will be eased and systems of inclusion/exclusion will be smoothed.[13]

Community participation as social capital and governance

Today, a new concept has entered public discourse, that of social capital. If it is tied to the idea of culture as a utilizable resource, it mainly refers to the ideas of non-economical resources and of networks (both formal and informal) that stem from relations of reciprocity based on mutual trust, shared norms and a common sense of belonging that facilitate cooperation and exchange between the members of a given social group.[5,16,49] This concept was incorporated in the work of the World Bank in 1993 (in its Social Capital Initiative), as it was seen as a means to better measure the impacts of social capital in development projects.

The infatuation with social capital parallels that with participatory methodologies, precisely at a time when many criticize the destructive social impacts of structural adjustment programs.[12,53] Social capital has appeared in studies on post-disaster reconstruction that explain how disaster-stricken groups are encouraged to draw on their social capital in order to rebuild their habitats when government responses are ineffective, lengthy or inadequate[9,10] (as Isabelle Maret and James Amdal explain in Chapter 6). Social capital can be taken as a new way of conceptualizing a community's available resources, but due to the array of often tautological and circulatory definitions that characterize it, it is not always easy to get a clear sense either of the concept or of its applicability.[46] As Kay puts it: 'Social capital is no more than a modern academic tag put onto age-old processes that permit a healthy community to function. The question is whether or not social capital can be used to generate communities' (page 167).[38] Nonetheless, in a history of concepts related to 'community participation', social capital remains of current interest.

To wrap up this overview, the authors of the third publication, *Participation: From Tyranny to Transformation*, explain that participation, after having been invested with different theoretical approaches, including that of social capital, refers now to the idea of the exercise of citizenship. Citizenship is to be taken as the normative framework that covers the notion of 'popular', 'local' or 'community' participation. This new orientation demonstrates the encounter between participation and questions relating to governance.[34] It offers an answer to the problems of the depoliticization of previous approaches. By emphasizing the rights of citizenship, participation becomes something much more substantial than a mere development technique. According to the authors, participation revives its transformational potential when it conjugates issues of governance and civic engagement, when it explicitly takes into account processes of social stratification and political economy and when it adopts a clear ideological posture anchored to a well-defined development theory. Linking participation to larger political changes and considering it as both a right and obligation of citizenship/belonging makes it possible again to uncover its emancipatory potential.

Together, these three commentaries offer important food for thought for reconstruction practitioners. Being aware of how 'community' and 'participation' tend to be idealized, how power operates in participatory projects and how governance issues traverse these initiatives linking local concerns to larger issues of political economy are important elements in designing reconstruction projects, especially when they are addressed to the less privileged people affected by a disaster. Indeed, many studies have demonstrated the extent to which the reconstruction of habitats is a highly social and political issue and how vulnerability-reduction initiatives directly affect development and people's livelihoods.[3,18,33,56]

Framing participation in post-disaster reconstruction

The literature on community participation is more abundant regarding projects that deal with the management, mitigation and evaluation of people's vulnerability to disaster and environmental risks[45,52] than on housing reconstruction initiatives per se – although some works have indeed addressed the subject, including research of a more sociological and anthropological nature.[44,49,51]

It should also be noted that beneficiaries' participation in reconstruction projects refers to one particular execution methodology among others. Under the label of participation there exists a variety of options.[20,22,37,50] In this chapter, beneficiaries' participation refers to the type of relations that are established between beneficiaries and NGOs, and particularly to the former's degree of involvement and control. It is now well established to say that participation in reconstruction projects is a good way for enhancing vulnerability reduction, technological transfer and sustainable development, but various authors have shown how these objectives can fail (see Chapter 2 in this volume).[37,50]

In her analysis of five different housing reconstruction methodologies following the 2001 Gujarat earthquake, Duyne Barenstein notes that different NGOs qualified as 'participatory' different approaches that were in fact very distinct from one another.[22] For some, participation was limited to the consultation of village elites; others consulted beneficiaries regarding the design of the houses, but their involvement finished there; others again called the beneficiaries' manual labour 'participation'. No doubt this multiple usage of the term 'participation' can be confusing. In order to clarify the issue, Duyne Barenstein qualifies as participatory an approach:

- in which the NGO takes a leading role;
- that does not involve professional contractors;

- in which the beneficiaries are involved at all levels of the project, from initial consultation in planning and design to construction.[22]

Taking a cue from her typology, I present a Salvadorian case study. I conducted about nine months of participant-observation fieldwork (from October 2001 to June 2002) in a particular reconstruction project addressed to fifty disaster-stricken families.

La Hermandad: the making of a new 'community'

Context and project logic

On 13 January 2001 an earthquake registering 7.6 on the Richter scale shook the small municipality of Lamaria,* causing limited deaths (twenty-three) compared to other areas in the country but destroying and damaging 4725 houses. Around 13,440 people were affected in Lamaria, which is more than half the town's population, in the sense that these people saw their houses either completely destroyed or partially damaged. Reconstruction of permanent housing in Lamaria started in May 2001.

La Hermandad is the name of a reconstruction site of fifty houses that was financed and managed by a European Chapter of the Red Cross in partnership with the Salvadorian Red Cross. It is located a few kilometres away from the centre of town and is linked to another very similar initiative, less than a kilometre away, that addressed 150 families (fifty of which were Red Cross beneficiaries; the other 100 were beneficiaries of an Italian NGO and a religious organization). Together these projects were building a 'model urbanization' that would reduce the physical and social vulnerability of the most vulnerable group of disaster victims, i.e. families that had never owned a house or a plot of land. Indeed almost all of them had been living in the temporary shelters erected shortly after the emergency period.

Among the fifty families in La Hermandad (Figure 9.1), close to a third were single mothers and all earned less than the minimum salary, established at US$97 per month at the time. The project started in May 2001 with the clearing up of a sugarcane field, and it was supposed to end in February 2002, but, due to various factors (in particular the longer-than-expected building process, as everything was done manually without any heavy machinery), it finished only in May 2002.

This participatory project required the manual labour of at least one adult member per family for a total of 160 hours per month. In exchange for their labour, and to supplement the lack of income, beneficiaries received monthly

* Names of people and places have been changed in order to preserve the confidentiality of certain information.

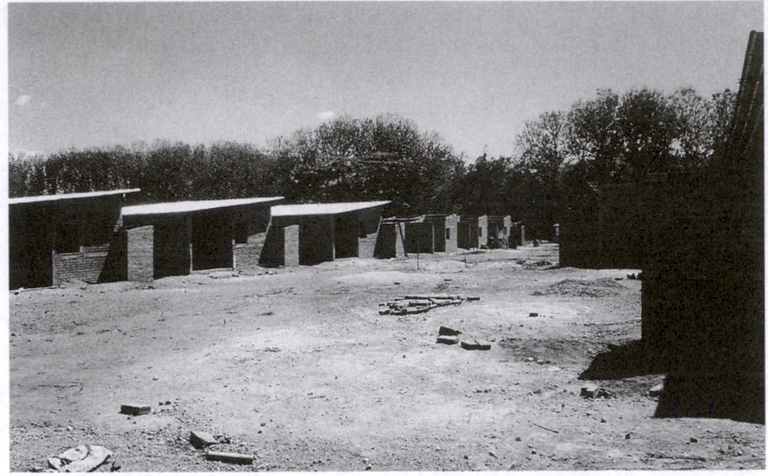

Figure 9.1 General view of La Hermandad under construction.

food rations distributed from the World Food Programme. Such 'food for work' projects were quite common in El Salvador after the earthquake. However, the real reward for people's labour was their access to private property in the form of an earthquake-resistant house of 40 square metres on a lot of 200 square meters – something none of the families could have afforded before the events. All of them had to live on the building site in the temporary shelters that had been distributed to them following the emergency period (Figure 9.2). These had to be regularly dismounted and reassembled according to the pace of construction.

No member outside the nuclear family was allowed to live on the site. In a context where poor people often rely on customary mutual aid networks and extended kinship ties, this restriction had negative consequences on many people's socioeconomic well-being.

Even though the project was qualified as participatory, the degree of beneficiary control remained limited: if at the start families were consulted on the general design of the houses, which followed a single standard model for all beneficiaries, their ulterior 'participation' was limited to their manual labour input. In this sense, the concept of participation does not correspond to Barenstein's definition. In addition, daily life was structured by a series of rules and regulations regarding number of working hours, surveillance tours and permits to leave the site during working hours. Two figures of authority were present: an engineer in charge of the technical aspects of reconstruction and a social worker whose mandate consisted of establishing social committees concerning the environment, risk analysis, food distribution and alphabetization, which were seen as giving an 'added value' to the project. The objective was to reinforce local capacities, those of women more particularly.

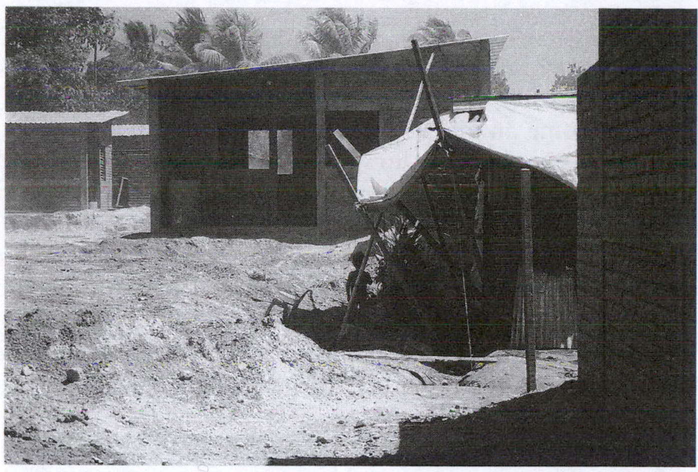

Figure 9.2 Houses under construction and temporary shelters.

A communitarian ideal framed the entire initiative; indeed, project leaders repeated time and time again, especially during the monthly general assemblies, that the families were there to form a new community – that thanks to their common labour, by appropriating the project, they had the possibility for a better life. Participatory work was promoted as the means *par excellence* to enhance the emergence of a community feeling. Access to a house worth US$4500 without contest represents an enabling opportunity unforeseen for poor families. But they were there for precisely that, to have access to private property, rather than to create a new community. And this is the source of many of the problems that arose. Between the official discourses and the daily practice of reconstruction, between project ideals and people's true motivations, there was a huge gap that translated itself into a series of conflicts. These conflicts were articulated in terms of:

- gender relations;
- socioeconomic markers;
- political initiatives;
- beneficiaries' own representation of the logic of the project.

In other words, in over a year's time, it was not a communitarian feeling that emerged between these families but rather an increasing process of differentiation and divisionism, which leads one to ask if things could have evolved differently. In what follows, the ways these processes manifested themselves are discussed.

Gender relations

At the level of gender relations, this project integrated around fifteen single mothers in a non-traditional female activity: house-building.

Gender has become an important policy element in post-disaster reconstruction.[23] Various works show how women's needs and their vulnerability are distinct from men's, but these should not be homogenized and nor should we consider women as victims of their culture.[36] The writings of Bradshaw[6] and Cupples[19] on women's participation in post-Mitch reconstruction in Nicaragua show interesting findings. In one of her studies, Bradshaw explains that women's participation, and particularly that of single women, did not necessarily entail an enhanced level of control of the process nor in their community.[6] Cupples' fieldwork revealed that women's experiences in reconstruction varied depending on the social context, i.e. on the degree of solidarity and social mobilization in each community after the disaster. She explains that in a locality named El Mirador, a 'community' created by a housing project (as in the case for La Hermandad), no sense of communitarian solidarity evolved but rather forms of personal interest and dependency on aid. Here, women's participation reproduced normative gender roles that marginalized them, because the division of labour assigned them to more 'gender appropriate' tasks (i.e. fetching water, sand and bricks). Compared to other more successful community experiences studied by the author, the case of El Mirador shows problems similar to those in my own case study.

In La Hermandad, single mothers were assigned to two working groups, one in charge of assembling the metal structures of the houses and the other dedicated to the concrete compaction for the foundations (Figure 9.3).

These women were proud of their contribution. But their daily contact with men on the site created a pervasive jealousy from other women whose male partners were working on the site. This is an example showing how identification with traditional and non-traditional gender roles may come into conflict. Between these two micro-groups, tensions and suspicions arose, accompanied by much gossiping that cannot be underestimated. As various ethnographies on Central American peasant culture have explained, gossip fills an important role of social control, as it expresses how a given behaviour is socially sanctioned or not.[35]

Friendship between sexes is not a customary 'cultural trait' of rural Salvadorian society. In La Hermandad the population was mixed, of both rural and urban origin. Many of the single mothers had lived in larger cities, working in *maquiladoras* (foreign-owned assembly plants in free-trade zones), and they were not shy to interact with men or even flirt with their co-workers on the site. And this was precisely the kind of behaviour other women would have no patience for. I cannot emphasize enough the divisive nature of all this talk, which endured for over a ten-month period and seriously hindered the emergence of a 'community feeling'. The active

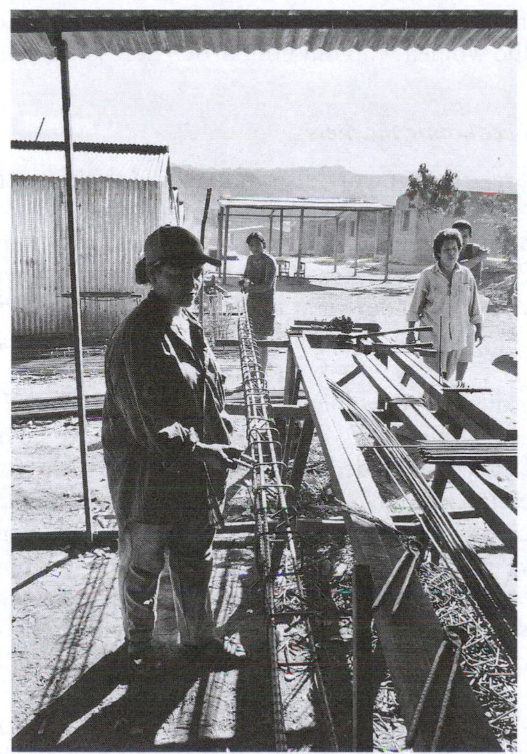

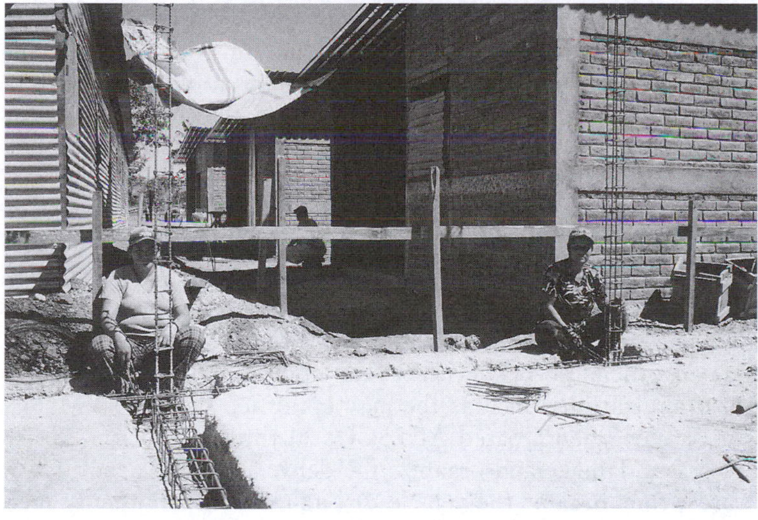

Figure 9.3 Women at work.

participation of certain women in the building process was not looked upon favourably by the women who did not participate.

Work and socioeconomic markers

More generally, relations at work also contributed to the creation of tensions between those who were considered dedicated workers by their superiors and those who were seen as lazy and unappreciative. Reputations were made, and some men labelled as sluggish and ungrateful were avoided by their co-workers, who did not want to be seen as '*problemático*' (a problem person) by the engineer. Again, this did not help in the creation of group solidarity.

The question of socioeconomic differentiation is telling. In the eyes of a foreigner, and at first glance, all these families seemed to belong to the same status. However, what extended fieldwork revealed is the way subtle processes of stratification form themselves. A process of economic differentiation unfolded, particularly as two women each decided to open a small shop, cook hot meals for the NGO masons and staff, and sell freshly made tortillas for the other residents. After a few months, their small businesses prospered so well that these women started to lend money to other beneficiaries, especially those for whom the lack of income was becoming more challenging as time passed. At the other extreme, seven families were entirely dependent on the monthly World Food Programme food distribution; and when these defaulted twice, they found themselves in a dire situation. The whole group could easily identify which were the 'most vulnerable' families. The growing polarity between the haves and the have nots created a lot of *envidia* (envy) among the families. These observations are not surprising; they remind us that within any social group, processes of differentiation emerge and evolve. In the very restricted space-time of reconstruction, they become accentuated, with lasting consequences.

Politics and power in La Hermandad

Another telling element concerns the residents' wish to create a Community Development Association (abbreviated to ADESCO in Spanish), which is a legally registered organization with elected representatives. An ADESCO serves as an official go-between between community members and other types of organizations, such as the mayor's office or NGOs. Many rural areas in Lamaria had created ADESCOs in the wake of the disaster in order to assess damage and organize the delivery of emergency assistance. Afterwards, they became the vehicle through which community members would discuss reconstruction and development options with various NGOs. Following from the previous discussion, this reflects the desire to establish a grassroots institution for local governance. Unfortunately, the project leaders did not consider this to be a good initiative, reasoning that it could eventually undermine their own authority. They stopped the families from following this path before the end of the building process, thus killing the one and only truly 'communitarian' initiative in La Hermandad.

Regarding the workers' perception of the logic of the project (remember that the project adopted a narrow vision of participation on a day-to-day basis, and the beneficiaries were far from exercising any control on the process), they were subject to a series of rules and the construction activities dominated all aspects of their lives. During the last months, people were exhausted and many had health problems; one family quit and quite a few men had left the site in search of salaried work, further slowing the process. Some would complain out loud and say that the project had nothing humanitarian about it and that the beneficiaries had been exploited as cheap labour. In these circumstances, people's participation did not lead to the emergence of a sense of community – at least, not during the reconstruction period.

It is interesting to compare this project with the one that occurred less than a kilometre away. There the NGOs in charge had decided to hire professional contractors for part of the building process, which led to much speedier completion; families moved into the houses around February–March 2002 and went back to their prior occupations. As for the promoters of the La Hermandad project, they confided that they were aware that they were not doing development work per se but that they were aiming to lay the 'material basis' of future sustainable development initiatives for a historically poor, vulnerable and marginalized group of people. During the project inauguration ceremony in June 2002, everybody got the impression that the project was a success: poor families had become homeowners, the quality of the houses was praised and the residents were compared to hundreds of other Salvadorian families still waiting for some form of reconstruction aid to repair their homes. The new residents of La Hermandad could say that the disaster gave them a new start in life.

However, in the context of a discussion on the merits of participation in post-disaster reconstruction, there is no doubt that participation could have taken on a different form.

Final comments

Post-disaster reconstruction programmes are not easy tasks. The desire to integrate participatory techniques and to enhance community participation in projects has much to commend it. But as the La Hermandad case shows, there are no guarantees that participation will benefit everybody; in this case it caused many conflicts and tensions between the new residents, and it did not empower them. Here, participation appeared to be 'tyrannical', but this does not mean that it is always bad by nature. The fact that beneficiaries did not form a prior community is a most important element in the equation. And so is the fact that in La Hermandad participation was limited to labour activities.

There is no one recipe that fits all contexts; successful community participation will depend on many factors. As Ian Davis[21] noted some thirty years ago, post-disaster reconstruction is a fundamentally social process, conjugating cultural, symbolic, political and economical dimensions. To be positive, participation must be sensitive to all these specificities and cannot be applied in a standardized fashion from one disaster to the next across the globe.

As various chapters in this volume show, many construction methodologies are available for post-disaster builders. With the growing body of research on the subject and the increased dialogue between the social and applied sciences, as well as between the building industry and development organizations, there is real potential for participation to become as empowering as some had hoped it to be. But for this to happen, participation ought not to be limited to its technical side alone; an apolitical application of participation cannot create sustainable livelihoods for the simple reason that disaster-stricken communities find themselves in highly politically charged contexts. A humanitarian emergency is not a neutral environment, nor is reconstruction. To find in participation a vector for social transformation, enough space and adequate means must be given to those populations so that they may express their agency as they see fit, which may mean, in certain cases, their refusal to participate. What Hickey and Mohan say about participation in development is also valid for reconstruction:

> New and promising ways forward are available. What is required is a greater level of honesty and clarity from both critics and proponents as to what form of participation is being debated; greater conceptual and theoretical coherence on participation; and more considered claims regarding its potential to transform the power relations that underpin exclusion and subordination. (page 21)[34]

Acknowledgement

Thanks to the Social Sciences and Humanities Research Council of Canada (SSHRC) and the Fonds de recherche sur la société et la culture (FQRSC) for their generous funding support for this research project.

10 User requirements and responsible reconstruction

Nese Dikmen

In the urgency of reconstruction, decision-makers tend to underestimate the need for a good fit between functional criteria (notably social and cultural) and the physical characteristics of the built environment. Traditional typologies of housing provide good indicators about cultural values, social rituals and community activities and should play a fundamental role in preserving the quality of life after disasters.

Tangible and intangible criteria for housing design

Housing design – even in "normal" conditions – is not an easy task, since, as Rapoport puts it, a house, apart from its social dimensions, aims to satisfy the basic and the most complicated needs of human beings; it is the central place of human existence.[8] Furthermore, housing becomes particularly important as a focus for the emotional, the personal and the symbolic; the primacy of these aspects shapes its form and in turn exercises important psycho-social impacts. In Rapoport's words, "Because building a house is a cultural phenomenon, its form and organization is greatly influenced by the cultural milieu to which it belongs."[7]

Reconstruction after natural disasters, as is well known, does not take place in "normal" conditions. Instead, a large number of decisions have to be made rapidly, frequently involving personnel from centralized authorities, whose daily experience is often far removed from the lifestyles of the intended beneficiaries; multiple contracts are let and a vast construction operation that often possesses few local characteristics is set in motion. This chapter explores one example and reveals its fundamentally flawed approach.

As Davidson explains in Chapter 5, the process of project initiation, development and design necessarily involves the following steps:

- identifying who the building will be used by (including social and cultural specificities, particularly regarding privacy);
- recognizing what users' activities will take place, and when (i.e. in any specific sequence); this is often called the functional programming;
- describing the conditions that are required for these activities to take place adequately (taking account of conditions created by the activities,

such as noise or odors); this takes the form of a more or less formalized performance specification or a specification of requirements;
- proposing a design and checking it against the requirements.

The challenge, therefore, is to ensure that the steps of this process (the specificities of the users' lifestyle) are properly taken into account, including the "soft" aspects, such as traditions and culture, as well as the more obvious "hard" ones derived from physiological requirements. (Here, "culture" refers to "the interactive aggregate of common characteristics that influence a group's response to its environment".)[5]

The requirements of tradition and culture that need to be respected

Demiröz states that house form is not only the result of physical factors or any single casual factor but is also the consequence of a whole range of socio-cultural factors in their broadest sense.[3] Thus social and cultural factors should not be eliminated from the housing reconstruction process. Oliver and Aysan suggest that:

> The house is often a significant indicator of the ways in which spaces are respected and utilized within a building: the degree of privacy or security that the dwelling affords, the number of people that occupy it, their domestic relationship and responsibilities to each other, and so on.[6]

According to Bayraktar and Aksu, there is no doubt that cultural differences between people living in different geographies lead to different expectations and demands about their houses.[2] Houses that are formed according to these dissimilar expectations and demands traditionally show unlike spatial and formal properties. In other words, this is – or should be – a design criterion for houses in urban and in rural areas alike.

It is a known fact that in rural areas where agricultural production is the mainstay of economy, a house also operates as the management centre of a small enterprise responsible for these agricultural activities.[4] Houses in rural areas reflect the economic dependence of their users. As Bayraktar and Aksu state, if the economy of the family depends on market gardening, spaces are needed to store the equipment used in the field and to store the crop.[2] However, if the economy of the family depends on animal rearing, cattle shed(s) or cattle sheds and hay barns are needed. Indeed

> Byres and stables, granaries and barns, mills and workshops all indicate the type of occupations which may be pursued. Each will be given land in an arrangement that is most appropriate to the successful functioning of its activities. These will obviously differ between pastoralists and agriculturalists, between mountain dwellers and fishing communities, or between sedentary peoples and nomads.[6]

It is important to realize that communities expect to re-establish themselves in a form that is close to their indigenous pattern after disasters.[3] (Isabelle Maret and James Amdal, in Chapter 6, emphasize that this expectation also applies to urban residents in post-Katrina New Orleans.) However, it is doubtful that measures of tradition and culture are taken into consideration during the design and application processes of post-disaster reconstruction projects. Thus the projects act as agents of (involuntary) change in the physical and social environments, especially for rural communities where individuals adhere strictly to their traditions. The change is large in scale, and the consequences are hazardous in most cases. As a result, the projects turn out to become interruptions in communities' social and physical environments. These problems are clearly illustrated in the case history that follows.

The 1995 Dinar earthquake and reconstruction period after the disaster

An earthquake with a magnitude of 5.9 shook the Dinar, Başmakçı, Dazkırı, Evciler and Kızılören districts of Afyonkarahisar province in Turkey on October 1, 1995. The earthquake severely damaged 2473 houses, moderately damaged 1218 houses and lightly damaged 2076 houses.[1] The disaster also caused nearly 100 deaths and over 200 injuries. Since most of the damage occurred in Dinar district, the disaster is referred to as the "Dinar earthquake".

The project as planned

The reconstruction project following the Dinar earthquake was initiated and controlled by the General Directorate of Disaster Affairs of the Turkish national government, with the support of the Directorate of Public Works and Settlement in Afyonkarahisar. It was decided to construct 5034 permanent post-disaster houses (2006 in the villages and 3028 in the district centers) and 1400 cattle sheds. A typical house plan with an area of 76.61 square meters and a plan for a cattle shed with an area of 50 square meters were selected from the archives of the Ministry of Public Works and Settlement to be constructed in the villages in the region.

Information about who these houses were originally designed for is not available. Probably, they were not designed for a specific user group. In general, post-disaster houses are designed by the architects of the General Directorate of Construction Affairs at any time when resources are available, and the plans are kept in the archives to be used in any region after a disaster. Earthquake resistance is considered during the design process of these houses; however, geographical and climatic conditions and local user requirements are not taken into consideration, since the houses are not designed for a specific region. Whenever a disaster strikes, some details of the plans selected for construction are modified. These modifications are mostly related to the climatic conditions of the disaster-affected region. For instance, wall thickness is changed and roof slope and thermal-insulation details are re-drawn.

The reconstruction project conducted in Dinar was funded by the Turkish government, and the beneficiaries received an interest-free loan, which they were obliged to pay back in 20 years. It was decided to proceed with a tendering process for this reconstruction project. According to this method, firms were hired for the construction of the buildings. There were 1234 permanent post-disaster houses and 873 cattle sheds constructed in 46 villages of Dinar district. Fifteen new settlements, consisting of 898 post-disaster houses, were erected in the area. Construction was completed in 1997, and the final acceptance of the buildings was performed in 1998, one year after completion, because, according to the tender process, the houses had to be used for one year and then controlled for any construction faults in the buildings.

Observations in the area 13 years after the earthquake

Information was gathered through interviews, questionnaires and observations on-the-spot.

- Officials of the General Directorate of Disaster Affairs, the General Directorate of Construction Affairs and the Directorate of Public Works and Settlement in Afyonkarahisar were interviewed to get information about the reconstruction project.
- Two field surveys including 12 villages in the region were done in the winter months of 2008. Observations were made in new and existing settlements; photographs of the post-disaster houses, cattle sheds, additional buildings, traditional houses and general views of the villages were taken.
- Observations were made of modifications to the post-disaster houses and cattle sheds, and additional buildings were observed during the first field survey; 11 samples were selected for the survey. The modified post-disaster houses and cattle sheds and additional buildings on the lots were measured. Then the buildings were drawn according to measurements, with the help of photographs taken.
- Next, an analysis was made in order to reveal types of and reasons for modifications, with the help of the drawings, photographs, data gained through the interviews and original plans of post-disaster houses and cattle sheds, taken from the archive of the General Directorate of Construction Affairs.
- Then the occupants of a number of post-disaster houses were interviewed, and a questionnaire was administered to a random sample of 372 permanent users of post-disaster houses, representing 30 per cent of the beneficiaries in the region. The study was completed in 30 villages where there were at least five post-disaster houses.

Four examples of the 11 samples mentioned above are described below.

In the villages of Dinar, the economy depends on agriculture. The traditional houses in the villages are the products of this economic dependency of the family, the physical conditions of the environment and the culture and lifestyles of their users. Figure 10.1 shows a traditional house where an extended family live and animal rearing takes place.

Surprisingly, observations of the post-disaster reconstruction project revealed that cattle sheds were provided to some of the families who do not rear animals; however, some families who did rear animals did not get them. As a result, beneficiaries who have animals constructed cattle sheds and villagers who do not own animals changed the function of the cattle sheds.

Post-disaster house 1

The economy of the extended family living in this house depends on animal rearing. Since a cattle shed was not provided to the family, they constructed two cattle sheds and a hay barn on their lot. The family, which consists of a father and mother and the family of the married son, lived in the post-disaster house for a few months; then they had to build a new house attached to the post-disaster house. A lean-to roof was added to the post-disaster house, and a bakery was constructed with the new house. The new buildings were constructed with indigenous materials and building techniques, without any engineering assistance (Figure 10.2). Figure 10.3 shows the plans of the buildings on the lot. The buildings represented with black are the original plans, whereas the parts in grey are the additional constructions.

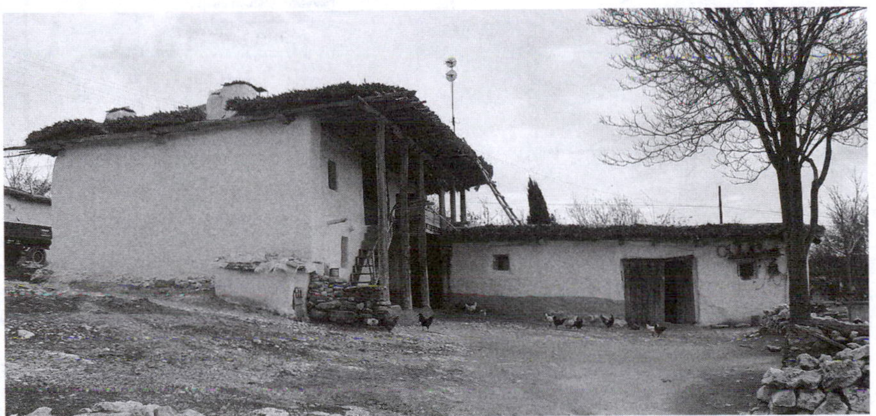

Figure 10.1 A traditional house in Karahacılı Village.

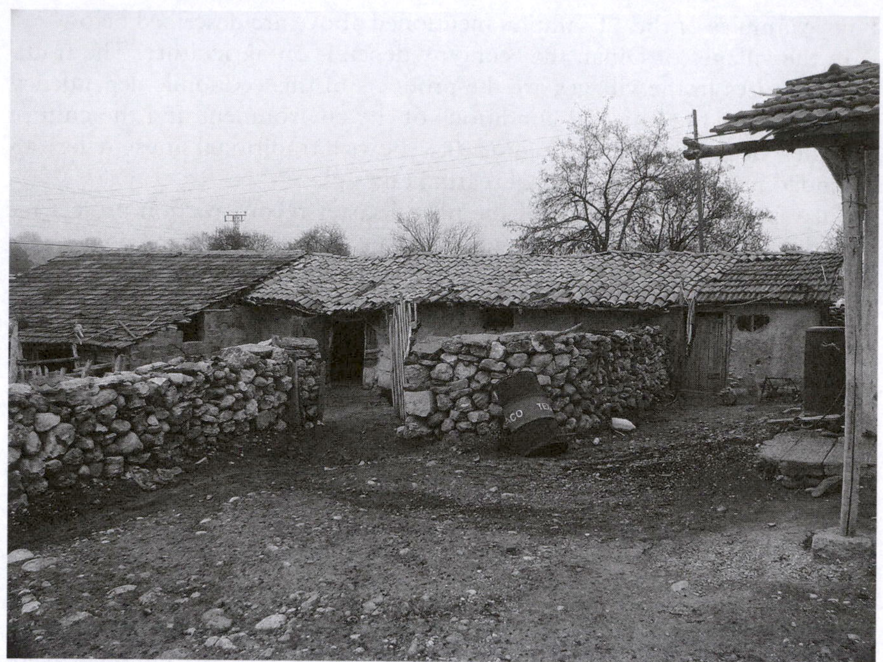

Figure 10.2 View of the cattle shed constructed by the user.

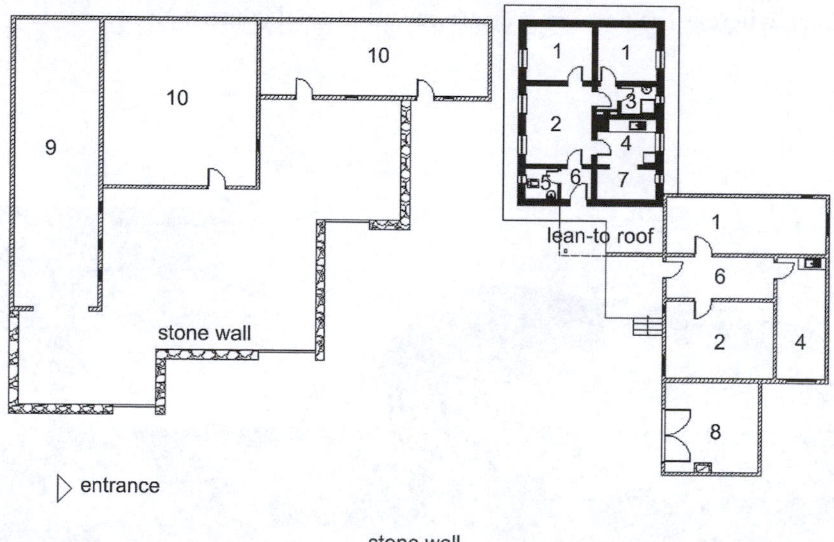

Legend: 1. Room; 2. Living space; 3. Bathroom; 4. Kitchen;
5. WC; 6. Entrance; 7. Store room; 8. Bakery; 9. Hay-barn; 10. Cattle shed

Figure 10.3 Plan showing the buildings constructed by the beneficiaries.

Post-disaster house 2

Users of this house have animals, and a cattle shed was provided to them. Compared to the original plan, a part of the cattle shed is used to serve as a hay barn and another part is used for storing coal. It was observed that the family uses the cattle shed as a hay barn and that they constructed a new cattle shed. The users also constructed a bakery attached to the cattle shed, which was provided by the government. In addition, there are open and semi-open spaces on the lot for the animals, and a lean-to roof was added to the post-disaster house (Figure 10.4).

Post-disaster house 3

A cattle shed was provided to the users of this house, who do not have animals. It was seen that a part of the cattle shed is being used as a bakery and the rest is being used for storage purposes. In addition, a lean-to was added to the roof of the post-disaster house (Figure 10.5 and 10.6).

Post-disaster house 4

This plan is representative of a number of houses in the region, since similar additions were observed in several of the settlements. Two rooms and a

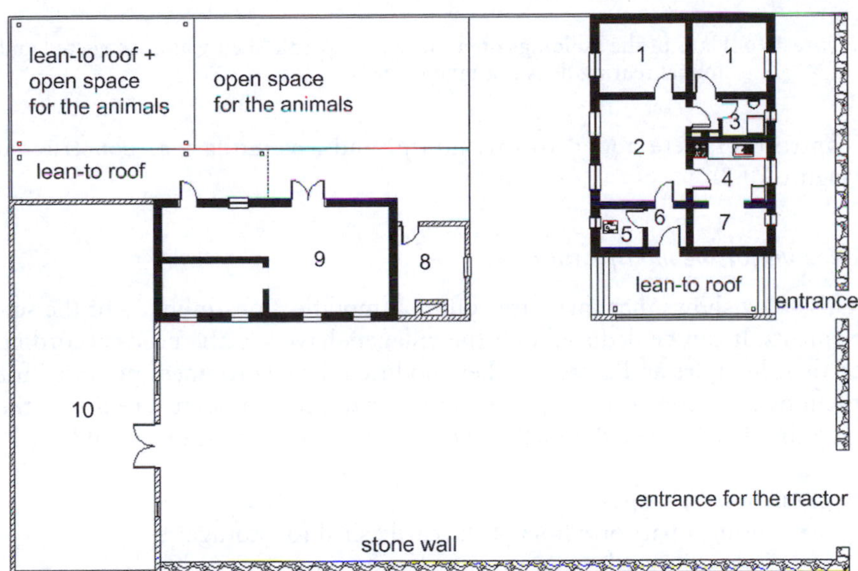

Figure 10.4 Plans of the buildings on a lot where animal rearing takes place.

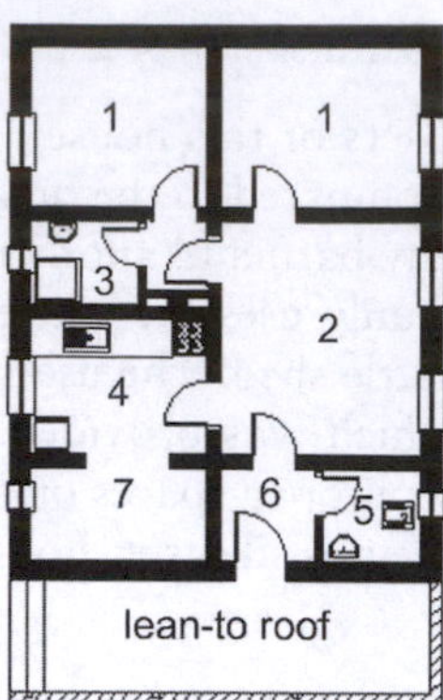

garden

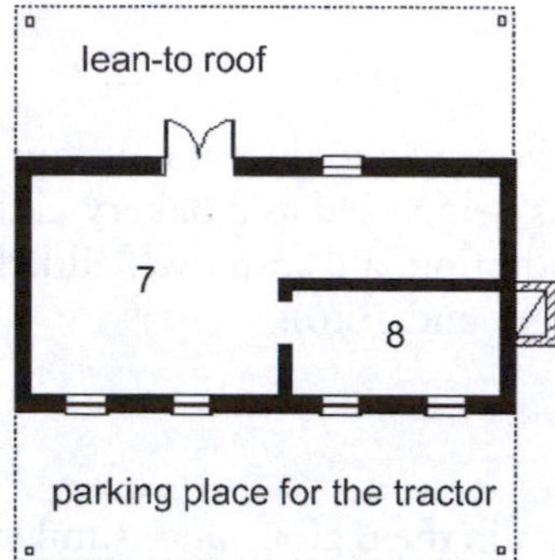

Legend: 1. Room; 2. Living space; 3. Bathroom; 4. Kitchen; 5. WC; 6. Entrance; 7. Store room; 8. Bakery

Figure 10.5 Plans of the buildings on a lot where a cattle shed was constructed and animal rearing does not take place.

lean-to roof were added to this house, and a veranda was constructed (Figure 10.7).

Reasons for the modifications

This study shows that there are common modifications in many of the settlements. It can be deduced that the villagers have specific needs according to their lifestyles and therefore they modified the environment provided for them by the reconstruction project in order to accommodate a return to the way they lived before the earthquake. Common modifications include:

- functional changes:
    - using a part or whole of the cattle shed for storage;
    - using the cattle shed as a hay barn;
    - using a part of the cattle shed as a bakery.
- additions to the houses:
    - lean-to roof;
    - rooms.

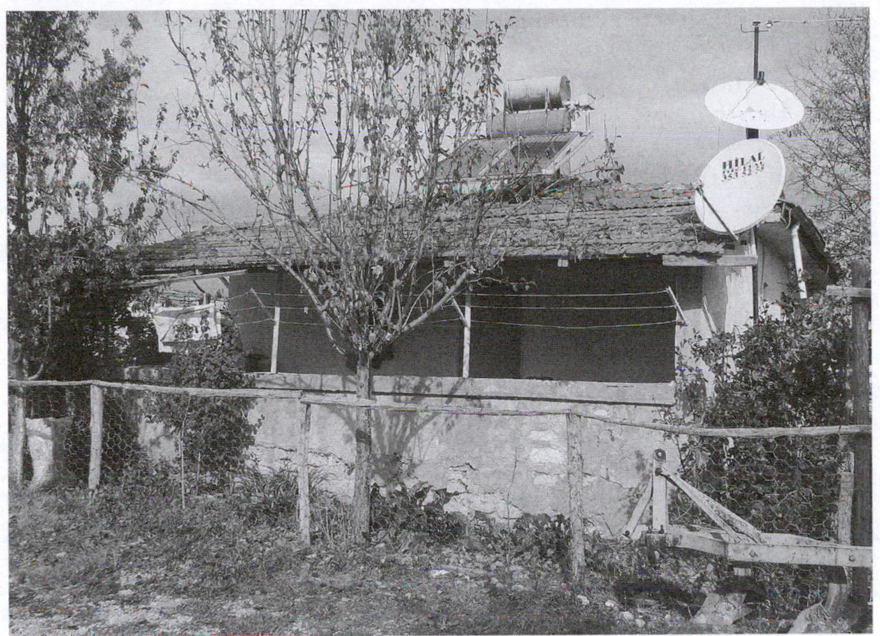

Figure 10.6 View of the lean-to roof.

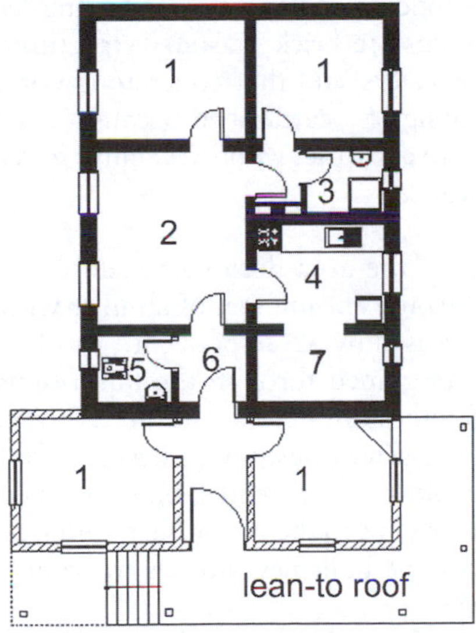

Figure 10.7 Rooms and lean-to roof added to the post-disaster house.

- newly constructed buildings:
    - bakery;
    - cattle shed;
    - hay-barn.

According to the data gained through the questionnaire, 99.5 per cent of the beneficiaries had a cattle shed, 99.2 per cent had a hay barn and 98.1 per cent had a bakery on their lot *before* the earthquake. These statistics, plus the list of newly built buildings in the area, demonstrate that most of the villagers need a bakery, a cattle shed and a hay barn to return to their way of life before the disaster. Traditionally villagers make their own bread, so they consider a space for this purpose during the construction of their houses. Since bakeries were not provided as a part of the post-disaster house nor as a separate building, some villagers constructed bakeries and some used a part of the cattle sheds for this purpose.

It was observed that none of the cattle sheds were used for their original function. Villagers who have animals generally use the cattle sheds as hay barns and they constructed cattle sheds for their animals. Villagers interviewed mentioned two reasons for not keeping their animals in the cattle sheds:

- First, villagers said that the cattle sheds were not big enough for their animals, so they felt they had to construct new sheds.
- The second reason concerns the construction materials used for the cattle sheds. These buildings are brick masonry structures with a reinforced concrete ceiling. Villagers said that concrete is not a suitable building material for the ceiling of a cattle shed because it is not healthy for the animals. They used to construct wooden ceilings for cattle sheds to allow the moisture to escape.

A number of villagers in the area decided to sell their animals after the earthquake for these reasons. The number of families who own animals after the earthquake has decreased by 32.86 per cent.

According to the data gained through the questionnaire, in the region 57.3 per cent of the families are nuclear and 42.7 per cent of the families are extended. The post-disaster houses were designed to be used by nuclear families so are not suitable for the extended ones. It was observed that some extended families added rooms to the post-disaster houses, some constructed additional storeys and some built new houses to be able to continue with their traditional lifestyle.

Villagers spend most of their time outside the house rather than inside. In front of their houses are important places to control the entrance of their land, to communicate with neighbors and to prepare food. Many of the users added lean-to roofs to the roofs of the post-disaster houses to create a space for these purposes.

Discussion

It is clear that the post-disaster houses constructed in the villages of Dinar do not meet all the needs of the users. The lifestyle of the villagers was apparently not considered during the decision-making process of the reconstruction project. Because of this, villagers spent effort and money to adapt the houses to their way of life. Since most of the villagers could not afford to use new building materials, generally the materials of the demolished buildings were used for the new additions. Some of the additional buildings are stone and some are sun-dried brick masonry structures that were not built according to any earthquake design code, which would cover important parameters for the construction of earthquake-resistant masonry structures, such as specifications of the building materials, length of the walls and placing of the doors and windows.

Even though some of the additions were constructed with contemporary building materials and techniques, they were not built by people who know about earthquake-resistant building principles, according to the Turkish earthquake design code. Consequently, the additions can even have negative effects on the earthquake performance of the post-disaster houses, which had been designed in accordance with the Turkish earthquake design code.

Reasons for the problems

The study of the post-disaster reconstruction project conducted in the villages of Dinar shows that traditional and cultural factors that gave form to the settlements in the area were not considered during the decision-making process. Since the earthquake occurred in winter, the authorities understandably tended to provide shelters to the victims as soon as possible. Because of that, decisions were made in a very short time so that the construction phase could be started as soon as the weather permitted.

In addition, for economic reasons, the post-disaster houses and the cattle sheds are not big enough. The Dinar project was funded by the Turkish government, and over 5000 houses and 1400 cattle sheds were constructed in the disaster-affected area. Because of the limited amount of money available, the construction of small buildings was preferred.

Another problem stems from difficulties in finding proper sites for the reconstruction. If the existing settlement is prone to future disasters and it is decided to relocate the disaster victims to a safer area, reconstruction generally takes place on lands that belong to the government. The beneficiaries do not pay for the land; they are only responsible for the cost of the houses. Because of that, the Turkish government does not provide large lots to the beneficiaries.

Nonetheless, this example shows that sometimes victims prefer to get post-disaster houses even if they know that the houses are not in accordance with their way of life, if only because houses built with contemporary building materials are attractive for them. Authorities also tend to provide post-disaster houses for those victims whose houses were only moderately damaged, because this approach is seen as an opportunity for rural development.

From the beneficiaries' point of view, post-disaster reconstruction projects are seen as the opportunity to get a free or very cheap house. They know that in the end they have to pay the government for the houses, but also they know that they have a chance to postpone the payment. Indeed, 13 years after the earthquake, 43 per cent of the beneficiaries had paid back less than half of the money to the government, 18.5 per cent did not know how much they had paid and 17.2 per cent of the beneficiaries had not paid anything. Some of these beneficiaries cannot afford to make the payment, but some do not care. Most of the beneficiaries do not know the total amount that they have to pay to the government.

Conclusions

Most of the problems related to the reconstruction project occurred due to the lack of detailed knowledge, on the part of the project initiators, about the villages and about the people who live in these settlements. Of course, some factors explain why those initiators preferred not to do research in the area before making the decisions, such as limited time and a limited number of people who can carry out research in the disaster-affected regions.

Problems are also related to the role of the government in the reconstruction project. There were a lot of responsibilities for government authorities and officials in a limited time after the disaster, leading them to ignore some factors that should be considered in reconstruction projects of this sort.

When a disaster strikes in Turkey, actions are necessarily taken according to the laws and regulations. Post-disaster reconstruction projects have to be initiated and controlled by the Ministry of Public Works and Settlements according to these laws and regulations. Sometimes other participants, such as private firms and beneficiaries, are involved in the projects. In the Dinar case, private firms were responsible for the construction of the buildings, and the beneficiaries were involved in the project only during the process of deciding on the locations of the new settlements.

This study shows that tradition and culture are among the most important factors that shape settlements, especially in rural areas. Family structure, economic dependence, number of family members, daily activities, etc. are considered while constructing houses under normal conditions in rural settlements. Since a post-disaster house is not (or should not be) different from a house except for in the construction speed, it is regrettable if the complex and intangible issues related to tradition and culture are not considered during the decision-making process.

The following suggestions are based on the investigation done in the Dinar villages and are made in order to increase the chances of success of future rural post-disaster reconstruction projects:

- Instead of constructing a large number of buildings and engaging considerable sums of money, beneficiaries can be encouraged and supported to repair and strengthen the less heavily damaged buildings. Thus they can use their own land and also the service buildings, such as bakeries and cattle sheds, provided of course that their site is not prone to future disasters.
- Investigation can be done in disaster-prone areas, and vulnerable buildings can be strengthened before a disaster occurs, so that losses due to future disasters can be prevented or they can at least be decreased.
- People in earthquake-prone areas can be trained about constructing earthquake-resistant buildings.
- Temporary houses can be provided to the disaster victims so that there can be more time to do research and make appropriate decisions on the permanent housing.
- Instead of providing plots with equal sizes for every beneficiary, sizes of the plots and the buildings to be constructed on them can be determined according to factors such as family size, economic dependence and number of animals owned by the beneficiary, etc.
- Regulations about the repayments for the buildings can be developed.
- Various sources of funding can be included in the projects.
- Agencies such as national and international NGOs and universities can be included in the post-disaster reconstruction projects from the decision-making process to the completion of the projects, so that more experts are available to do research on the subject and also so that those who have experience in reconstruction projects can share the responsibilities and carry out the needed investigations in the affected regions.
- Time spent in the upfront activities of functional analysis is essential to avoid the sorts of problems encountered in the Dinar village reconstruction, particularly if the decision-makers are not inherently familiar with local conditions and traditions.

Acknowledgments

This study was supported by TÜBİTAK (The Scientific and Technological Research Council of Turkey) Grant No. 106K256, awarded to N.D. for the research project "An Investigation on the Post-Disaster Reconstruction Project Conducted and the Post-Disaster Houses Erected in Dinar After the 1995 Earthquake."

11 Space and place after natural disasters and forced displacement

Roger Zetter and Camillo Boano

Post-disaster reconstruction initiatives often concentrate on building houses. They rarely focus on recuperating a sense of domestic and public space and place that is crucial for the long-term recovery of affected populations. The result exacerbates the feelings of loss and deprivation among survivors who could beneficially be enabled to contribute to the decision-making processes concerning their built environment, their spaces and places.

Disasters are well known for causing or exacerbating homelessness. Less known is the fact that they also provoke the emergence of what many analysts call 'placelessness' (a term often used to describe the loss of the sense of place). Previous chapters of this book have already explained that post-disaster interventions often neglect important cultural and social characteristics that are embedded in indigenous housing, such as housing layouts, the design of external spaces (and the sense of place they create) and attributes of the built environment related to location. Unfortunately, inappropriate outcomes frequently increase or reproduce pre-disaster vulnerabilities, constituting unsustainable resettlement strategies.

This chapter argues that space and place are rarely recreated in responses to forced displacement – such as often occurs with post-disaster reconstruction (but it is also applicable to post-conflict displacement). It provides a comprehensive understanding of the complexity of needs associated with space and place, as well as their symbolic and socio-cultural specificity in post-disaster environments. This study shows that sustainable post-disaster reconstruction requires: (i) a coherent understanding of space and place; (ii) a clear articulation of the processes linking relief, rehabilitation and development in the production of space and place; (iii) the consideration of institutional constraints at the national and international levels to achieve integrated responses; and (iv) the recognition of rights-based approaches to the articulation of space and place.

Space and place in post-disaster housing and post-conflict relocation

As was explained in Chapter 4, government agencies and humanitarian groups sometimes relocate affected populations to temporary shelters or camps in order to facilitate the delivery of humanitarian assistance and to ensure their security. But as Zetter and Boano point out, this process of secondary displacement further fragments the relationship between people and their familiar habitual environments.[53] Often this not-so-temporary relocation is conducted against the will of those directly affected, who, as Kälin notes, would prefer instead to stay close to their properties or to immediately return.[25]

Even worse, relocation sometimes magnifies pre-disaster patterns of socio-economic vulnerability. The result is the disruption of the fragile but crucial relationship between the house as a material commodity and its spatial and social importance.

As discussed in previous chapters, common reconstruction practices often focus on short-term emergency provision and on narrowly conceived 'bricks and mortar' outputs. They are often driven by top-down approaches to project delivery and include little understanding of local vernacular styles of shelter and building technologies. These shortcomings are exacerbated by the fragmented institutional framework of donors and humanitarian agencies and by the political imperatives of rehousing disaster-affected populations as rapidly as possible.

The fractured relationship between space and place – in other words, the homelessness and placelessness of displacement – presents particular challenges for both post-disaster and post-conflict shelter interventions. A significant reconceptualisation of current approaches is proposed – one that is based on a better understanding of the complex meaning of 'home' – simultaneously situating the meanings and experiences of home in their relative cultural and social environments.

Elusive terms

Recognising semantic confusions is an essential first stage in achieving this understanding. In fact, *shelter* (and housing) juxtaposed with *forced migration* activates contradictory meanings: one is associated with the groundedness and finiteness of buildings, the constitution of space and place; the other represents uprootedness, forced mobility and transience.

The term 'house' and its related words 'dwelling', 'home', 'residence' and 'shelter' hold different meanings.[34] However, Skotte and other authors have demonstrated that, in the world of emergency relief programmes, they are used as if they were synonyms.[40] Adding to this confusion, there is an abundance of micro-terminology at the project and practice levels. For example, the Office of the UN High Commissioner for Refugees (UNHCR) uses the terms *camps*, *dispersed settlements*, *reception and transit centres*, *self settled camps* and *planned camps*,[48] while Jalali prefers the term *tent cities*,[24] Hansen and Oliver-Smith use *resettlement sites*,[18] and Boano uses *relocation sites*.[3]

A similar semantic confusion also pervades short-term responses. For the UNHCR, *emergency shelter* typically involves the supply of temporary shelter materials such as tents and plastic sheeting,[48] but the term also elides with the notions of *temporary shelter, collective buildings* and *mass shelter* (as in collective buildings, including the use of public buildings such as mosques, churches, schools, empty buildings or specially built accommodation). Others, such as Lambert and Pougin de la Maisonneuve, use the term *temporary living centres*,[28] while Corsellis and Vitale prefer the new term *transitional shelter*, which 'provides a habitable covered living space, over the period between a disaster and achieving a durable shelter solution.'[9]

Despite extensive cultural variation, there are few other concepts so widespread and easily understood across the world as 'home'.[11] But from the early philosophical works of Heidegger,[20] Bachelard[1] and Tuan[44] to more recent studies by Dovey,[13] Benjamin,[2] Rapoport[36] and Porteous and Smith,[33] the enduring tensions between the words 'house' and 'home' speak of the underlying complexity and elusive meaning of these terms. A central concern is the debate around the material and the social representation of housing. This debate is well captured by Saegert's assertion that

> Not only is it [home] a place, but it has psychological resonance and social meaning. It is part of the experience of dwelling – something we do, a way of weaving up a life in a particular geographical space. (page 287)[39]

Yet for many decades, the approaches that have driven post-disaster housing reconstruction have defined the house in narrow physical terms, a materialistic definition contested by many researchers such as Rakoff[35] and Tuan.[45] Similarly, Kemeny proposes a dualistic analysis of the house that challenges the reductionist view of the house as just a building.[27] He identifies space as a salient characteristic in two senses: the internal spatial organisation of dwellings and their social use, and the spatial organisation of the dwelling within the locality. The point here is that beyond the cultural specificity of home and space, it is important to recognise that the everyday practices, material cultures and social relations that shape *home* on a domestic scale resonate far beyond the household.

Hyndman identifies the 'exclusiveness' of the house-space.[23] In one sense, the house may be a physical structure in which one feels a unique sense of belonging, attachment or even sanctuary from the more public world outside – an exclusive private and privatised space. But the house is also exclusive in another sense: it is a space that literally excludes certain people or groups from entering, occupying or possessing. Articulating this point in a different way, Bachelard writes that home is 'our corner of the world ... our first universe, a real cosmos in every sense of the word' (page 23).[1]

Davis's assertion, in the post-disaster context, that 'shelter must be considered as a process, not as an object'[10] echoed Turner's contention of 'housing as a verb'[46] and drew early attention to this 'product or process' dichotomy. This opened up the call for more culturally sensitive approaches to home making or re-making in the aftermath of disasters. Notably, this focused on the need to consider vernacular technologies and culturally bounded experiences.[14,21]

A better understanding of space would help to accomplish the integrative task of linking social and material needs in housing reconstruction projects and programmes. On the one hand, Boano[3] and Skotte[40] argue for a better appreciation of the outward-looking characteristics, focusing on the home as 'a centre' (a place of refuge, freedom, possession, shelter and security). On the other hand, they draw attention to inward-looking features, focusing upon home as 'identity' (family, community, attachment, memory and nostalgia, community structure and relationships).

The materiality of 'house' and the definition of place

> By almost any definition community implies existence of a place, – a physical place made up of land, buildings, and public space.[38]

Disaster displacement and destruction are forms of albeit temporary but often protracted homelessness. However, the relationship between home and homelessness is more complex than the simple presence or absence of home and the physical adequacy of the shelter.[26] While for many people home can mean the location where one 'dwells' and which provides opportunities to claim a sense of belonging and a context (as Heidegger[20] suggested long ago), Kellett and Moore argue that it is as much about the house being placed in a particular social world.[26] For Skotte it is a location in a particular livelihood system,[40] and for Saegert it is the locus where the main activities of daily life are conducted and thus imbued with symbolically charged values.[39]

Canter has also expressed this sense of belonging to a place by arguing that home-as-place is the anchor that binds the experiential entities of physical enclosure, social relations and psychological feelings, reinforcing the way in which place mediates social life.[6] On similar lines, Gupta and Ferguson also emphasise how the material form of the house, its particular physical location and the meanings invested in them combine to form emotional and sentimental bonds between people and a place.[17]

However, places can also be terrains of power that may dominate people by their location, built-form and symbolic meanings.[30] Indeed, people and communities are inextricably linked to a given territory, in what Connolly refers to as 'a politics of place.'[8] Similarly, we should not forget that places are not fixed and static phenomena; they are made by people who ascribe qualities to the material and social things gathered there. The home both as an entity and as a place is in a constant process of consolidation, transformation and adaptation. Both de Certeau[12] and Etlin[16] draw attention to the fact that place-making is not just the domain of the powerful or of design professionals; place-making is also a process where ordinary people create a bounded, identified, meaningful, named and significant place. This is particularly significant in the context of post-disaster reconstruction.

In other words, housing must convey and impart a sense of place and location in all its complexity. Accordingly, the loss of place through disaster or conflict has potentially devastating implications for individual and collective identity, memory and history – and for psychological well-being.

Reflecting on current practice, Zetter summarises the contemporary debate on post-disaster and post-conflict housing in the following terms:

> [...] physical projects and technocratic deliverables are thus the means not the ends of interventions which operate at multiple levels. Crucially, reconstruction programmes for the built environment must be conceived within a strategic framework of interventions ... rather than a simple and linear asset-replacement strategy. The multiple objectives encompass: (i) physical and psychological health including protection from the elements and a feeling of home and community, (ii) privacy and dignity for families and for the community, (iii) physical and psychological security, and (iv) livelihood support. (page 160)[52]

To be without a place of one's own – *persona non locata* – is to be almost non-existent. For those permanently forced from their homes and places by conflict or disasters, the challenge of making new homes and places in relocation projects is far more complicated.[33]

Place and space in post-disaster shelter and settlement: main challenges

A fundamental change in orientation is required, moving away from 'bricks and mortar' solutions – the physical dwelling – towards a broader social and economic dimension of housing. Understanding home as a significant type of space and place, no longer limiting it to a dichotomy of 'house' as a physical structure and 'home' as a social, cultural and emotive construct, helps tie the physical components to the social, cultural and emotive ones. This approach allows an understanding of homes as nodes located both within networks of social relations and at the centre of a dynamic interplay with surrounding places.

Space and place assume their significance in four crucial areas of shelter policy development and project implementation:

- enriching a narrowly technical approach to housing by moving beyond one-dimensional perceptions of space and place;
- overcoming artificial boundaries between relief and development programming;

- addressing the institutional constraints on an integrated approach;
- embracing rights-based needs.

There is a proliferation of manuals in this area. The Sphere guidelines,[41] the UNHCR guidelines[47] and the United Nations Office for the Coordination of Humanitarian Affairs (OCHA) manual[49] provide ample detail of the design of post-disaster *dwellings*.

The following examples of post-disaster reconstruction in Sri Lanka, India and Indonesia (Aceh) after the 2004 tsunami clearly illustrate how space and place lie at the core of the reconstruction problem. These examples are drawn from a range of research and consultancy assignments conducted between 2005 and 2008 but also build on longer-term research in post-conflict and post-disaster settings. Specifically, the cases discussed here are all post-disaster reconstruction projects developed by different NGOs in:

- Sri Lanka: Mandanai relocation site in Thirukkovil, with 303 houses built by Ceylon Tobacco, BASF/Habitat, Forut; Kolavil resettlement site in Alayadivembu, with 100 houses built by the Methodist Church; Siribopura I in Hambantota, where Singapore – SL Buddhist Research Society built 150 houses as part of a 700-unit development funded by a range of donors; Ganesh Rajah and Sothilingam in Kalmunai, with 68 houses built by Italian Coopi and People's Church.
- India: projects at Vondh and Bhachao, where 1400 houses were built by the Government of Gujarat.
- Indonesia: projects in Banda Aceh and Aceh Besar, built by the Aceh and Nias Rehabilitation and Reconstruction Agency (BBR).

Loss of space and place in post-tsunami Sri Lanka, India and Indonesia: some examples

Settlement layouts often result in a rigid grid, which hinders the development of a sense of community, as just described. In the case of the Kolavil resettlement site in Sri Lanka, the layout follows just such a design approach, supposedly in order to accommodate as many houses as possible. No attention is paid to communal spaces. Figure 11.1 illustrates the typical way in which concepts of space and place are sacrificed in post-disaster housing developments, where no attention is given to a comprehensive spatial design. Instead, the design adopts a standard and rigid physical format creating a monotonous layout, permitting few, if any, options for individual adaptation and little scope for economic livelihood activities, representing a narrow, mechanistic view of what housing really encompasses.

Figure 11.2 illustrates the ways in which infrastructure services and facilities pose additional spatial and design layout challenges. In both sites, the technical solutions had negative impacts on the private open areas. The

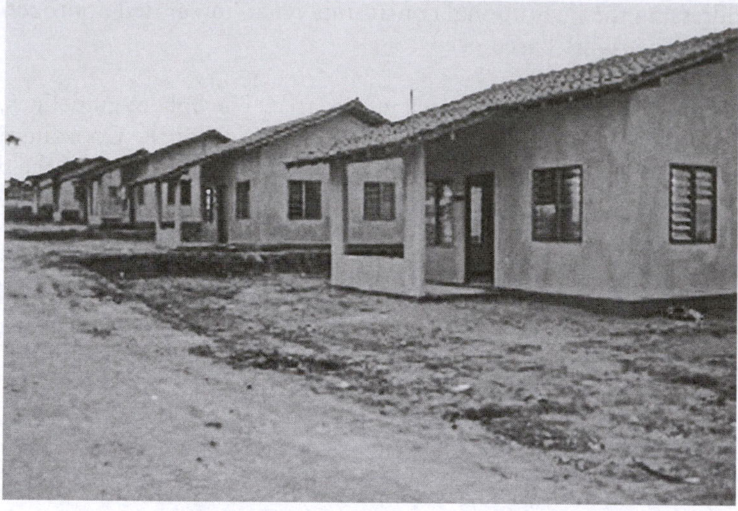

Figure 11.1 Typical example of the 'rationalistic' approach to post-disaster housing design. Mandanai resettlement in Thirukkovil, Sri Lanka.

solution in Kolavil (Figure 11.2, top) was to create wells. Despite technical problems due to a low water table, well construction was less invasive in terms of space and scale impacts, and therefore it was a more appropriate design response than that used in Thirukkovil (Figure 11.2, bottom). In the latter project, on-plot provision of a rainwater-harvesting system was a valuable sustainable solution to the problem of providing water; but the large water tanks, combined with the dominant on-plot latrines, erode the sense of cohesive space and make infeasible the use of the plot (for growing supplementary food, for example).

Often, very limited space available between units or simply the lack of attention to design details hampers appropriate provision of sewage systems. This results in bad maintenance and may increase neighbourhood tensions. Figure 11.3 shows such constraints imposed by space limitations and negligence to detail in Sri Lanka and Aceh. In the case of Sri Lanka (Figure 11.3 top), very limited space available between units hampered the provision of appropriate sewage systems resulting in inappropriate maintenance and in conflicts over the use of space. The Aceh project (Figure 11.3, bottom) shows the very typical results of inefficient and uncoordinated planning and design processes, where housing and infrastructure are planned as if they were separate components.

The examples in Figure 11.4, both in Aceh, show in contrast a more carefully designed layout of housing and infrastructure that respects technical needs for flood protection and is appropriate for local conditions; some attempt is made to create place and to increase a sense of community, as well

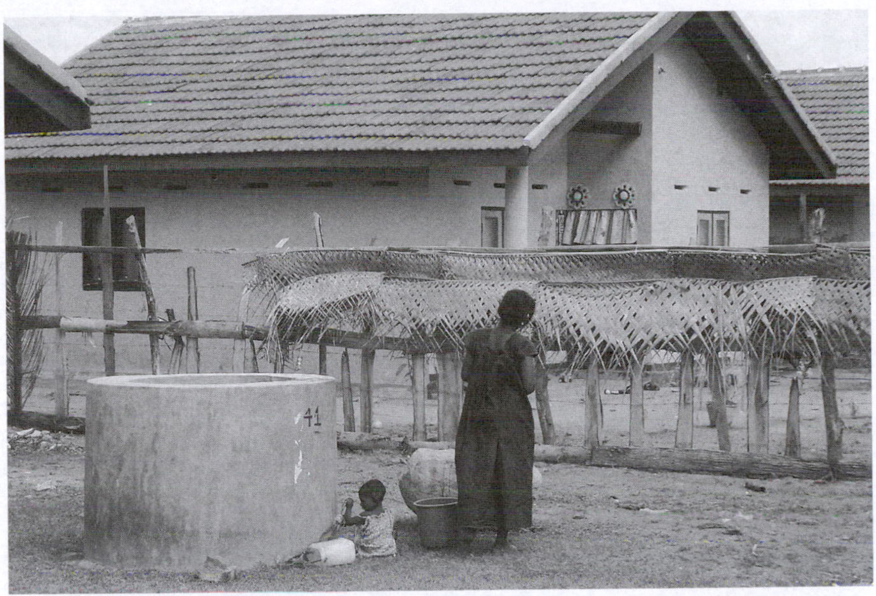

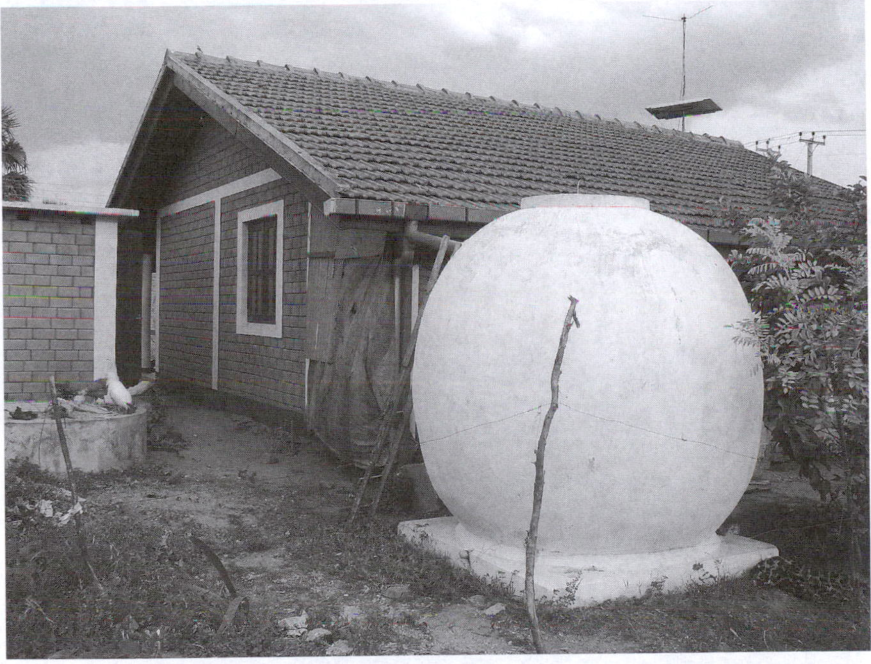

Figure 11.2 Designing layouts in relation to infrastructure needs – domestic water supply. **Top:** Kolavil resettlement scheme in Thirukkovil, Sri Lanka. **Bottom:** Thirukkovil resettlement scheme in Sri Lanka.

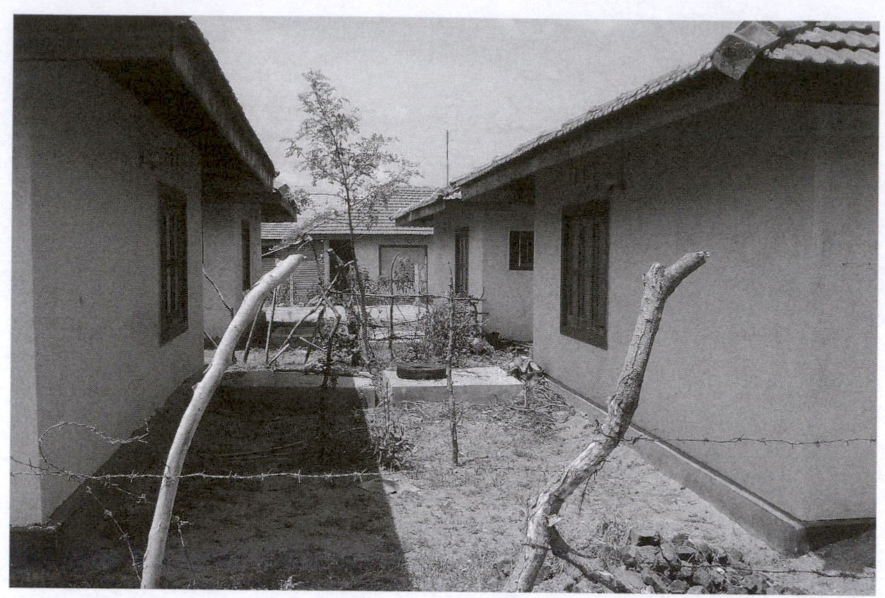

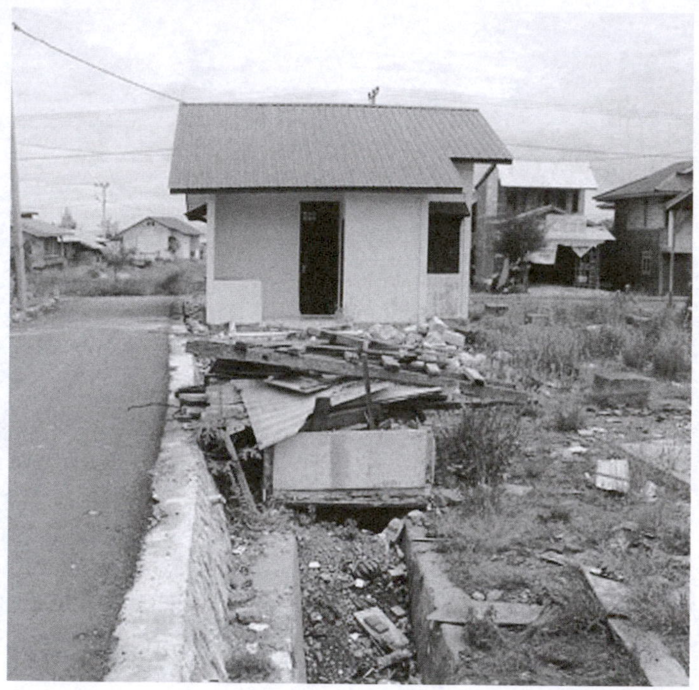

Figure 11.3 Designing layouts in relation to infrastructure needs – sewage disposal. **Top:** Mandanai II resettlement scheme in Thirukkovil, Sri Lanka. **Bottom:** House on sewage canal, Aceh (photo: Duyne Barenstein).

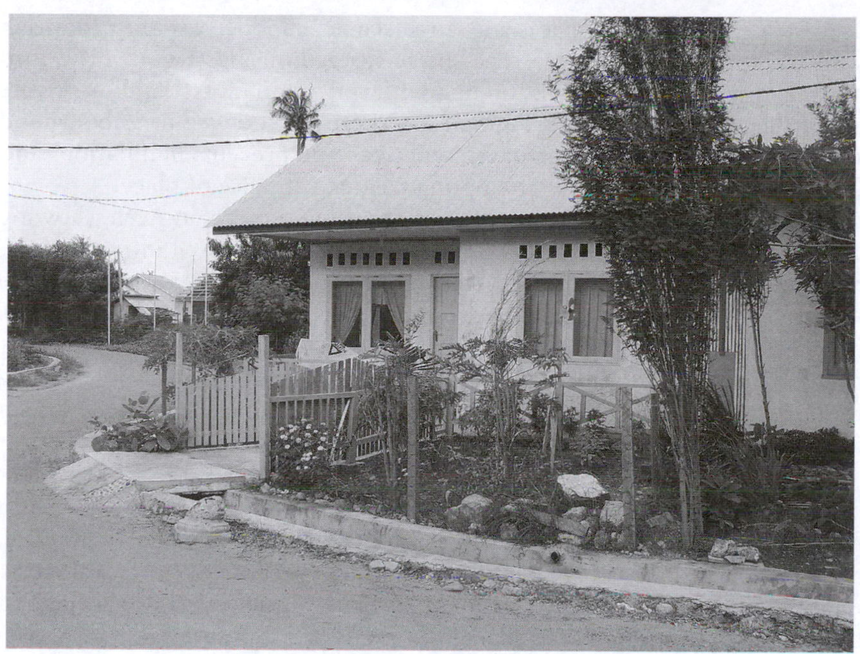

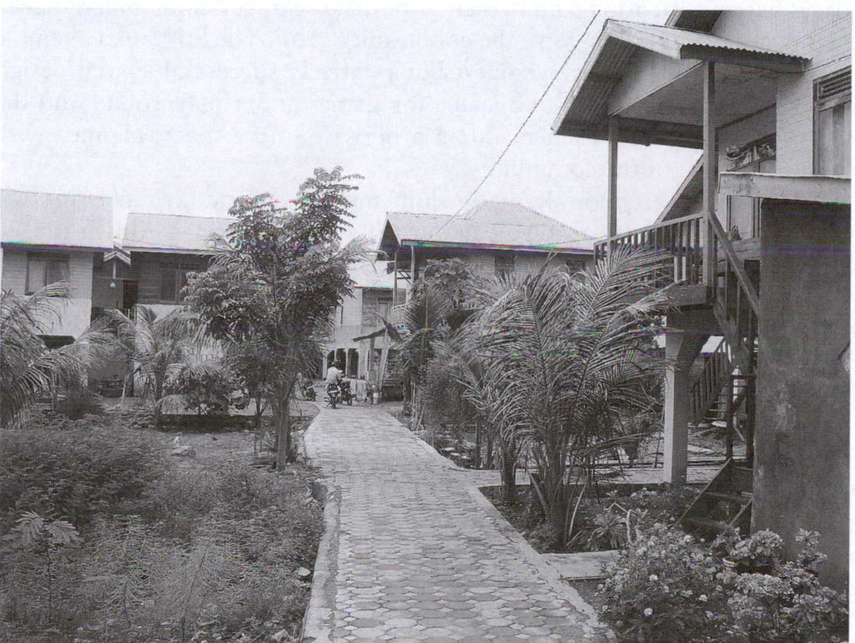

Figure 11.4 Successful layout design coordinating housing and infrastructure. **Top:** Single-storey house in resettlement scheme in Aceh. **Bottom:** Streetscapes, Aceh (photo: Duyne Barenstein).

as to create intermediate spaces and 'streetscapes' conducive to the pedestrian scale as well as to traffic use. The single-storey housing (Figure 11.4, top) illustrates appropriate designs, though with very small plots, that link private and public spaces. Likewise, Figure 11.4 (bottom) shows a neighbourhood streetscape, which provides a paved walkway and prevents inundations and floods while simultaneously attempting to create a sense of place.

Figure 11.5 contrasts two resettlement housing projects in Aceh, showing how site selection, in this case in relation to the provision of infrastructure, must be taken into consideration in the design process. Both projects recognise the need to provide culturally appropriate stilt houses. However, the units illustrated in Figure 11.5 (top) are constructed with no foresight with respect to flooding. Inappropriate site selection and the lack of landscape planning for flood prevention result in the neglect of place-making. The scheme shown in Figure 11.5 (bottom) illustrates more careful site selection.

Public and community spaces are normally conceived of as a by-product of planning design without specific attention to their fundamental role in community life and the creation of a sense of identity with place. In practice, this lack of attention often results in void spaces because of the lack of community involvement in their use, inappropriate site selection or shortage of funds for completion. These challenges are illustrated in Figure 11.6. The case of Vondh (Figure 11.6, bottom) shows neglected public and community spaces with no attention paid to their potential use by the community; indeed their planning did not involve the community at all. The Sri Lanka example (Figure 11.6, top) shows a modest but relatively successful spatial design with the simple provision of a space for games and a playground and the provision of colourful elements in an otherwise empty space, planned with the involvement of the community.

The creative search for alternative housing designs and layouts is another major challenge and can result in very poor outcomes. As illustrated in Figure 11.7, Ganesh Rajah and Sothilingam, both post-tsunami resettlement projects in Karaithivu Division in Sri Lanka, have adopted a semi-detached housing layout on two floors, which is shared by two families. The objective of the choice of two-storey housing was to increase density and thus to house more families in very small areas (1.06 acres in Ganesh Rajah and 1.82 acres in Sothilingam, totalling 68 units). But the solution is not culturally suitable for families used to living in single-storey buildings with space for family and social activities. The change to an unfamiliar pattern of space design has had several negative results, including difficulties in using internal space within the dwellings (since the units are small and the upper floor units have no plots). There is increased competition over the use of common spaces, already very small in scale in comparison with pre-disaster provision, leading to increased tensions between members of the community and also potentially resulting in a lack of maintenance.

Site selection and location, for both temporary and permanent settlement, have significant ramifications for the design of space and place. Poorly chosen

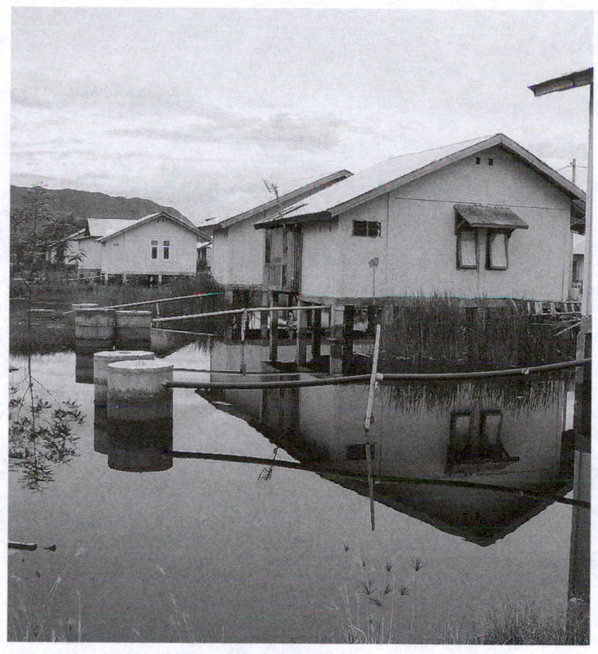

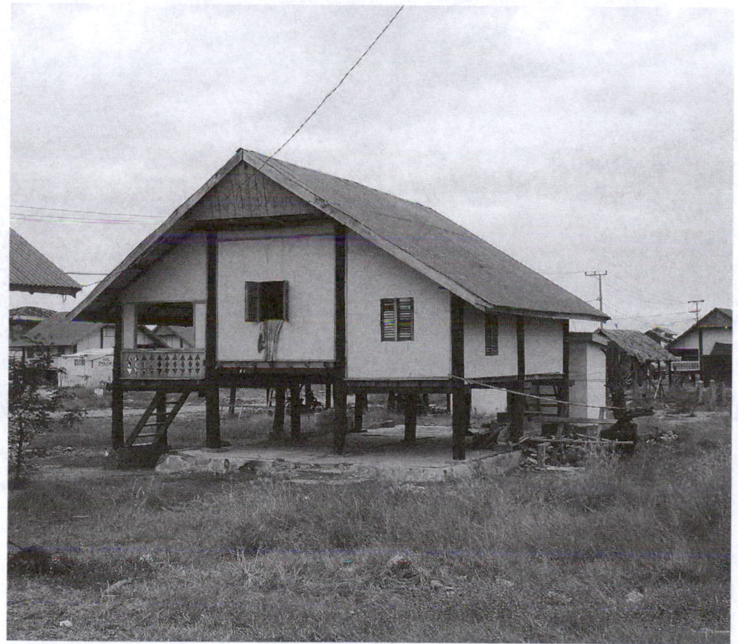

Figure 11.5 The challenge of site selection in relation to infrastructure provision.
Top: Houses in flooded areas, Aceh (photo: Duyne Barenstein).
Bottom: Stilt house in Aceh.

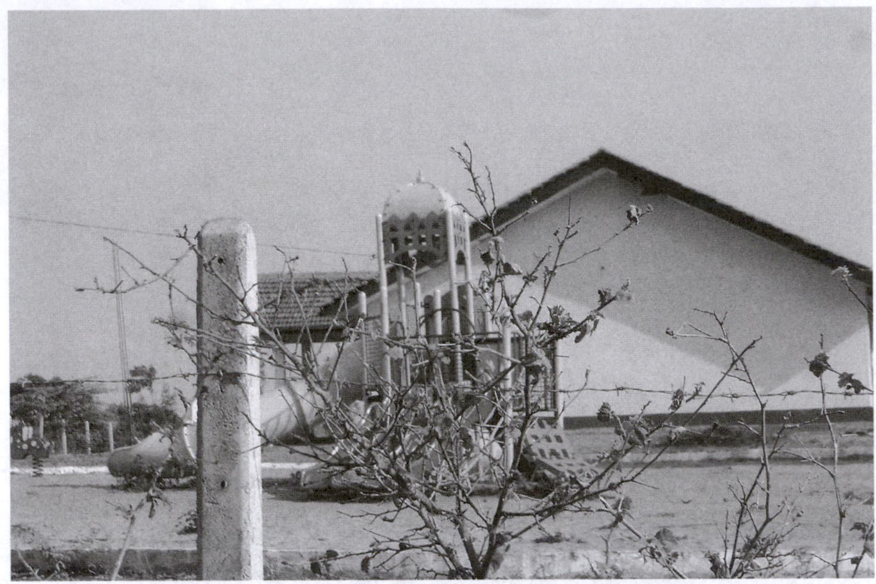

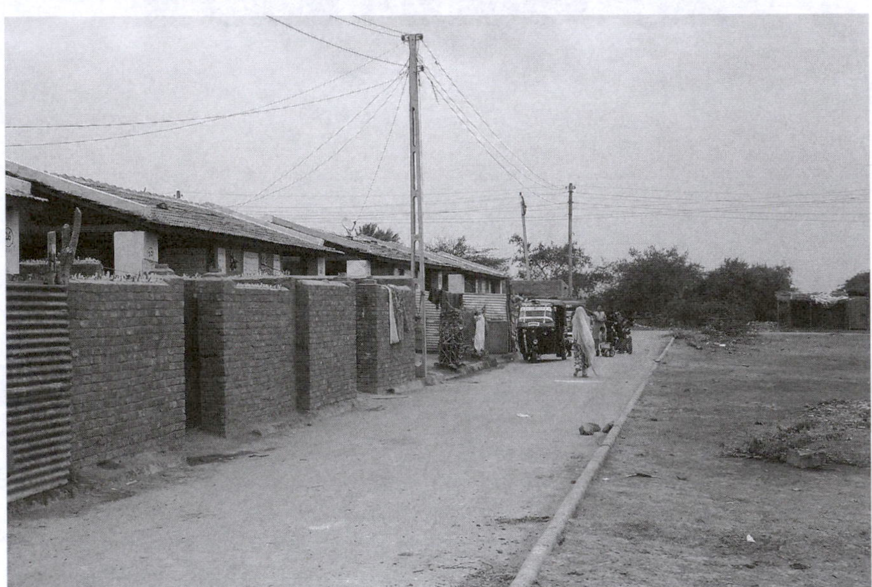

Figure 11.6 Designing public space and place. **Top:** Siribopura I resettlement site in Hambantota, Sri Lanka. **Bottom:** Vondh resettlement site in Gujarat, India.

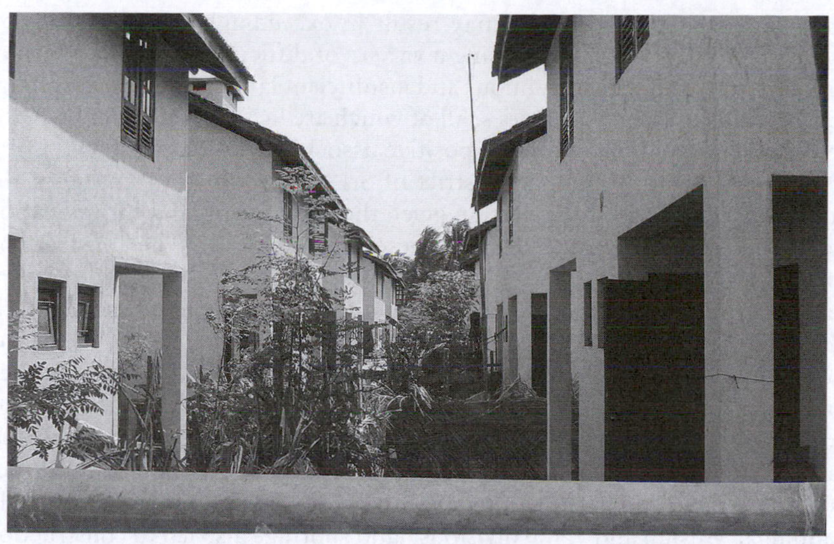

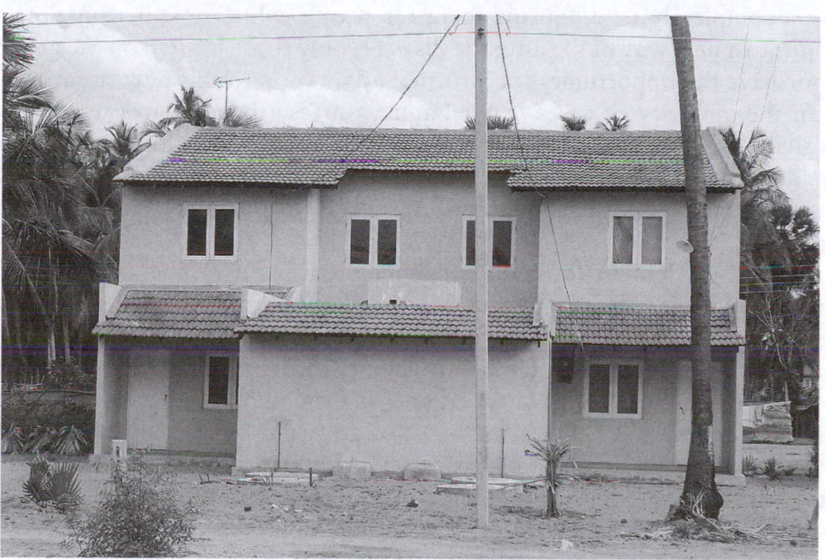

Figure 11.7 Culturally inappropriate housing design. **Top:** Ganesh Rajah housing scheme in Kalmunai, Sri Lanka. **Bottom:** Sothilingam housing scheme in Kalmunai, Sri Lanka.

sites with hostile topography may result in exceedingly high densities on small amounts of flat land, causing a variety of difficulties, such as a lack of privacy, stress-inducing conditions and insufficient land around the dwellings for informal and public activities, all of which are factors which diminish the sense of space and the otherwise positive associations with home.

Figure 11.8, in the Ampara district of Sri Lanka, illustrates some of the consequences of poor site selection given the shortage of land for relocation of those displaced by the tsunami. These pressures led to the construction of multi-storeyed apartment buildings. Despite proximity to the place of origin of the displaced people, the design imposes a completely new lifestyle to which the residents find it difficult to adjust. The outcomes are the reduction of individual space (the flats are relatively small – 45 to 55 m^2); limited provision of individual plots of land and thus limited scope for adaptation and small-scale income-generating activities, except for those living on the ground floor; limited open space; high proximity to other families and thus lack of privacy; and poor maintenance of narrow common service areas. In Kalmunai Muslim and Tamil divisions, land shortage also led to construction of multi-storeyed apartment buildings as illustrated in Figure 11.9, constituting a completely new housing form for people who are still struggling to adjust to a new way of life after the disaster; only those located on the ground floor have the opportunity for informal adaptation to this new situation.

In the majority of cases in Sri Lanka, on resettlement sites where land availability was not an issue, the housing typologies were culturally appropriate and provide, as Figure 11.10 illustrates, sufficient space for livelihoods, small gardening and space adaptations such as the opening of small business activities.

Finally, settlement location can have significant impacts on how the sense of place is created and thus on the levels of satisfaction that displaced people feel. Figures 11.11 and 11.12 exemplify how the selection of sites for relocation of post-tsunami settlements in Sri Lanka was often made without feasibility studies or social and environmental impact assessments. The key criterion was the availability of government-owned land so as to avoid lengthy land-acquisition processes. Although neglected in the case of Sri Lanka, once land is identified, it is crucial to take into account issues such as distance from people's sources of livelihood, markets and services, as well as the quality of soil and availability of water. If these factors are neglected, the resettlement sites may be perceived by their inhabitants to be remote, either because they are a significant distance from the original homes and jobs (up to 15 km in the case of Sri Lanka) or because they are poorly served by roads, public transport and water infrastructure. These outcomes must be avoided in order to promote the sense of community attachment to new settlements and in order not to undermine the creation of place in the terms conceptualised earlier.

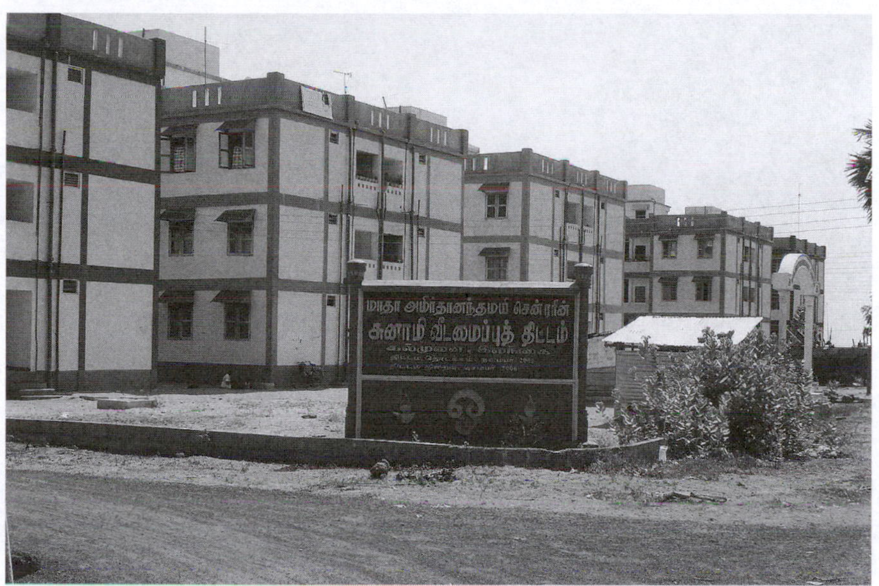

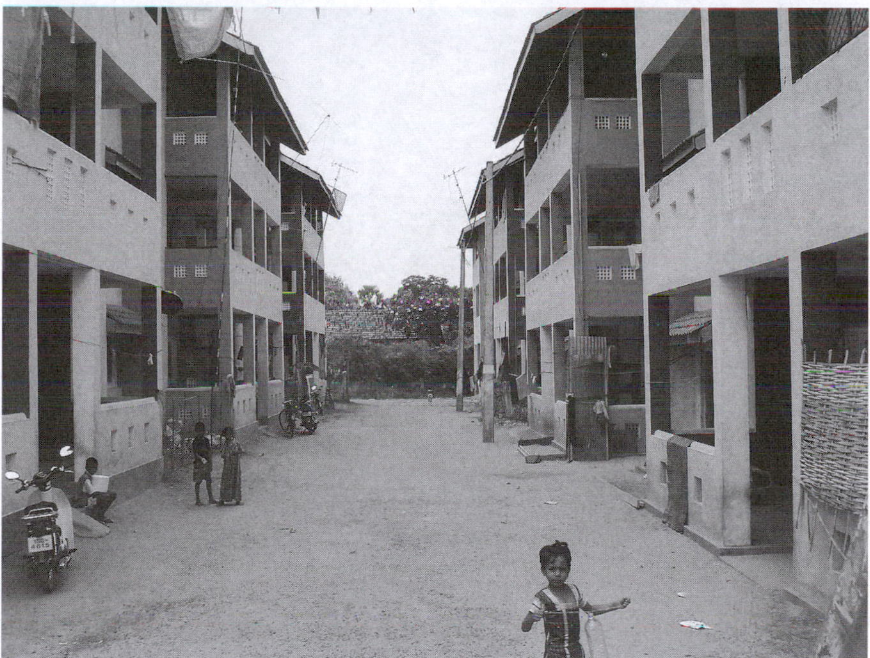

Figure 11.8 The design constraints imposed by poor site selection and land shortages. **Top:** Periyaneelavanai resettlement sites in Kalmunai, Sri Lanka. **Bottom:** Islamabath resettlement sites in Kalmunai, Sri Lanka.

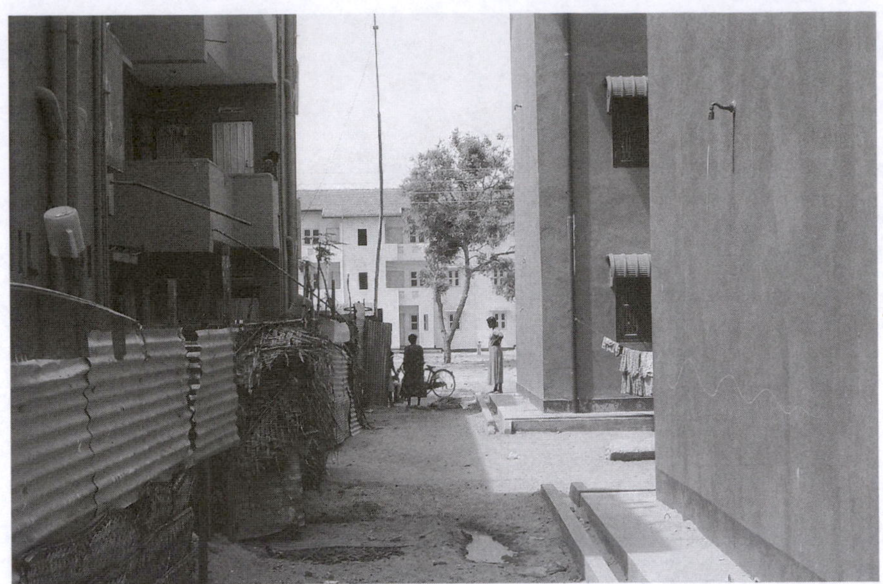

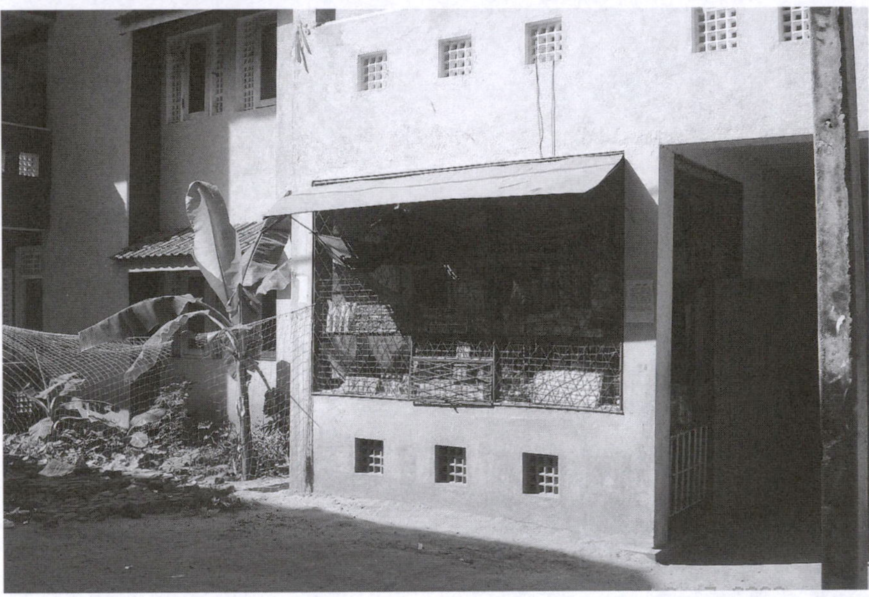

Figure 11.9 Adaptations to housing types. **Top:** Periyaneelavanai MHP resettlement site in Kalmunai, Sri Lanka. The photo shows ground-floor adaptation to this new situation, with the development of tiny plots or small income-generating activities eroding pubic spaces. **Bottom:** Islamabath resettlement sites in Kalmunai, Sri Lanka. The photo shows ground-floor adaptation of small income-generating activities in the house veranda.

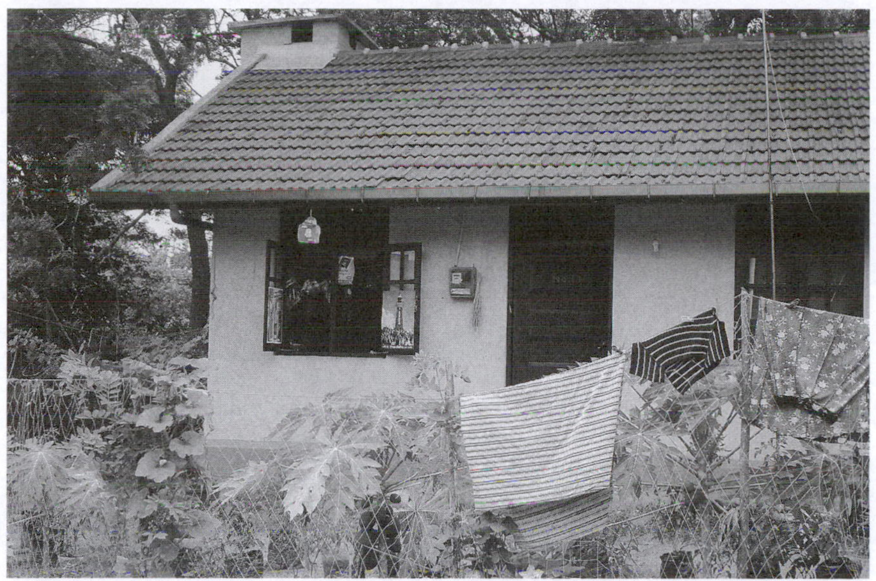

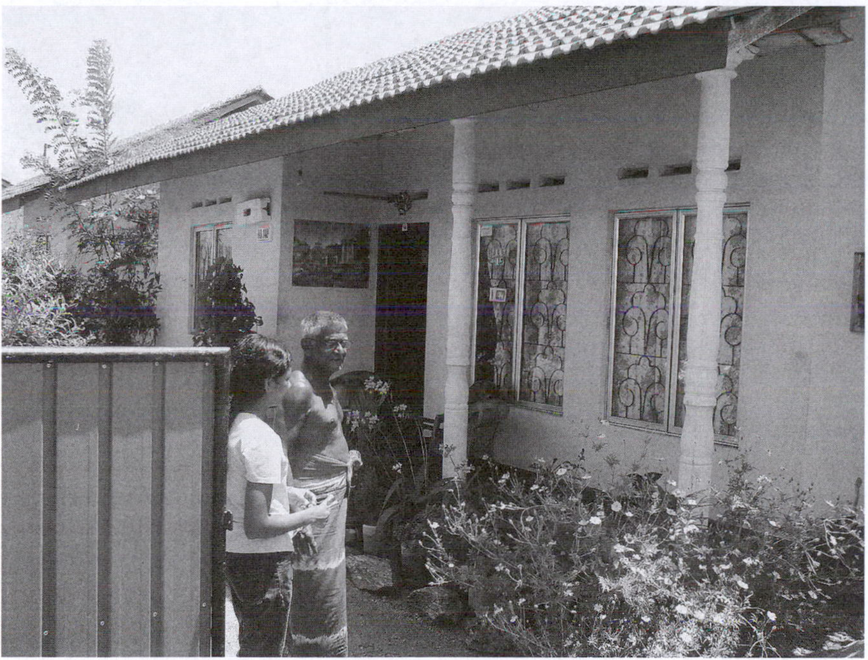

Figure 11.10 Culturally appropriate housing design. **Top:** Medagama resettlement site in Hambantota, Sri Lanka. **Bottom:** Siribopura I resettlement site in Hambantota.

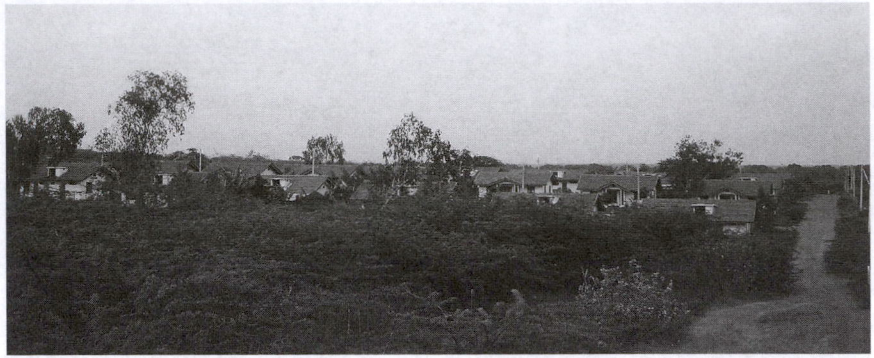

Figure 11.11 The impact of settlement location. Uhapittiagoda, remote resettlement site in Ambalantota, Sri Lanka.

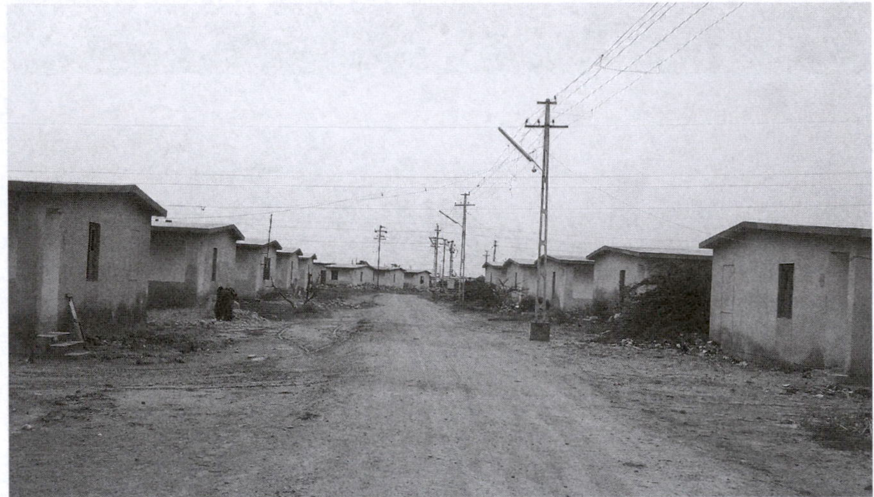

Figure 11.12 Vondh resettlement site in Gujarat, India.

Linking relief, rehabilitation and development

Establishing the linkage between emergency relief and the longer-term development needs of forcibly displaced populations is a core principle in designing space and place in post-disaster housing. The continuity of housing processes in disaster responses, the so-called *relief-to-development continuum* or *relief-and-reconstruction complex* discussed in the literature – for example Zetter,[51,52,54] Macrae,[29] Harmer and Macrae[19] – poses complex conceptual questions and operational challenges, because shelter serves both emergency and permanent needs. As has been argued in Chapters 1 and 2 of this book, host governments and international humanitarian assistance agencies have found it exceptionally difficult to tackle the continuum. By adopting short-term, pragmatic responses, they frequently compromise long-term needs. Post-disaster housing can provide a critical link, particularly with the participation of the beneficiaries in the decision-making process concerning their future living environments.

It is often assumed that displacement is a temporary phenomenon, pending a sustainable solution through a return home or assisted resettlement. However, temporary structures and their communities stay in place far longer than anticipated and often become unintended 'semi-durable' physical assets that, for better or for worse, serve longer-term recovery and development objectives. Familiar outcomes like this must be foreseen and incorporated in post-disaster shelter strategies.

These dynamic dimensions of housing and home-making in effect link the emergency and development phases of post-disaster reconstruction. They should be fully incorporated into the design criteria and spatial planning for rehousing the displaced. The ways to achieve this objective are to ensure that appropriate technologies and culturally appropriate design solutions are preferred over imported, standardised and capital-intensive ones; that collective and creative participatory processes and action-oriented implementation are preferred over top-down and centralised modes of action; and that coherent and comprehensive planning is preferred to creating mass-produced housing and public spaces and layouts determined by infrastructure technology alone.

In short, the housing sector should be a catalyst for relief *and* development interventions which, as El-Masri and Kellet point out, can lead to effective sustainable development, particularly if the affected population is involved.[15] Relief *and* development occur both simultaneously and as a continuum, not as distinct and sequential phases as predicated by much current practice.

Institutional constraints on an integrated approach

Many of the challenges of creating housing environments that provide sustainable space and place are symptomatic of the wider challenge of creating coordinated institutional and strategic response frameworks (see Chapter 5 for a detailed argument on this subject). A recent OCHA manual emphasises the importance of embedding this institutional cohesion from the initial crisis through to recovery, transition and continuum.[49]

The need to address institutional constraints is evident in several ways. First, this need arises because of the diverse characteristics of the shelter and settlement sector. Post-disaster shelter interventions must be structured in a way that intersects different programme arenas (for example, community strategies and livelihoods) and different spatial and operational scales (from field-level projects to national recovery and development strategies).

Next, housing (re-)construction is an ongoing process in most societies, especially for forcibly displaced populations, not simply an end-state package delivered by humanitarian agencies. This continuity lends further weight to the need for humanitarian institutions to better integrate the 'relief-to-development continuum' discussed above as a central core of their post-disaster reconstruction strategies. A holistic approach is essential.[52]

Third, the challenge of achieving a more integrated approach is apparent at different institutional levels. At the national level, there is frequently a lack of institutional capacity, for example special national agencies, to tackle shelter and housing-related issues for people displaced by disasters. Similarly, there is limited national capacity to monitor and evaluate displacement and housing reconstruction. Weak national-level capacity to involve affected communities and consult them in planning and policy-making also needs to be addressed, and it reflects the broader weaknesses of governance structures and state fragility in those countries most prone to disasters and conflict. Telford and Cosgrave provide telling evidence of the post-tsunami failure to implement effective participation by local populations in the reconstruction process.[43]

These national-level limitations mirror even greater challenges evident at the international level. The Humanitarian Response Review (HRR) in 2005 has addressed some of the problems that intergovernmental agencies have experienced in coordinating and managing post-disaster responses by defining principles and practices for better coordination,[32] also noted by OCHA.[49] The search for better coordination is mirrored in coalitions of organisations such as USAID and Interaction.[50]

The HRR process designated two distinct 'clusters' for the sector: the International Federation of the Red Cross (IFRC) now leads on shelter responses in natural disasters, while UNHCR leads on shelter and camp management in conflict situations. Despite some operational benefits from these recent initiatives,[42] it could be argued that a more effective way forward is to recognise that many settlement responses are transferable between these two displacement scenarios and should form a comprehensive process of intervention.[5] This new formulation actually introduces a sectoral division and inhibits a generic learning-from-experience process. Moreover, institutionalising this division only makes sense if we accept that natural disasters are truly *natural*. But – as explained in Chapter 1 – the differential impacts on affected populations are part of a wider process of socio-economic differentiation that is highlighted by disasters, thus reinforcing the case for shared learning across both natural disaster and conflict-driven displacement.[7,31]

Finally, the interplay between the limited institutional capacity of national governments and the dominant and competing interests of multilateral organisations and donor agencies is problematic. This further compounds the problems of the poor coordination and implementation of shelter policies for displaced populations. Thus, in order for space and place to be better designed, indeed to successfully achieve the wide range of objectives that the shelter sector is expected to deliver, renewed efforts are needed to ensure coordinated agency planning at all levels and the reconciliation of conflicting mandates.

A rights-based approach to shelter and settlement

Disaster (and conflict) situations are periods of rapid social transformation where the rights of the affected vulnerable populations are most under threat. The growth of rights-based approaches to humanitarian intervention resonates with the role of the shelter-and-settlement sector in disaster and conflict situations.[4,41] A rights-based agenda entitling the displaced to temporary shelter or enabling them to repossess and return to their homes is one of the most important developments in recent peace-building efforts.[22]

Rights-based interventions should ensure that the design of spaces and places is far more responsive to the needs of the affected populations. The design modalities should involve not only the protection of rights such as gender equality, freedom of movement, reducing vulnerability and meeting utilitarian needs such as the preservation of dignity and privacy, but also the representation and involvement of affected populations in decision-making about reconstruction and resettlement in displaced and return settings, including, for example, principles for design and layout; the production and construction of space and place; and land rights, especially in repatriation or resettlement.[41,47]

Addressing these rights can help to ensure that the post-disaster coping capacity of communities will be strengthened in both the short and long term.

A way forward

The design of shelters and settlements that are responsive to the wide range of needs and values for populations resettled or returning after disasters is a complex task. This chapter challenges the dominant approach, in which housing is conceived as a mono-dimensional and standardised physical artefact, constructed as a reactive, top-down, technology-driven and 'end state' product. This pragmatic reductionism adopted by the international humanitarian community results in lower-order measurable outputs such as contract completions, costs per housing unit and number of buildings restored. But this approach is viable neither as a short-term emergency response nor as a permanent, sustainable solution. All too often this sort of response actually compounds impoverishment, social disarticulation and the loss of livelihoods.

The increasing awareness of these negative outcomes calls for a wide-ranging response. Addressing the poor conceptualisation of housing, notably around the principles of designing space and place, is a critical factor in formulating such a response. It requires a more profound conceptual understanding of housing as a complex functional resource; as a cultural symbol and social artefact; as an object of economic value; and as part of a wider community expressed through the spatial design of settlements. In essence, a far more coordinated and integrated approach is required – one that links the art of designing space and place to the wider needs that shelter fulfils in terms of the social, cultural and rights-based aspirations of disaster-displaced populations. In this way, the long acknowledged link between a dwelling place, personal well-being and identity finds both a theoretical explanation and practical solutions through the design of space and place.

Design for post-disaster reconstruction involves satisfying material needs and resolving competing social requirements through a process of active participation by the occupants and the *mediation* of 'professionals'. Walls and joists can be arrayed so that a building stands up, but occupants must also be able to see space that suits their needs and that the process of (re-) construction also ensures the formation of 'place'. Thus the design process is simultaneously the production of physical form, the creation of social, cultural and symbolic resources, and also the outcome of a negotiative/ facilitative process. Such an approach fundamentally reconceives the role of the 'technical aid workers'. They are not, in Roy's pointed phrase, the 'innocent professionals',[37] but they are involved in a process that requires them to reflect upon what they produce through both material *and* discursive practices.

Bringing these arguments together, an integrated and multidimensional reconceptualisation of post-disaster housing reconstruction is represented in Figure 11.13. This symbolic outline understands post-disaster shelter and settlement responses to be the integration of four critical components. These components must be continuously articulated through time – three broad time periods/phases of post-disaster recovery are identified – but they have differential importance at different phases; this is represented by the relative sizes of the symbols.

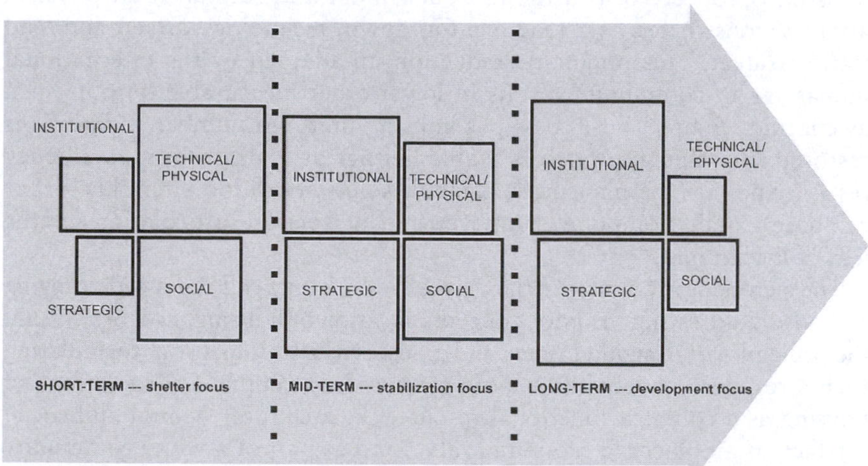

Figure 11.13 Operational framework for housing reconstruction.

The four dimensions are:

- The *institutional dimension*: this links housing provision to the arena of policy and governance. The need to ensure far better institutional coordination of all the stakeholders involved in the design and delivery of post-disaster shelter programmes is essential here. At the same time, intervention processes should safeguard the rights of resettled communities, as well as returnees and those who have remained behind, by ensuring they have critical inputs into the design and development of housing policies and into space selection. It is, of course, fundamental to safeguard policy parameters such as location, building standards and planning regulations and to ensure that housing projects provide security of title and tenure.
- The *social dimension*: this is related both to the house understood as a social space and to the interface between occupiers and communities in the production of place. This layer is crucial to ensuring the interaction between the physical artefact of house and the social dimension of households, community and locality. Strengthening local capacities and ensuring sustained participation at all stages of the design and reconstruction process is a high priority. Such empowerment can help to avoid standardisation of places and the rationalistic production of spaces, which can lead to unsuitable typologies and domination by imported spatial attributes.
- The *technical/physical dimension*: this is related to the house itself as a physical object and to all the technical requirements, from building materials to construction mechanisms. Attention must be focused on the use of local construction skills and materials, on allowing for better maintenance, sustainability, enabling incremental upgrading and expansion. It embraces the use of traditional construction techniques that allow the involvement of owners, local builders and small contractors in the construction process, maximising the local economic value of the reconstruction programme. Moreover, attention should be dedicated to place-making processes and community strategies for redeveloping livelihoods and tightening social relationships through the production of shared public and semi-public spaces that are culturally sustainable.
- The *strategic dimension*: this dimension is related to the house as a strategic resource and economic multiplier. Fundamental is the fact that housing reconstruction should directly support and link into economic objectives and policies, at local and regional levels, in regenerating building materials and housing components industries and in re-establishing construction labour markets that generate income to support the livelihood needs of local populations. Conceiving housing and physical assets strategically is thus fundamental in adopting a wider livelihoods approach in the reconstruction.

This integrated and multidimensional model shows an attempt to move from a top-down and project/relief-based approach to a balanced-assets approach. In this model, relief and development occur simultaneously and as a continuum, based on the integration of the four key components. Thus the three operational phases are not distinct and sequential but serve to highlight those phases where *different* dimensions might have a *different* priority, but, crucially, they always coexist and cohere with each other.

12 The importance of institutional and community resilience in post-disaster reconstruction

Lee Bosher

Still shocked by deaths and losses, residents, politicians, professionals and organisations are particularly sensitive to issues concerning disaster mitigation and prevention after a disaster. However, reconstruction and prevention strategies should be closely linked because post-disaster interventions are not only an opportunity to rebuild but also an opportunity to reduce the vulnerabilities of the population.

Towards a holistic approach to resilience

The ability of the built environment to withstand the impacts of extreme events and to meet the needs of urban populations during the aftermath of a disaster is a key element in how society can recover from traumatic events. Many efforts to deal with natural hazards have focused on changing the physical attributes of structures, while less attention has been paid to effecting needed change within specific social, political, cultural and economic environments.[20] The consequence is that the people who were the intended beneficiaries of apparent advances in both technical knowledge and policies have sometimes become steadily more vulnerable.

This observation raises two key issues, which are as pertinent for high-income nations as they are for low-income nations.

The first issue can be considered as a reactive strategy and is related to the rehabilitation and reconstruction of areas affected by extreme events. When a disaster strikes, market forces tend to establish pressures to reconstruct built assets (such as water supplies, transportation networks, healthcare facilities and commercial buildings) as quickly as possible.[17] The attempt to hastily minimise post-event economic losses, to reduce social impacts and arguably to improve political ratings inevitably hampers efforts to implement the issues identified from previous disasters.

The second issue is related to more proactive strategies and particularly to the mitigation of hazards through a number of approaches such as local capacity building, sound urban/rural planning and disaster-risk-reduction initiatives. In considering these issues, this chapter highlights why a holistic approach to resilience is important, in that socio-political aspects of resilience are as important as the physical aspects, which are typically the focus of technocratic approaches to dealing with disasters. Evidence from India is presented to demonstrate how ill-thought-out and overly technocratic approaches to post-disaster reconstruction can severely impinge upon efforts to attain social resilience as well as physical resilience.

Resilience

The United Nations' International Strategy for Disaster Reduction has defined 'resilience' as:

> The capacity of a system, community or society potentially exposed to hazards to adapt, by resisting or changing in order to reach and maintain an acceptable level of functioning and structure. This is determined by the degree to which the social system is capable of organising itself to increase this capacity for learning from past disasters for better future protection and to improve risk reduction measures. (page 340)[24]

This holistic concept of resilience is important because it integrates the physical (both built and natural) and socio-political aspects, and goes some way to illustrating how multi-faceted the concept of resilience is. The socio-political aspects are arguably as important for the attainment of resilience as the physical aspects. For instance, it has been suggested that to attain a more resilient built environment, a more resilient infrastructural context – with regards to the professions and the structures and processes that govern construction activity – is also required.[8] Therefore, it has been posited by Bosher that:

> a resilient built environment should be designed, located, built, operated and maintained in a way that maximises the ability of built assets, associated support systems (physical and institutional) and the people that reside or work within the built assets, to withstand, recover from, and mitigate for the impacts of extreme natural and human-induced hazards. (page 13)[4]

If built assets are affected repeatedly by particular hazards, there is a pressing need to learn lessons from them and replace or retrofit the original structure(s) with an improved version that is more resilient (in social, physical and economic terms). In many wealthier nations, buildings are designed using certain standards that are effectively enforced and they are thus less vulnerable to major structural damage. For instance, the starkest failure of many structures during severe earthquakes can be found in countries where most of the construction is semi-engineered or un-engineered.[20] It has been suggested by Petal, *et al.* that in many developing parts of the world:

> modern forms of construction, perceived as 'development' and 'progress', have undercut the value of traditional apprenticeships, degraded traditional construction and demanded technical knowledge and skills that builders have not yet acquired. The lack of formal educational opportunities combined with high illiteracy make it challenging to communicate knowledge and techniques. (page 194)[20]

In recent years, advances have been made to embed physical resilience into long-term developments; for instance, nations such as Peru, Turkey and, to a certain extent, India have developed guidelines to mitigate for some hazards, such as the earthquake-resistant design of adobe or non-engineered construction. Such initiatives are important, but it should be noted that in studies of risk perception, Asgary and Willis have found that 'safety measures enforced without considering people's preferences fail to be adequately adopted in practice' (page 613).[2] In the same way, a close examination of economic and social realities in less economically developed countries is critical to understanding the continued construction of highly vulnerable built assets in the face of natural hazards.[4,10]

It might be thought that communities would give careful consideration to location before starting to build, particularly avoiding known seismic areas or sites that are subject to, or can be affected by, other hazards such as floods and landslides. However, for many people in developing countries, there is no choice about where they live – the benefits of a location outweigh the costs. People grow accustomed to a low-probability risk and they accept it; the hazard is perceived as being unavoidable or an 'act of God' and natural hazards are familiar aspects of everyday life.[26]

As explained in Chapter 1, people have different capacities to avoid or cope with disasters; in other words, they have differing *vulnerability*. Vulnerability is 'the characteristics of a person or group and their situation that influence their capacity *to* anticipate, cope with and recover from the impact of a natural disaster' (page 11).[26] People's vulnerability is generated by social, economic and political processes that influence how hazards affect people in varying ways and with different intensities.[26] Therefore, the outcome of a disaster is shaped both by the physical nature of the hazard and the vulnerability of people who are involved (e.g. why people live in dangerous locations and unprotected buildings and the lack of disaster preparedness at particular places at particular times). The human influences upon the causes of disasters are too often overlooked because sometimes these influences can be discrete and driven by very different socio-economic factors. For example, in many high-income countries, people like to live near rivers (and are prepared to pay for the benefit in many cases) for the aesthetic and recreational benefits that rivers can offer. Therefore, a flood event that occurs in the non-tidal stretch of the Thames in southern England, for example, inundating people's homes, businesses and lifelines, will typically be referred to as a 'natural disaster', but the flood event manifests itself as a disaster because members of this sort of society have chosen to build in such locations.

Socio-economic factors that affect people's exposure to hazards can manifest themselves differently in low-income nations, with key factors being related to poverty (low access to assets), marginalisation (poor access to public facilities) and powerlessness (low access to political and social networks).[3] These factors have an influence on the choices that people have regarding where they can live; for instance, landless squatters live on the flood plain of the Buriganga River in Dhaka, Bangladesh, and informal slums (*favelas*) are situated on the steep landslide-prone hills of Rio de Janeiro in Brazil. These factors also influence the levels to which people can provide themselves with adequate shelter for protection from local conditions; therefore geographic proximity and exposure to hazards will affect levels of individual and social resilience.[26] Consequently, unlike the case of higher-income nations where many people choose to live in areas that are exposed to hazards, in low-income countries it is more the case of a 'lack of choice' that forces people to live in areas that are exposed to hazards.[4]

After disastrous events, residents often feel that their only choice is to rebuild their houses with unreinforced methods, thus leaving their new homes just as vulnerable as those that were originally damaged or destroyed. Petal, *et al.* have noted that this might be because hazard-resistant designs are perceived to be too expensive, to rely on materials that are not available through the local market or to demand a level of construction skill that has not been developed within the local population.[20] Thus there should be a form of construction based on hazard-resistant building design that is specifically aimed at benefiting the poor. For example, Jigyasu describes an increase in the vulnerability of local communities after the Latur 1993 earthquake in India, where sustainable recovery interventions were poorly planned and implemented.[12] Therefore, it is argued here and in a number of other chapters in this book that a 'community-based' imperative is needed in which construction and design professionals learn to share their knowledge with, and at the same time learn from, the users of the structures. This knowledge exchange would yield a bottom-up demand for safe construction and voluntary compliance with standards, and there would be public, government and private-sector expectation and support for enforcement.[20]

A case from South India

Andhra Pradesh is the third largest state in India, covering 275,000 km^2, and bordering the Bay of Bengal. It is also one of the world's most cyclone-prone regions. Historically, tropical cyclones have been the cause of large-scale losses of human life, livestock, crops, property and infrastructure in Andhra Pradesh, with serious adverse effects on the local and regional economies. Despite the threat that cyclones and floods pose to the livelihoods and lives of millions of people, many inhabitants remain in the area through poverty and lack of choices, striving to live in regions that are dominated by mangrove swamps, brackish rivulets, aquaculture tanks and paddy fields.[22]

For the purposes of this study, the district of East Godavari was selected for research (Figure 12.1) because of the tropical cyclone (07B) disaster that affected the area in November 1996 and the subsequent vulnerability-reduction initiatives undertaken by the Andhra Pradesh state government and local non-governmental organisations (NGOs). These vulnerability-reduction initiatives included the construction of community cyclone shelters, storm-warning systems, improved evacuation measures, hazard mapping and enhanced community preparedness through education programmes in cyclone-prone areas.[19,22]

Research was undertaken as part of a study conducted in Andhra Pradesh between February 2002 and September 2003. The study was focused on the investigation of the social and institutional aspects of vulnerability and resilience to disasters in Andhra Pradesh. Cartographic surveys of eight case-study villages and over 200 questionnaire surveys, 24 semi-structured interviews and five focus-group meetings were undertaken with village inhabitants, local and regional government officials and personnel working for local NGOs involved with disaster-management-related activities.

It was observed that the provision of basic needs such as shelter, drinking water, education and healthcare facilities can be strained at the best of times but the situation after a disaster is typically much more desperate.[3]

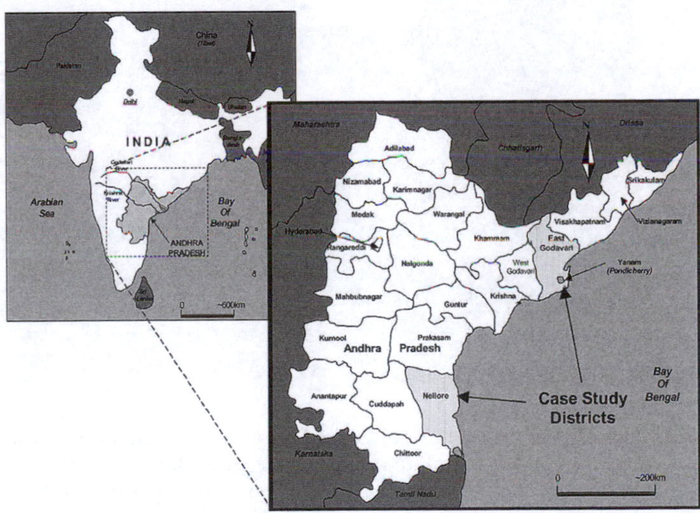

Figure 12.1 Location of Andhra Pradesh and the case-study districts. Andhra Pradesh is the third largest state in India, covering 275,000km². Bordering the Bay of Bengal, it is located in one of the world's most cyclone-prone regions.[3]

However, when a disaster strikes, market forces and political influences tend to establish pressures to reconstruct built assets as quickly as possible.[17] Some of these hasty developments can result in built assets that are inadequate for their intended purposes. Figure 12.2 shows a cyclone shelter and community healthcare centre that was constructed in a fishing village in Andhra Pradesh, India. This shelter was built in 1997 in the aftermath of a tropical cyclone that affected the village the previous year; the photograph was taken in 2001. The cyclone shelter was not destroyed by an extreme natural event but by poor construction practices, inadequate materials and little or no maintenance, and it is testament to the problems associated with the hasty construction of built assets. It is not unreasonable to suggest that the aforementioned cyclone shelter was destroyed by a human-induced disaster: a technocratic approach that did not engage with the local community and wasted finite and valuable resources.

A similar example was found in a neighbouring village (Figure 12.3); the case was not as extreme as that shown in Figure 12.2, but the cyclone

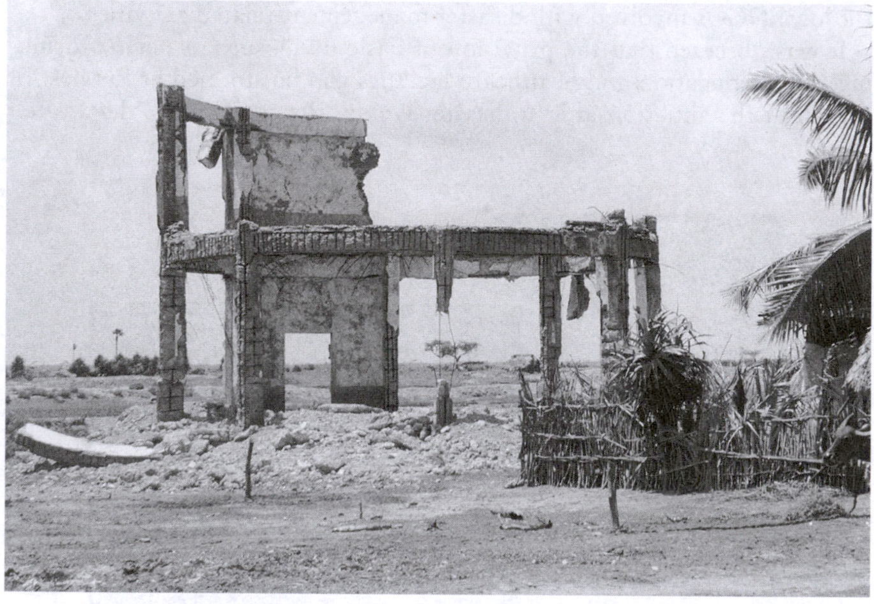

Figure 12.2 Shell of cyclone shelter devastated by poor construction, inappropriate materials and inadequate maintenance. A cyclone shelter in East Godavari, Andhra Pradesh that was built during 1997 in the aftermath of a tropical cyclone that affected the village the previous year; the photograph was taken in July 2001. The cyclone shelter was not destroyed by an extreme natural event but by poor construction practices, inadequate materials and little or no maintenance, and is testament to the problems associated with the hasty construction of built assets.

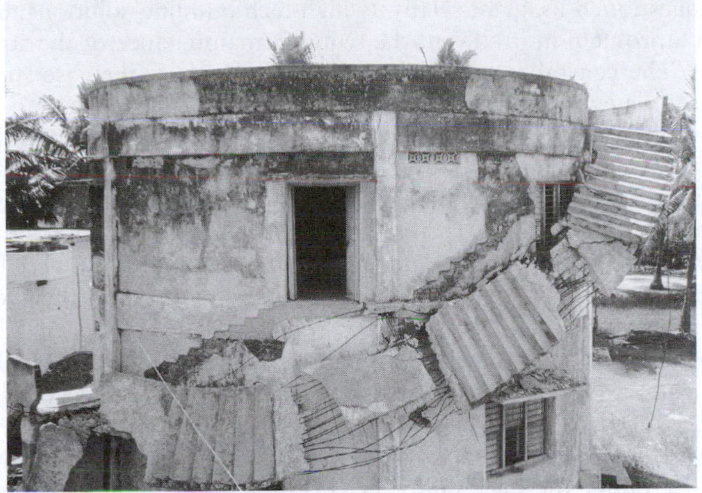

Figure 12.3 Another example of a poorly constructed cyclone shelter and community centre. This cyclone shelter in East Godavari, is another example of an important local asset that has been made redundant through poor construction practices, inadequate materials and little or no maintenance.

shelter (that was also used as a community centre and makeshift school) was rendered just as useless.

What is important to acknowledge is that it is not only the inability of these cyclone shelters to function and benefit the local communities that is a problem; it is also the psychological impact of such 'technological failures' on the local community, as this account illustrates:

> When the government came to build the cyclone shelter cum community centre the other villagers and I were very happy. We thought that the government would then also provide us with boreholes for safe drinking water, a small school or health centre and a decent road. When the cyclone shelter started to crack and then fall to pieces we were frightened to use the structure, it was useless, it was unsafe. It was then that we considered whether the government was more interested in being seen to help us than actually helping us. You will not be surprised to hear that we still do not have any safe drinking water, sanitation, school or health centre.
>
> Interview with village elder in East Godavari

Some of the key problems that were observed during this study included:

- Technocratic approaches that resulted in low (or typically non-existent) consultation with the local communities (for further discussion on this, see Twigg[23] and Petal, *et al.*[20]).

- Unquestioned usage of relatively high-tech building solutions: this was not a problem in itself, but the required maintenance of the structures was. The coastal region of Andhra Pradesh where the case study was located is exposed to an extremely saline atmosphere that can quickly damage concrete structures. Therefore, such structures will require high levels of maintenance, but the local community was not given suitable training to provide such maintenance to the cyclone shelters. A director of a local NGO said, 'as soon as some superficial cracks appeared on the surface of the building, the locals did not want to use them because they feared that the building would collapse; in most cases their concerns were proved right.'
- Use of low-quality materials: numerous accounts relayed that the concrete mix was created using seawater and sand from the beach. This is a concern because it has been well reported that seawater is inappropriate for use in structural concrete (see Kaushik and Islam[14] and Neville[18]).
- Design faults: the steel reinforcements used in the cyclone shelters were not sufficiently embedded within the concrete, so when the superficial cracks exposed them, the saline air quickly caused the steel to rust and fail structurally (see Neville[18]).
- Development that contributed to a substantial debt burden for low-income families: so-called 'cyclone-resistant housing' (Figure 12.4, bottom) was subsidised by local NGOs and the state government, with the recipients contributing approximately 10–20 per cent of the final cost of 40,000–50,000 Indian rupees (IR), which at the time of the research was equivalent to US$1000–$1250. The costs incurred by the recipients therefore ranged from IR4,000 to IR10,000. However, a large proportion of people in the case-study areas were earning a daily average wage of IR60 (approximately US$1.50), and therefore many needed to borrow the money from local money lenders, who tended to charge disproportionately high interest rates.[3]
- Inappropriate designs and materials for the local climatic conditions: traditionally, the most common houses in the case-study villages were very basic huts that were constructed by the inhabitants from locally sourced materials such as mud, wood and palm fronds (Figure 12.4, top). These structures are very vulnerable to the high winds and heavy precipitation that is typically associated with tropical cyclones and therefore afford scant protection for the inhabitants and their possessions during such events (but compared to more technocratic solutions, such structures are nonetheless relatively inexpensive to reconstruct after a cyclone has occurred).

The Andhra Pradesh state government and local NGOs were involved in the construction of 'cyclone-resistant housing' (see Figure 12.4, bottom, for an example of a semi-detached two-house design). While such structures could indeed protect the inhabitants from the effects of severe tropical cyclones

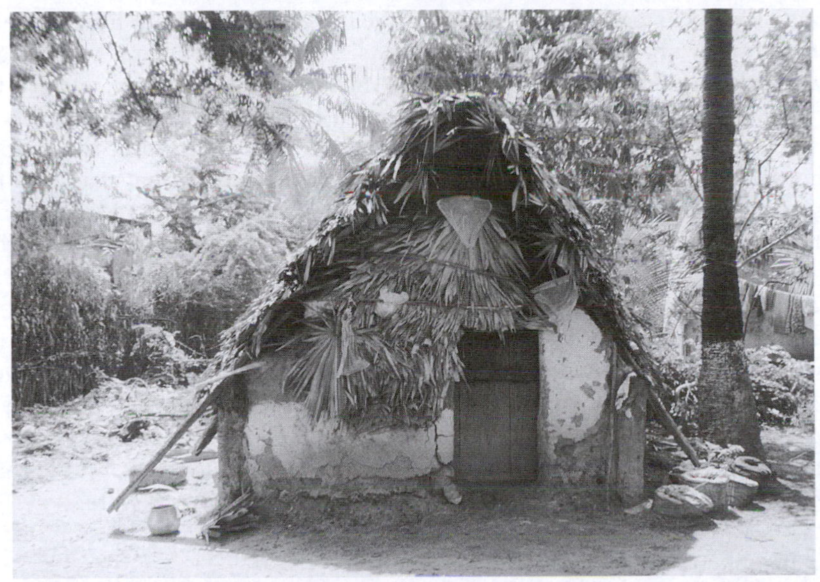

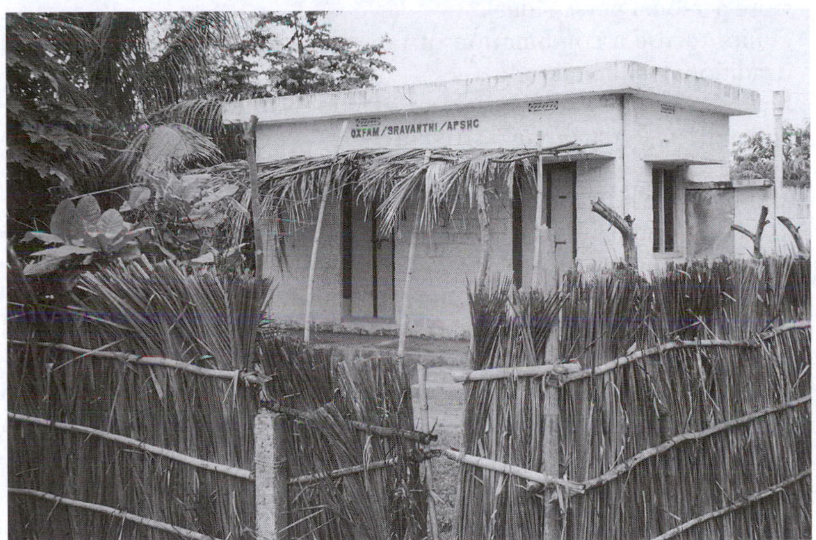

Figure 12.4 Traditional 'kutcha' and modified formal unit. **Top:** The 'kutcha' hut is the most common house type in the case study villages. These houses are typically constructed by the inhabitants from locally sourced materials such as mud, wood and palm fronds. **Bottom:** The 'Cyclone-resistant house', with an improvised veranda, is subsidised by local non-governmental organisations and the State government, with the recipients contributing approximately 10–20 per cent of the final cost of 40,000–50,000 Indian Rupees.[3]

(that may occur once every five to 10 years), these concrete houses were generally very uncomfortable to live in for significant proportions of the year, such as during the hot season (April to August, when they were referred to as ovens) and also during the cooler season (November to January, when they were referred to as damp ice boxes). A large proportion of the people who owned 'cyclone-resistant housing' had tried to adapt the structures to improve their utility by adding bamboo verandas (see Figure 12.4, bottom, for an example), canopies on the roof and even entire huts on the side (for living and sleeping in while the cyclone-resistant house was predominately used to store possessions).

During September 2003, five focus-group discussions and a vast range of rudimentary sketches were undertaken with respondents from two villages in East Godavari; during these discussions, the respondents were asked what types of housing they would find most suitable to live in. The key criteria that the villagers prioritised for defining the type of house design (note that protection from tropical cyclones was not one of the criteria) were:

- flexible use of enclosed and open spaces;
- safety from theft and robbery (including incorporation of a safe box to store personal possessions);
- ability to use a combination of different materials and technologies (traditional and modern);
- flexibility to provide a variety of functions and uses through possible adaptations to the original structure.

It is interesting to note that these four key criteria were also identified, along with 10 other criteria, during in-depth studies on informal housing projects undertaken in South America and Turkey.[15]

After many iterations of design and even more glasses of *chai* (sweet milky tea), the consensus of opinion regarding the most appropriate type of house that would meet their everyday needs fell somewhere between the low-cost basic *kutcha* hut and the relatively expensive 'cyclone-resistant house'. Figure 12.5 illustrates the type of house that the respondents decided would most meet their everyday needs but also afford a degree of protection against tropical cyclones (not drawn to scale).

The house illustrated in Figure 12.5a is essentially six vertical columns (which could be constructed of steel-reinforced concrete or timber) located on a raised concrete platform, with further reinforced concrete or timber bars providing bracing for the roof (which could be made out of traditional and locally available thatching materials such as grass/straw/wood).

Some of the interesting design features of this 'locally designed' house were:

- The four external walls of the house are left open so that the home owners can use locally available materials such as mud daubed on wood or

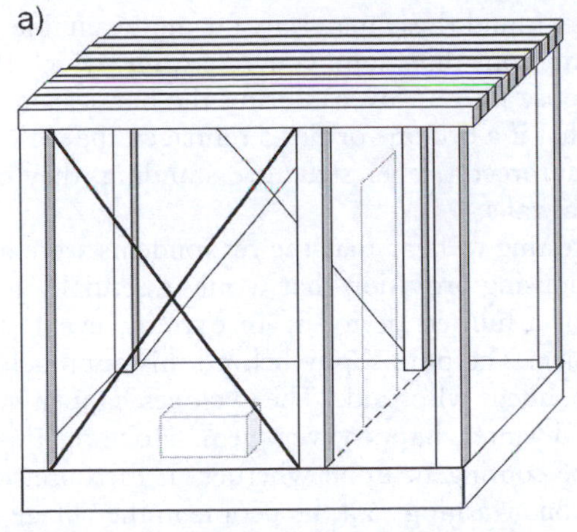

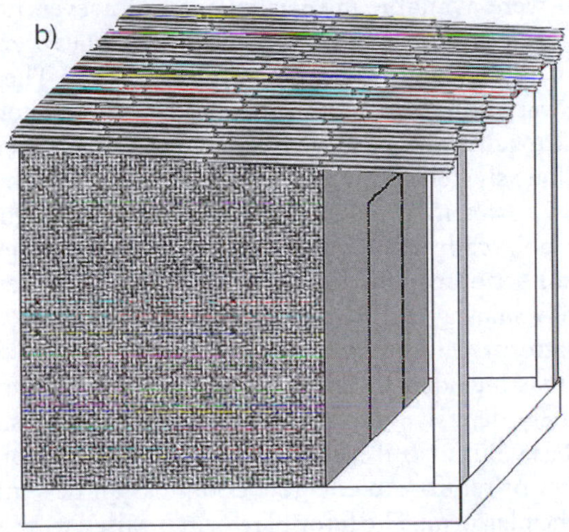

Figure 12.5 Basic illustration of the house that the village respondents designed. The type of house that the villagers decided would most meet their everyday needs but also afford them a degree of protection against tropical cyclones; **a**) illustration of the basic structure of the house built upon a raised concrete plinth; **b**) illustration of the finished house using locally available materials such as mud daubed on wood or bamboo matting, or adobe brick as infill for the walls.

bamboo matting, or adobe brick as infill (as illustrated in Figure 12.5b). The villagers found these materials far more suitable for the prevailing climatic conditions than solid concrete walls, which they felt tended to 'turn the house into an oven' during the hot season. The respondents explained that if a cyclone or flood damaged the walls but left the main concrete reinforced/timber structure standing, they could quite easily rebuild such walls.

- It was interesting to hear that the respondents were advocating an approach to housing provision that would essentially render their homes unusable for a limited period if an extreme event such as a tropical cyclone struck. The philosophy behind this approach was summed up by one respondent who said, 'The cyclones happen very rarely but the summers and winters happen every year.' However, this approach would obviously be contingent upon whether, at the onset of extreme events such as cyclone warnings, all the people in the village were able to seek shelter from the cyclone. In the villages where the focus groups were undertaken, there were no constraints on people in using the cyclone shelters that were available in their villages. However, in some villages (typically multi-caste agricultural villages) two issues were raised about the ability of all the villagers to use a cyclone shelter. These issues were: a) everyone was allowed to take shelter in a cyclone shelter but there was insufficient capacity; and b) some people in the village were not allowed to use a cyclone shelter because they were excluded on the lines of caste (with 'lower' castes in some cases being excluded by the numerically weaker but politically and economically stronger 'higher' castes) and gender (a number of men voiced their objections to the female members of their family sharing facilities with 'strange men'; also see Rashid[21]).
- The floor platform includes a watertight sunken recess that can be locked. This recess was included in the design proposed by the respondents as a type of safety deposit box where valuables could be stored not only on a daily basis but also if a disaster struck. The platform is designed so that timber or reinforced concrete columns can be sunken into holes located on the platform. The floor platform is raised to protect the house from the flooding that can regularly occur during the monsoon season. In a part of India where rights over land ownership can be contested in post-disaster situations (also see Chapter 7 for a more in-depth discussion on land-rights issues), the floor platform could also provide proof of land ownership (for example, via an embedded and unique identification number).
- The roof can be extended (using reinforced concrete or traditional thatching materials) over the door to provide a veranda that affords protection from the extreme elements and also acts as extended accommodation during the hot season (as illustrated in Figure 12.5). The village respondents also felt that the basic structure could provide a base 'module' to which more 'modules' could be added if the financial

circumstance allowed (i.e. the structure was adaptable and flexible to meet the family's needs and future aspirations).

It should be noted that this design is not being endorsed as a universally appropriate solution for cyclone-resistant housing, though this design was crafted by a wide range of villagers, male and female, young and old, who felt the design was suitable for them for the context in which they live. The criticality of context-sensitive post-disaster reconstruction is explained in more detail in various chapters of this book. The key caveats that should be considered in the potential success of such a design are related to a) the use of suitable materials in the preparation of any concrete; b) the high-quality design of any reinforced components; c) the provision of suitable training on construction and maintenance for the local population; and d) affordability. In support of these design considerations, it would also be important that access to a cyclone shelter be made available for all communities.

It is interesting to note that this design does not fully conform either to the typical *kutcha* hut or to the relatively high-cost 'cyclone-resistant house'; it arguably falls within the middle ground between traditional and high-tech. It is also important to appreciate that there can never be a 'one size fits all' solution to hazard-resistant housing or post-disaster reconstruction, and that is why knowledge of the local context and full involvement of local stakeholders is an essential component in the attainment of resilience. It should be added that local participants should not be only the most powerful/richest members of the local communities; a concerted effort should be made to involve the most marginalised members of society, who are typically also the most vulnerable (an argument also explained by several contributors to this book and by Bosher[3]). Ideally, these considerations should not wait until a disaster has occurred before they are acted upon. 'Pre-disaster' is the key window of opportunity for appropriate development that is attuned to the needs of local communities while also integrating the principles of disaster risk reduction.

The way forward

Many efforts to deal with natural hazards have focused on changing the physical attributes of structures, while less attention has been paid to effecting needed change within specific social, political, cultural and economic environments.[20] The consequence is that the people who are the intended beneficiaries of apparent advances in both technical knowledge and policies have sometimes become steadily more vulnerable. For example, it is often suggested that poverty breeds fatalism with regard to disasters. However – as explained in Chapter 2 – when informed choices are permitted with regard to building, most people tend to incorporate *affordable* safety features.[16] In contrast, people who have homes built for them – without consultation, without information and without choice – are likely to adopt a fatalistic view of the product.[20] This tragic irony suggests the necessity for a community-based approach to construction for disaster risk reduction. It is in view of these concerns that a more 'holistic approach' to post-disaster reconstruction is required.

A 'holistic approach' to post-disaster reconstruction is an approach that utilises, in a socially, culturally, financially and technically appropriate manner, the 'middle ground' between the 'top-down' technological approaches and the 'bottom-up' or traditional approaches to the construction of buildings (Figure 12.6).

Interfaces between top-down and bottom-up considerations

Figure 12.6 is a simplified representation of a very complex set of issues that will need to be considered if a more holistic approach to post-disaster reconstruction is to be attained. It is the interface between the top-down and bottom-up factors that constitutes the holistic approach; these context-specific factors will now be explained.

Threats and impacts of natural hazards and the root causes of social and physical vulnerability

Research in the field of natural hazards was dominated for many years by a focus on the physical processes and on the conditions caused by extreme

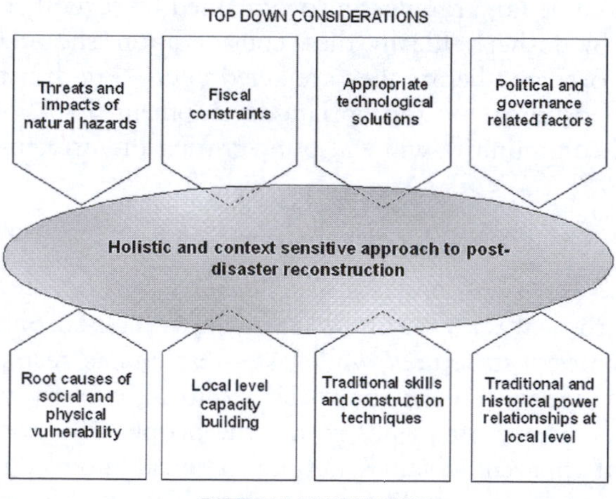

Figure 12.6 A holistic approach to post-disaster reconstruction. A simplified representation of what is a very complex set of issues that will need to be considered if a more holistic approach to post-disaster reconstruction is to be attained. It is the interface between the top down and bottom up factors that constitutes this holistic approach.

events, while socio-economic and political processes were excluded from the analytical framework. This view tended to divorce the 'disaster events' from 'everyday life', thus missing the links between the two.[7,9,25] However, studies and policy over the last 20 years has shown that understanding the social and economic forces that govern societies and create vulnerability should have the same emphasis as understanding the physical processes. It has been this paradigm shift that has contributed to the move away from the reactive attributes of 'disaster management' towards the more proactive 'disaster risk management' (DRM) approach that should now be 'mainstreamed' into developmental initiatives.

Fiscal constraints plus local-level capacity building

The resources required to reduce levels of vulnerability are finite and it is essential that agencies assess which members of society they should provide assistance to and in what ways the assistance should be provided.[6] For instance, it has been demonstrated that establishing networks with certain social institutions can help to increase people's coping strategies and therefore their resilience.[1,3,5] Jigyasu states that five main issues and challenges are evident in the context of rural communities of South Asia for reducing their disaster vulnerability through building local knowledge and capacities. These are:

1 loss of material and land resources (from rural communities);
2 loss of traditional skills;
3 cultural incompatibility of external interventions;
4 increasing social and economic inequity; and
5 weakening of local governance.[11]

Therefore, where building standards are not enforced, hazard-resistant construction will become common only if appropriate technology is locally available, widely known, easy to adopt with limited training and education, competitively priced or low-cost and culturally accepted (also refer to Chapters 2 and 3).[11] While the finances made available for long-term development and post-disaster reconstruction are likely to be constrained, it is essential to assess which institutions are effective in helping to build capacity within communities, particularly for the most vulnerable people.

Appropriate technological solutions incorporating traditional skills and construction techniques

Jigyasu presents a case for avoiding the categorisation of traditional and scientific knowledge into mutually exclusive domains.[13] Rather, attempts should be made to reconcile the two; science can enable traditional knowledge systems to be easily understood by the professionals, and traditional knowledge enables scientific concepts to be translated into modes of communication that are locally understood. The theoretical attractiveness of this proposition is obvious, but its practical realisation requires an open-mindedness on the part of built-environment professionals and local communities to embrace traditional/contemporary methods, and it also requires the safeguarding of traditional skills and knowledge while ensuring that they are informed by scientific understanding of future hazards. However, overcoming these challenges is necessary to safeguard and diffuse the knowledge of traditional techniques that have demonstrably led to hazard-resistant buildings (and to more appropriate site selection) in the past. Adapting and reapplying this knowledge will ensure that it evolves in a way that accords with the changing nature of threats, since it will benefit from information provided by the involvement of those with knowledge of the local context.[8]

Political and governance-related factors incorporating traditional and historic power relationships at the local level

Bosher concluded that the main factors that appear to influence levels of vulnerability (to a wide range of hazards) in the coastal regions of Andhra Pradesh were caste, gender, the type of village the respondents inhabit and their involvement with community-based organisations (CBOs) and NGOs.[3] The research showed that there appears to be a hierarchy of vulnerability based along the lines of caste classification, with the 'highest' castes being the least vulnerable and the 'lowest' castes being the most vulnerable. This observation was also made regarding levels of education and the quality of housing, in that the 'lower castes' obtained the lowest levels of education and tended to live in basic shelters on marginal land.

It was concluded that many of the respondents in the study were poor, marginalised and powerless *because* they are low caste; therefore they were the most vulnerable *because* of their status within society. Bosher and co-authors suggest that caste is a dominant social institution that influences levels of vulnerability because it not only affects the most vulnerable respondents' current levels of vulnerability but it also means that their ability to change their circumstances is restricted through enduring caste-defined inequalities concerning access to the resources that might help them to increase their levels of resilience.[5] Of course it is not caste per se that has these effects but the stigma, status and social processes that inevitably accompany it.

Therefore it is important to not only be aware of the prevailing macro-level political issues but also to be attuned to localised power struggles and how these can impinge upon efforts to improve social resilience. For instance, conducting an analysis of social institutional roles from a local perspective will give developmental and vulnerability-reduction agencies and practitioners a better understanding of the socio-political structures of the communities with whom they work. The intention is that the interventions they initiate in the future will be better targeted and ultimately be more appropriate and sustainable than they have been in the past.

Towards interventions that are holistic and contextually appropriate

This chapter has presented a (not unusual) case of how ill-thought-out and overly technocratic approaches to post-disaster reconstruction can severely impinge upon efforts to attain not only physical resilience but also social resilience. It has been stated that such approaches can be constrained due to a number of factors, such as poor consultation with the local communities, the imposition of inappropriate technology, low levels of construction skills within the local community to maintain certain types of structures and ultimately an insufficient understanding by many development agencies of what the recipients of post-disaster assistance actually need.

Undertaking focused and participatory research aimed at understanding the needs and limitations on the local people made it possible to find out what the local communities actually needed. In the Andhra Pradesh case, the house design that was developed by a wide range of villagers, male and female, young and old, was suitable for the context in which they live and was therefore not a standard or transferable solution. What has been important to recognise is that although time and effort is required, it is essential to adopt a more holistic approach to post-disaster reconstruction: a contextually appropriate approach that embraces the interfaces between the top-down and bottom-up issues.

Acknowledgements

The author is grateful to the Flood Hazard Research Centre, Middlesex University, for financing this study and to Edmund Penning-Rowsell, Sue Tapsell, Peter Winchester and Sarah Bradshaw for advice and support throughout the duration of the research that has contributed to this chapter. In addition, the author would like to thank the individuals and organisations that provided valuable assistance during field work in Andhra Pradesh. Most importantly, the author would like to extend heartfelt gratitude to all the villagers involved in this study for their time, patience, hospitality and generosity. The research was undertaken to more clearly understand the nature of socio-economic vulnerability and resilience in the context of social interactions.

13 From complexity to strategic planning for sustainable reconstruction

Gonzalo Lizarralde, Cassidy Johnson and Colin Davidson

Attempts to simplify the problem of post-disaster reconstruction, reducing it to technical issues, building design, choice of materials, etc., rarely produce positive results. Instead, the challenges have to be tackled and understood within their real and full complexity. Understanding this complexity and mastering it through a systems approach is necessary to improve reconstruction practices, as it leads to understanding the interrelations between the various processes involved in a reconstruction project and thence to developing an appropriate organization.

Understanding and tackling complexity

The previous chapters in this book amply show that post-disaster reconstruction has many levels of complexity – politico-social complexity, economic complexity, technical complexity, organizational complexity and functional complexity:

- politico-social complexity – because of the large numbers of stakeholders, their different origins and cultures and their not-so-converging priorities (without mentioning their often-hidden agendas);
- economic complexity – because of the structures of financing through international and national public entities and the demands of private-sector fund-raising, added to the complexity of deciding how much to invest in immediate relief or in sustainable development;
- technical complexity – because of the need to choose between imported and local building methods, within several timescales and within the contexts of available skills and technologies, and within the constraints of climate and logistics;
- organizational complexity – because decisions have to be taken and activities initiated rapidly and coherently, in the best interests of the affected communities; various actors with different organizational cultures, and sometimes limited experience, have to work together, often without a clear project leader;
- functional complexity – because housing requires much more than the creation of houses; successful human habitats require multiple services

and public and private spaces of different natures and different uses.

In situations of such multi-level complexity, some way to tackle the interlocking problems is necessary, and it must translate into coordinated action plans for each of the involved parties – even if there is no obvious "project leader."

This sort of situation calls for a systems approach to problem definition and to problem-solving; the systems approach helps to get a handle on the complexities and to support the decision-making processes of the many stakeholders.

The systems approach

As defined by Hall,[2] a *system* is a set of elements having relations between them and their attributes, and the key to the systems approach lies in choosing the class of elements to be attended to and the kinds of relationships that are of interest in a given context. In other words, a given complex situation can be considered as a system from a number of different points of view. In the five complexities just mentioned, for example, one can understand a situation and its participants in political and social terms (these are the "elements" in the definition of a system) and then consider the relationships, which, for better or for worse, anticipate how they do (or might) interact for the reconstruction challenge. Similarly, the same situation can be differently described in terms of economics, techniques, organizational patterns and functional patterns. For example, in Chapter 11, Roger Zetter and Camillo Boano pick up on the politico-social and organizational complexity of reconstruction programs, describing the challenges of integrating strategies of local, national and international institutions into one coordinated response. In a systems approach, each one of these entities can be conceived of as part of the same system (working toward the same goal), and their relations and roles can be understood as part of the system. In Chapter 12, Lee Bosher points out the need for professionals engaged in reconstruction to understand traditional and historic power relations at the local level.

In this way, each level of the general complexity is powerfully apprehended in terms not so much of the individual parts that make up the system (which are many and heterogeneous) but rather in terms of the patterns of parts (which are few) and the relationships between them, which can be formal (explicitly chosen and defined) or, no less important, informal (those relationships that do not correspond to legal or administrative responsibilities).

However, because of the very fact that there are several levels of complexity within the reconstruction task, it is important that some enriched systems approach allows them to be seen together, since one view of a system (the politico-social view, for example) is closely tied into the others (the economic, technical, functional and organizational views, in this instance). Here, another concept borrowed from the world of systems engineering can help, and that is the notion of *environment*.

Every system exists in an environment, and, by definition, the environment of a system is the set of objects that lie *outside* the system but (a) that are directly or indirectly affected by a change of the system (sometimes in almost imperceptible manners); or (b) which affect the system if they change.[2] There are two types of environments: one close (or immediate) environment to the system over which the project participants have influence and one larger environment over which they do not have any significant influence. For example, the immediate neighbors of a given project are part of a close environment; the project participants can influence (mediate, negotiate, convince, persuade, etc.) these neighbors. On the other hand (again by way of example), a major economic crisis in the Western world is part of the larger environment of the economics of a project, with almost certain financial repercussions on any post-disaster program or projects; however, architects, engineers and other stakeholders cannot significantly influence political or macro-economic conditions for the benefit of their project.

Furthermore, again taking as an example the same economic level of complexity, the complexities at the other levels (politico-social, technical, functional and organizational) are part of the environment of the economic level. To take another example, in reference to Chapter 7, as described by Graeme Bristol, the reconstruction of the fishing villages after the tsunami was largely affected by the environment outside the project, that is to say, by the international markets and thus the private developers looking to invest in and capitalize on tourism in the area. Participants in the reconstruction projects were eventually able to influence this environment (i.e. how much land the developers could claim) through perseverance in their struggle and involvement of actors from the state.

Project risks

The practical question is: How can this systems approach actually help with decision-making in the realities of post-disaster reconstruction?

In practice, the systems approach serves the decision-maker in three ways. First, it enables the complexities to be apprehended more easily, since the number of variables (controllable or uncontrollable) can be reduced to essentials, and second, it enables the complexities to be woven together across the habitual boundaries of direct responsibilities and corresponding disciplines. Last, it provides the decision-maker with a framework to understand possible influences on the project, allowing her/him to reduce the risk of oversights.

As we have seen, project participants exercise a direct influence over the system and its immediate environment and on its inherent risks, but no influence over risks that come from the larger environment (a political change in the Western world, for instance). Stakeholders can, however, anticipate those negative risks and prepare for them through three alternatives: (i) avoid the risk (avoiding the characteristics of the project that make it vulnerable to the risk); (ii) transfer the risk (sharing the risk or transferring it to other project participants who are better prepared to deal with it); or (iii) mitigate the risk (by assuming that it might occur but trying to reduce its negative effects and associating it with contingency plans aimed at dealing with those effects).[4] For example, Rohit Jigyasu, in Chapter 3, explains how providing a rigid design package is a high-risk manner to propose a new technology, as it is unlikely to be adopted by the beneficiaries. Instead, this risk can be greatly mitigated by developing the technology along with project participants, thus ensuring that the technology is appropriate and that the delivery mechanisms are institutionalized at the same time.

Consider also the example of community participation as described by Alicia Sliwinski in Chapter 9. As was shown, community participation is often reduced to nil or to sweat labor; in reality, there is a spectrum of levels of potential community participation, which can be equated with levels of community involvement in the necessary stages of reconstruction: project organization, project financing, project design and project construction/implementation[5] (Isabelle Maret and James Amdal show, in Chapter 6, that in the case they describe, communities are often doing all of these). A decision-maker trained in the systems approach will then:

1 avoid confusing the *objective* of the project (e.g. provide for sustainable economic recovery and wellbeing) with the possible *methods* to achieve it (e.g. decentralizing the collection of information about the real needs and expectations of affected residents) or with the available tools (e.g. transferring responsibility over decision-making to residents themselves so they can individually choose among a series of alternatives that are enhanced or facilitated by the project);
2 recognize that the performance of the project depends as much on the performance of the system itself as on the influences it might receive from the environment (the trained decision-maker will therefore identify and prepare for the risks that might negatively affect the implementation of a participatory approach);
3 understand that the important aspect is not so much composed of the elements of the system itself (construction materials, plots, building codes, reconstruction guidelines, control agencies, etc.) but of the relationships between them: the capacity of municipalities, for example, to influence residents to adopt building codes in subsequent additions made to their core units.

In practice, and taking the same example, this also means that difficult questions concerning the level of community participation can be meaningfully assessed and compared with alternatives that might include additional external resources. The emerging decision on this subject can then be checked against economic, social or cultural variables – all the while, the organizational openings (or constraints) that bear on the questions under consideration can be reviewed.

As we have seen in Chapter 8 and Chapter 2, owner-driven reconstruction (or user-driven reconstruction, as some prefer to call it) is more successful than contractor-oriented procurement strategies. This is precisely because owner-driven reconstruction distributes the responsibilities (and thus the project risks) among as many actors as there are beneficiaries involved. This strategy intelligently avoids the risk of beneficiaries' acceptance (or refusal) of the project and shares the risks of delays and cost over-runs with all the beneficiaries involved. It also allows for maximum variety and multiplicity of solutions to the individual problems, reducing almost to nil the chances of mistakes in designing once and for all the individual units of any construction project, as was the case in Dinar, Turkey (described by Nese Dikmen in Chapter 10). Owner-driven reconstruction avoids the dangers associated with centralized decision-making in the building industry – an industry that is largely characterized by high levels of uncertainty.

From tactical to strategic planning

As we have seen in the chapters of this book, decision-makers in reconstruction projects often make the same mistakes over and over again. This apparent short memory is not exclusive to the reconstruction sector. It is also well known by actors of the building industry and by project managers.

In fact, project managers of the building sector often identify two types of management actions: tactical planning, which concerns the decisions made within the boundaries of one single project, and strategic planning, which – by going beyond the boundaries of any one project – is concerned with making decisions that permit anticipating the position of a project (or of an organization, for that matter) in the mid- and long-term future and in the corresponding environments. Project managers also know that lessons learnt at the tactical level are rarely transferable to other projects or contexts. Various reasons explain this difficulty: (i) every project is unique and therefore knowledge useful for one project is not automatically transferable to another; (ii) actors change from one project to another, so the temporary multi-organizations[1] of the building sector do not easily allow for knowledge and experience to be kept and capitalized in the way it can be in other industries and corporations (where work is performed by relatively permanent teams); (iii) contexts change from project to project and so does the pertinence of the lessons themselves; (iv) project budgets and timelines rarely anticipate resources and time to collect, interpret, classify and distribute information derived from the lessons learned; and (v) project-based organizational cultures often neglect the importance of transferring knowledge between projects. It is for all these reasons that project managers also know of the importance of decision-making at the *strategic* level.

At first glance, strategic thinking seems to contradict the very functioning of the construction and reconstruction sectors (sectors that work on a project-by-project basis). However, even though the project teams are temporary and unique for each project, various actors of the reconstruction sector work consistently on various projects over and over again. National cooperation agencies, major funding bodies such as the World Bank and international banks, international agencies such as the Red Cross or the Red Crescent and various national and international NGOs are part of this group. Despite the fact that collective knowledge is often dispersed after the temporary multi-organization responsible for any given project is dissolved, these higher-level organizations are potentially capable of collecting knowledge and lessons learned and applying them in subsequent projects.

These organizations are also potentially capable of conducting systemic studies of a reconstruction problem and of collecting knowledge that can be transferred to subsequent projects, *prior* to taking irreversible steps such as actually launching a building project. Inevitably, some broad-scope studies have to be performed rapidly post-disaster – unless adequate upfront planning has been done (which is preferable). And here again is a systemic decision that should be (or should have been) made: *should* one and *how can* one plan for a disaster that is likely to occur but that nobody can really foresee in timing, location and extent (with the possible exception of hurricanes, which occur seasonally and regionally with sinister regularity).

These broad-scope studies relate primarily (a) to identifying the stakeholders, their characteristics, requirements, rights and powers; and (b) to designing the organization that enables them to contribute, as best as possible, to the reconstruction tasks (see Chapter 5 for an expanded discussion on organizational design). NGOs, for example, can plan strategically and thus recognize their strengths and weaknesses in a given present environment and those that will change in the future – are they experienced with urban planning and construction, for example? Or, do they represent a particular cultural slant? Chapter 4 discusses how this can be applied for governments doing strategic planning for temporary housing – for example, making procurement arrangements with suppliers or designating land to be held available for temporary housing.

Despite, or perhaps because of, the rigor required by the systems approach, it is reasonable to suggest that instead of "starting from scratch" in planning for post-disaster reconstruction, there should be some mechanism that ensures that hard-won experience is made available in a totally disinterested way to organizations and entities faced with an impending catastrophe.[3] In a sector that is largely characterized by uncertainty, a stable supportive mechanism of this sort (which has to be created at the international and also at the national level) must be designed so that information drawn from experience and also explicit and tacit knowledge can be gathered, stocked, organized and made available as needed. However, the creation of such sources of information and experience is no substitute for each participant (institution or group of individuals) adopting a systematic approach to solving the disaster-induced problems, however urgent they may be.

In addition to proposals for mechanisms for stocking experience-based information derived from earlier disasters and earlier reconstruction efforts, access to abundant information to help decision-making *immediately after* a disaster is of paramount importance. In this context, it is noteworthy that popularized information technology (internet and social-networking sites) can be, and have been, used to generate rapid multi-layered information extremely fast. Lea Winerman[6] explains how affected people and their relatives can spread literally up-to-the-minute information about the real extent of an emergency; she quotes examples of research into the ravages of the forest fires in California in 2007 and the earthquake in Sichuan in 2008.

Comparing this emerging resource with the habitual approach to post-emergency information, Winerman[6] writes specifically about official post-disaster information that "the system, with a clear top-down chain of command, views communication with the public as a one-way street: information is supposed to flow from officials to the public via warnings sent out to the public." However, and quite differently, social networking can be mobilized because "when people are under threat, perceived or actual, they go into this intensified information seeking period [...] and these days, they are increasingly doing so through social networking sites. But social-network users often end up bypassing the authorities – a tendency that has left officials scrambling to use this information and integrate it into traditional responses."

Participation by the affected population is now assuming an added dimension; mechanisms to take advantage of it have to be devised and recorded for best use in a rapidly changing environment.

References

1 Rebuilding after disasters: from emergency to sustainability

1 Arnstein, S.R., 1969. A ladder of citizen participation. *Journal of the American Institute of Planners*, 35 (4), 216–24.

2 Beatley, T., 2003. Green urbanism and the lessons of European cities. *In* R. LeGates and F. Stout, eds. *The city reader*. 3rd ed. London: Routledge, 399–408.

3 Blaikie, P., *et al.*, 1994. *At risk: natural hazards, people's vulnerability and disasters*. London: Routledge.

4 Cafered, 2000. *Editorial Noticias (News editorial)*, 25 January, p. 15. Bogotá: Federación Nacional de Cafeteros de Colombia.

5 Choguill, M.B.G., 1996. A ladder of community participation for underdeveloped countries. *Habitat International*, 20 (3), 431–44.

6 Davidson, C., *et al.*, 2007. Truths and myths about community participation in post-disaster housing projects. *Habitat International*, 31 (1), 100–15.

7 Davidson, C., Lizarralde, G. and Johnson, C., 2008. Myths and realities of prefabrication for post-disaster reconstruction. *In 4th international i-Rec conference on post-disaster reconstruction: building resilience, achieving effective post-disaster reconstruction* [pdf], 30 April – 2 May, Christchurch. Montreal: i-Rec. Available at http://www.grif.umontreal.ca/i-Rec.htm [Accessed 10 August 2008].

8 Fijalkow, Y., 2002. *Sociologie de la ville (Urban sociology)*. Paris: La découverte.

9 Gendron, L., 2007. Trop pauvre pour construire cheap *(Too poor to build cheap)*. *L'Actualité* [online], July. Available at http://www.lactualite.com/shared/print.jsp?content=20070531_154113_600& [Accessed 15 June 2007].

10 Hewitt, K., 1997. *Regions of risk: a geographical introduction to disasters*. London: Longman.

11 Imperadori, M., 2006. L'armadillo®: a new low-cost ready to build house system. *In* D. Alexander, *et al.*, eds. *Post-disaster reconstruction: meeting stakeholder interests*. Florence: Florence University Press, 393–403.

12 Jigyasu, R., 2000. From 'natural' to 'cultural' disaster: consequences of post-earthquake rehabilitation process on cultural heritage in Marathwada region, India. *In International conference on seismic performance of traditional buildings* [online], 16–18 November, Istanbul. Available at http://www.icomos.org/iiwc/seismic/Jigyasu.pdf [Accessed 15 January 2009].

13 Johnson, C., 2007. Impacts of prefabricated temporary housing after disasters: 1999 earthquakes in Turkey. *Habitat International*, 31 (1), 36–52.

14 Johnson, C., Lizarralde, G. and Davidson, C.H., 2006. A systems view of temporary housing projects in post-disaster reconstruction. *Construction Management and Economics*, 24 (2), 376–8.

15 Keivani, R., and Werna, E., 2001. Refocusing the housing debate in developing countries from a pluralist perspective. *Habitat International*, 25 (2), 191–208.
16 Kellett, P., and Franco, F., 1993. Technology for social housing in Latin America. *Habitat International*, 17 (4), 47–58.
17 Lizarralde, G., 2004. *Organizational design and performance of post-disaster reconstruction projects in developing countries*. Thesis (PhD). Université de Montréal.
18 Lizarralde, G., 2008. The challenge of low-cost housing for disaster prevention in small municipalities. *In 4th international i-Rec conference on post-disaster reconstruction: building resilience, achieving effective post-disaster reconstruction* [pdf], 30 April – 2 May, Christchurch. Montreal: i-Rec. Available at http://www.grif.umontreal.ca/i-Rec.htm [Accessed 10 August 2008].
19 Lizarralde, G., and Root, D., 2007. Ready-made shacks: learning from the informal sector to meet housing needs in South Africa. *In CIB world building congress: construction for development*, 14–17 May, Cape Town. Cape Town: CIB, 2068–2082.
20 Lizarralde, G., and Root, D., 2008. The informal construction sector and the inefficiency of low-cost housing markets. *Construction Management and Economics,* 26 (2), 103–13.
21 Lizarralde, G., and Massyn, M., 2007. Unexpected negative outcomes of community participation in low-cost housing projects in South Africa. *Habitat International*, 32 (1), 1–14.
22 Low, I., 2006. Negotiating extremes: global condition, local context. *Digest of South African Architecture, 2005–2006*. Cape Town: The South African Institute of Architects and Picasso Headline, 9–10.
23 Maskrey, A., 1989. *Disaster mitigation: a community based approach*. Oxford: Oxfam.
24 Phillips, B., 1996. *City lights: urban-suburban life in the global society.* New York: Oxford University Press.
25 Porter, M., 2003. The competitive advantage of the inner city. *In* R. LeGates and F. Stout, eds. *The city reader*. 3rd ed. London: Routledge, 277–89.
26 Putnam, R., 2003. Bowling alone: America's declining social capital. *In* R. LeGates and F. Stout, eds. *The city reader*. 3rd ed. London: Routledge, 105–13.
27 Quarantelli, E.L., 1995. Patterns of shelter and housing in US disasters. *Disaster Prevention and Management,* 4 (3), 43–53.
28 Rossi, A., 1999. *The architecture of the city*. 10th ed. New York: Opposition Books.
29 Sassen, S., 2001. The impact of the new technologies and globalization of cities. *In* R. LeGates and F. Stout, eds. *The city reader*. 3rd ed. London: Routledge, 212–20.
30 Schoenauer, N., 1994. *Cities, suburbs, dwellings in the postwar era*. Montreal: McGill University.
31 Stallen, M., Cabannes, Y. and Steinberg, F., 1994. Potentials of prefabrication for self-help and mutual-aid housing in developing countries. *Habitat International*, 18 (20), 13–39.
32 Turner, J.F.C., 1977. *Housing by people: towards autonomy in building environments*. New York: Pantheon Books.
33 Tzonis, A., and Lefaivre, L., 2003. *Critical regionalism*. New York: Prestel.
34 United Nations Department of Humanitarian Affairs – UNDHA, 1992. *Glossary: internationally agreed glossary of basic terms related to disaster management.* Geneva: UNDHA.
35 United Nations Disaster Relief Organization – UNDRO, 1982. *Shelter after disaster: guidelines for assistance*. New York: UNDRO.
36 United Nations International Strategy for Disaster Risk Reduction – UN/ISDR,

2009. *UNISDR terminology on disaster risk reduction* [online]. Geneva: UN/ISDR. Available at http://www.unisdr.org/eng/terminology/terminology-2009-eng.html [accessed 26 January 2009].

37 Wegelin, E., and Borgman, K., 1995. Options for municipal interventions in urban poverty alleviation. *Environment and Urbanization,* 7 (2), 131–52.

38 Wheeler, S., 1998. Planning sustainable and livable cities. The impact of the new technologies and globalization of cities. *In* R. LeGates and F. Stout, eds. *The city reader*. 3rd ed. London: Routledge, 486–96.

39 Wisner, B., 2001. Risk and the neoliberal state: why post-Mitch lessons didn't reduce El Salvador's earthquake losses. *Disasters: The Journal of Disaster Studies, Policy and Management*, 25 (3), 251–68.

2 Post-disaster low-cost housing solutions: learning from the poor

1 Bhatt, V., and Rybczynski, W., 2003. How the other half builds. *In* D. Watson, A. Plattus and R. Shibley, eds. *Time-saver standards for urban design*. New York: McGraw-Hill, 1.3.1–1.3.11.

2 Brand, S., 1994. *How buildings learn: what happens after they're built*. New York: Penguin.

3 Davidson, C.H., Johnson, C., Lizarralde, G., Dikmen, N., and Sliwinski, A., 2007. Truths and myths about community participation in post-disaster housing projects. *Habitat International*, 31 (1), 100–15.

4 Davidson, C., Lizarralde, G. and Johnson, C., 2008. Myths and realities of prefabrication for post-disaster reconstruction. *In 4th international i-Rec conference on post-disaster reconstruction: building resilience, achieving effective post-disaster reconstruction* [pdf], 30 April – 2 May, Christchurch. Montreal: i-Rec. Available at http://www.grif.umontreal.ca/i-Rec.htm [Accessed 10 August 2008].

5 Feng, V., Russell, A. and Potangaroa, R., 2008. Can houses learn? *In 4th international i-Rec conference on post-disaster reconstruction: building resilience, achieving effective post-disaster reconstruction* [pdf], 30 April – 2 May, Christchurch. Montreal: i-Rec. Available at http://www.grif.umontreal.ca/i-Rec.htm [Accessed 10 August 2008].

6 Ferguson, B., and Navarrete, J., 2003. A financial framework for reducing slums: lessons from experience in Latin America. *Environment and Urbanization,* 15 (2), 201–16.

7 Kellett, P., and Tipple G., 2000. The home as a workplace: a study of income generating activities within the domestic setting. *Environment and Urbanization*, 12 (1), 203–13.

8 Lizarralde, G., 2004. *Organizational design and performance of post-disaster reconstruction projects in developing countries*. Thesis (PhD). Université de Montréal.

9 Lizarralde, G., 2008. The challenge of low-cost housing for disaster prevention in small municipalities. *In 4th international i-Rec conference on post-disaster reconstruction: building resilience, achieving effective post-disaster reconstruction* [pdf], 30 April – 2 May, Christchurch. Montreal: i-Rec. Available at http://www.grif.umontreal.ca/i-Rec.htm [Accessed 10 August 2008].

10 Lizarralde, G., and Boucher, M.F., 2004. Learning from post-disaster reconstruction for pre-disaster planning. In *2nd international conference on post-disaster reconstruction: planning for reconstruction*, 22–3 April, Coventry. Coventry University, 8-14–8-24.

11 Lizarralde, G. and Massyn, M., 2007. Unexpected negative outcomes of community participation in low-cost housing projects in South Africa. *Habitat International*, 32 (1), 1–14.

12 Lizarralde, G., and Root, D., 2007. Ready-made shacks: learning from the

informal sector to meet housing needs in South Africa. *In CIB world building congress: construction for development*, 14–17 May 2007, Cape Town. Cape Town: CIB, 2068–2082.
13 Lizarralde, G., and Root, D., 2008. The informal construction sector and the inefficiency of low-cost housing markets. *Construction Management and Economics,* 26 (2), 103–13.
14 Simon, H., 1996. *The sciences of the artificial.* Cambridge, MA: Massachusetts Institute of Technology University Press.
15 Turner, J.F.C., 1977. *Housing by people: towards autonomy in building environments*. New York: Pantheon Books.

3 Appropriate technology for post-disaster reconstruction

1 Arya, A.S., 2002. *Guidelines for repair, restoration and retrofitting of masonry buildings in Kachchh earthquake affected areas of Gujarat*. Ahmedabad: Gujurat State Disaster Management Authority.
2 Freire, P., 2007. *Pedagogy of the oppressed.* New York: Continuum.
3 *Hunnar Shaala foundation for building technology and innovations, Bhuj, India* [online], 2007. Available at http://hunnar.org/projects.htm [Accessed 15 August 2008].
4 Jigyasu, R., 2002. *Reducing disaster vulnerability through local knowledge and capacity: the case of earthquake prone rural communities in India and Nepal.* Thesis (Dr. Eng). Trondheim: Norwegian University of Science and Technology.
5 Jigyasu, R., 2005. Disaster: a "reality" or "construct"? Perspective from the "East". *In* R.W. Perry and E.L. Quarantelli, eds. *What is a disaster? New answers to the old questions.* Philadelphia: Xlibris Corporation, 49–59.
6 Jigyasu, R., 2008. Structural adaptation in South Asia. *In* L. Bosher, ed. *Hazards and the built environment.* London: Taylor & Francis, 74–94.
7 Langenbach, R., 2001. A rich heritage lost, the Bhuj, India, earthquake. *Cultural Resource Management Magazine,* 24 (8), 33–4.
8 Mistry R., Dong, W. and Shah, H., eds., 2001. *Interdisciplinary observations on the January 2001 Bhuj, Gujarat earthquake. World seismic safety initiative and Earthquakes and megacities initiative* [pdf]. Available at http://www.rms.com/publications/Bhuj_EQ_Report.pdf [Accessed 4 April 2009].
9 Oanda, 2008. *The currency site: foreign exchange services and trading* [online]. Available at http://www.oanda.com [Accessed 2 August 2008].
10 Quebral, N., 2001. Development communication in a borderless world. *In National conference-workshop on the undergraduate development communication curriculum: new dimensions, bold decisions,* 23 November, University of the Philippines Los Baños. Los Baños University Press, 15–28.
11 United Nations Development Programme – UNDP, 2001. *From relief to recovery – the Gujarat experience.* [pdf] New York: UNDP. Available at http://www.preventionweb.net/english/professional/publications [Accessed 28 July 2008].
12 University of Colorado, 2009. *Gujarat earthquake January 2001* [online]. Available at http://cires.colorado.edu/~bilham/Gujarat2001.html [Accessed 4 April 2009].
13 Unnati Organisation for Development Education, 2006. *Owner driven housing process post earthquake reconstruction programme: Bhachau.* [pdf] Ahmedabad: Unnati. Available at http://www.unnati.org/books.html [Accessed 6 January 2009].

4 Planning for temporary housing

1 Alexander, D., 1986. *Disaster preparedness and the 1984 earthquakes in central Italy*. Natural Hazards Center working paper no. 55. Boulder, CO: University of Colorado.

2 Arslan, H., and Cosgun, N., 2008. Reuse and recycle potentials of the temporary houses after occupancy: example of Duzce, Turkey. *Building and Environment,* 43 (5), 702–9.

3 Comerio, M., 1998. *Disaster hits home: new policy for urban housing recovery*. Berkeley, CA: University of California Press.

4 Dandoulaki, M., 1992. The reconstruction of Kalamata City after the 1986 earthquakes: some issues on the process of temporary housing. *In* Y. Aysan and I. Davis, eds. *Disasters and the small dwelling: perspectives for the UNIDNDR*. London: James and James, 136–45.

5 Davis, I., 1978. *Shelter after disaster*. Oxford: Oxford Polytechnic Press.

6 Geipel, R., 1982. *Disasters and reconstruction: the Friuli (Italy) earthquakes of 1976*. London: George Allen and Unwin.

7 Geipel, R., 1991. *Long-term consequences of disasters: the reconstruction of Friuli, Italy in its international context, 1976–1988*. New York: Springer-Verlag.

8 Hirayama, Y., 2000. Collapse and reconstruction: housing recovery policy in Kobe after the Hanshin great earthquake. *Housing Studies,* 15 (1), 111–28.

9 Johnson, C., 2002. What's the big deal about temporary housing? Types of temporary accommodation after disasters: an example of the 1999 Turkish earthquake. *In TIEMS 2002 international disaster management conference*, 15–17 May, Waterloo. University of Waterloo.

10 Johnson, C., 2007. Impacts of prefabricated temporary housing after disasters. *Habitat International,* 31 (1), 36–52.

11 Johnson, C., 2007. Strategic planning for post-disaster temporary housing. *Disasters: The Journal of Disaster Studies, Policy and Management,* 31 (4), 435–58.

12 Johnson, C., Lizarralde, G. and Davidson C.H., 2006. A systems view of temporary housing projects in post-disaster reconstruction. *Construction Management and Economics,* 24 (2), 367–78.

13 Maki, N., Muira, K., and Kobayashi, M., 1995. Emergency housing supply after the great Hanshin-Awaji disaster. In *4th Japan-United States workshop on urban earthquake hazard reduction,* 17–19 January, Osaka. Tokyo: Institute of Social Safety Science, 235–8.

14 Quarantelli, E.L., 1995. Patterns of shelter and housing in US disasters. *Disaster Prevention and Management,* 4 (3), 43–53.

15 Tomioka, T., 1997. Housing reconstruction measures from the great Hanshin-Awaji earthquake. *In 5th United States/Japan workshop on earthquake hazard reduction*, 15–17 January, Pasadena, CA. Oakland, CA: Earthquake Engineering Research Institute, 37–57.

16 United Nations Disaster Relief Organization – UNDRO, 1982. *Shelter after disaster: guidelines for assistance*. New York: UNDRO.

17 United Nations Office for the Coordination of Humanitarian Affairs –UN/OCHA, 2008. *Transitional settlements and reconstruction after natural disasters* [pdf]. Geneva: United Nations. Available at http://www.sheltercentre.org/library/Transitional+settlement+and+reconstruction+after+natural+disasters [Accessed 15 January 2009].

5 Multi-actor arrangements and project management

1 Ardie, A., 2008. NGOs and post-disaster reconstruction – solving logistics problems with clear policies. *Ethical Corporation Magazine* [online], June. Available at http://www.ethicalcorp.com/content.asp?ContentID=4229 [Accessed 24 June 2008].
2 Conklin, J., 2006. Wicked problems and social complexity. *In* J. Conklin, ed., *Dialogue mapping: building social understanding of wicked problems*. New York: Wiley Management Science, 3–41.
3 Davidson, C.H., 1988. Building team. *In* J.A. Wilkes and R.T. Packard, eds. *Encyclopedia of architecture: design, engineering & construction*, vol. 1. New York: John Wiley and Sons, 509–15.
4 Flack, J., 2008. Security in an uncertain world. *Nature*, 453, 451–2.
5 Johnson, C., Lizarralde, G. and Davidson, C.H., 2005. Reconstruction in developing countries – a case for meta-procurement. *In International symposium of CIB Working Commission W92, procurement systems: the impact of cultural differences and systems on construction performance*, 8–10 February, Las Vegas. Tempe, AZ: Arizona State University PBSRG, 87–97.
6 Katsanis, C.J., and Davidson, C.H., 1995. Horizon 2020: how will North America build? *International Journal of Architectural Management Practice & Research*, 9, 146–62.
7 Masterman, J.W.E., 2002. *An introduction to building procurement systems*. London and New York: Spon Press.
8 Mohsini, R., and Davidson, C.H., 1991. Building procurement – key to improved performance. *Building Research and Information*, 19 (2), 106–13.
9 Mohsini, R., and Davidson, C.H., 1992. Determinants of performance in the traditional building process. *Construction Management and Economics*, 10 (4), 343–59.
10 Project Management Institute, 2004. *A guide to the project management body of knowledge*. Newtown Square, PA: Project Management Institute.
11 Rittel, H.W.J., and Webber, M.M., 1973. Dilemmas in a general theory of planning. *Policy Sciences*, 4, 155–69.
12 Simon, H.A., 1996. *The sciences of the artificial*. 3rd ed. Cambridge, MA: MIT Press.
13 Syarief, A., and Hibino, H., 2003. Evaluating the semantic approach through Horst Rittel's second generation systems analysis. *Journal of the Asian Design International Conference* [pdf]. Available at http://www.idemployee.id.tue.nl/g.w.m.rauterberg/conferences/CD_doNotOpen/ADC/final_paper/014.pdf. [Accessed 15 June 2008].
14 United Nations Economic Commission for Europe – UNECE, 1959. *Government policies and the cost of building*. Geneva: UNECE.

6 Stakeholder participation in post-disaster reconstruction programmes – New Orleans' Lakeview: a case study

1 City of New Orleans, 2007. *Dr Kevin Stephens testified today before a U.S. House of Representatives' Subcommittee* [press release], 13 March. New Orleans: City of New Orleans.
2 Gordon, C., 2005. Bush rhetoric evokes other Gulf. *Newsday* [online], September 16. Available at http://www.newsday.com/news/nationworld/nation/ny-usbush164427986sep16,0,5174051.story [Accessed 20 September 2005].
3 *Greater New Orleans Community Data Center* [online], 2008. Available at http://www.gnocdc.org [Accessed 12 January 2009].
4 Louisiana Association of Business and Industry, 2006. The recovery continues.

LABI Enterprise [pdf], 31 (2), 15. Available at http://www.labi.org/assets/docs/news/JuneEnterpriseWeb%2006.pdf [Accessed 14 September 2007].

5 Louisiana Recovery Authority, 2006. *Governor Blanco, LRA and Workforce Commission launch $38 million workforce training program focused on sectors with highest demand.* Baton Rouge, LA: Louisiana Recovery Authority. Available at http://www.lra.louisiana.gov/index.cfm?md=newsroom&tmp=detail&articleID=294 [Accessed 12 January 2009].

6 Manyena, S.B., 2006. The concept of resilience revisited. *Disasters: The Journal of Disaster Studies, Policy and Management*, 30 (4), 434–50.

7 Maugh, T., and Kaplan, K., 2007. Katrina leaves permanent scar on forests. *Los Angeles Times* [online], 16 November. Available at http://www.latimes.com/news/la-sci-trees16nov16,0,685072.story?coll=la-home-center [Accessed 14 December 2007].

8 Nelson, M., Ehrenfeucht, R., and Laska, S., 2007. Planning, plans, and people: professional expertise, local knowledge, and governmental action in post-Hurricane Katrina New Orleans. *Cityscape,* 9 (3), 23–52.

9 Pelling, M., 2003. *The vulnerability of cities: natural disasters and social resilience*. London: Earthscan.

10 Vale, L.J., and Campanella, T.J., 2005. *The resilient city: how modern cities recover from disaster*. New York: Oxford University Press.

11 Vogel, C., *et al.*, 2007. Linking vulnerability, adaptation, and resilience science to practice: pathways, players, and partnerships. *Global Environmental Change,* 17 (3–4), 349–64.

7 Surviving the second tsunami: land rights in the face of buffer zones, land grabs and development

1 Asian Coalition for Housing Rights, 2005. Housing by people in Asia. *Newsletter of the Asian Coalition for Housing Rights* [pdf], (16), August. Available at http://www.achr.net/000ACHRTsunami/Download%20TS/ACHR%2016%20with%20photos.pdf [Accessed 10 January 2009].

2 Asian Coalition for Housing Rights, 2006. Tsunami update Thailand: 18 months later. *Newsletter of the Asian Coalition for Housing Rights* [online], June. Available at http://www.achr.net/000ACHRTsunami/Tsunami%20Update%2016/01Update.html [Accessed 10 January 2009].

3 Centre for Policy Alternatives – CPA, 2006. *Landlessness and land rights in post-tsunami Sri Lanka: report commissioned by the IFRC* [pdf]. Colombo, Sri Lanka: CPA. Available at http://www.cpalanka.org/research_papers.html [Accessed 10 January 2009].

4 Community Organizations Development Institute – CODI, 2006. CODI fact sheet. *People's leadership in disaster recovery: rights, resilience and empowerment international workshop*, 30 October – 1 November, Phuket, Thailand.

5 Cuny, F.C., 1983. *Disasters and development*. New York: Oxford University Press.

6 De Silva, C., 2005. *Tsunami recovery in Sri Lanka: housing* [online]. Sri Lanka: World Bank. Available at http://web.worldbank.org/WBSITE/EXTERNAL/COUNTRIES/SOUTHASIAEXT/0,contentMDK:20751445~pagePK:146736~piPK:146830~theSitePK:223547,00.html [Accessed 10 January 2009].

7 Ekachai, S., 2005. Tsunami aftermath/help or hurt. *Bangkok Post* [online], 2 March. Available at http://www.karencenter.com/showstateless.php?id=987&comm=det [Accessed 10 January 2009].

8 Elias, D., 2005. *Education for sustainable development in action: another day in paradise? A place for indigenous people in protected areas, Thailand* [online]. Bangkok: UNESCO. Available at http://www.unescobkk.org/natural-sciences/

featured-projects/a-place-for-indigenous-people-in-protected-areas-thailand/newsevents/education-for-sustainable-development-in-action-another-day-in-paradise/ [Accessed 10 January 2009].

9 Fitzpatrick, D., 2008. *Women's rights to land and housing in tsunami-affected Aceh, Indonesia. Asia Research Institute, Aceh working paper no. 3* [pdf]. Singapore: National University of Singapore. Available at http://www.ari.nus.edu.sg/docs/downloads/aceh-wp/acehwps08_003.pdf [Accessed 10 January 2009].

10 Kälin, W., 2005. *Protection of internally displaced persons in situations of natural disasters. A working visit to Asia by the representative of the United Nations Secretary-General on the Human Rights of IDPs, 27 February to 5 March* [pdf]. Geneva: Office of the United Nations High Commissioner for Human Rights. Available at http://www.brookings.edu/fp/projects/idp/20050227_Tsunami.pdf [Accessed 10 January 2009].

11 Klein, N., 2007. *The shock doctrine: the rise of disaster capitalism*. New York: Henry Holt and Company.

12 Kraus, E., 2005. *Wave of destruction: one Thai village and its battle with the tsunami*. London: Satin.

13 Narumon, A., 2005. *Moken – their changing huts and village*. Bangkok: Chulalongkorn University Social Research Institute (quote from page 1).

14 Oxfam International, 2006. *The tsunami two years on: land rights in Aceh. Oxfam Briefing Note* [pdf], 30 November. Oxford: Oxfam International. Available at http://www.oxfam.org.uk/resources/policy/conflict_disasters/bn_tsunami2years.html [Accessed 10 January 2009].

15 PBS Online News Hour, 2006. Renewed violence in Sri Lanka raises fears of return to full-scale war. *PBS online news hour* [online], 15 June. Available at http://www.pbs.org/newshour/updates/asia/jan-june06/srilanka_06–15.html [Accessed 10 January 2009].

16 Robinson, G., 1993. *Shock therapy: restoring order in Aceh, 1989–1993*. London: Amnesty International.

17 Roosa, J., 2005. The tsunami and military rule: Aceh's dual disasters. *Counterpunch* [online], 12 January. Available at http://www.counterpunch.org/roosa01122005.html [Accessed 10 January 2009].

18 Saroor, S., 2006. Tsunami: what went wrong in NE Sri Lanka. *The South Asian* [online], 15 January. Available at http://www.thesouthasian.org/archives/2006/tsunami_what_went_wrong_in_ne.html [Accessed 10 January 2009].

19 Shanmugaratnam, N., 2005. Challenges of post-disaster development of coastal areas in Sri Lanka. Consultative workshop on post-tsunami reconstruction experiences of local NGOs, 23 November, Colombo [pdf]. Aas, Norway: Norwegian University of Life Sciences. Available at http://www.sacw.net/peace/ChallengesPostdisasterShanNovember2005.pdf [Accessed 10 January 2009].

20 Sinitchkina, S., 2005. Tsunami and Aceh conflict resolution. *Inventory of conflict and environment case studies* [online], (165), November. Washington DC: American University. Available at http://www.american.edu/ted/ice/tsunami-aceh.htm#three [Accessed 10 January 2009].

21 Sukarsono, A., 2005. Tsunami-hit Indonesia coast to get buffer zone. *ReliefWeb* [online], 7 February. Available at http://www.reliefweb.int/rw/rwb.nsf/db900SID/DDAD-69DUXH?OpenDocument [Accessed 10 January 2009].

22 Tourism Concern, 2008. *Tsunami of tourism* [online]. London: Tourism Concern. Available at http://www.tourismconcern.org.uk/index.php?page=tsunami-of-tourism [Accessed 10 January 2009].

23 United Nations Development Programme – UNDP, 2006. *Tsunami-hit Thai Muslim community granted land rights in a national park* [online]. Bangkok: UNDP-Thailand. Available at http://www.undp.or.th/newsandevents/2006/news-060307.html [Accessed 10 January 2009].

24 Wijetunge, J., 2006. Two years on: how safe are we from a future tsunami? *The Sunday Times* [online], 31 December. Available at http://sundaytimes.lk/061231/Plus/014_pls.html [Accessed 10 January 2009].

8 Who governs reconstruction? Changes and continuity in policies, practices and outcomes

1 Abhiyan, 2005. *Coming together: a document on the post-earthquake rehabilitation efforts by various organisations working in Kutch*. Bhuj: United Nations Development Program/Abhiyan.
2 Anath Pur, K., 2007. Rivalry or synergy? Formal and informal local governance in rural India. *Development and Change*, 38 (3), 401–27.
3 Asian Development Bank, United Nations Development Program and World Bank, 2005. *India post-tsunami recovery program: preliminary damage and needs assessment* [pdf]. Available at http://www.adb.org/Documents/Reports/Tsunami/india-assessment-full-report.pdf [Accessed 12 January 2009].
4 Aysan, Y., and Davis, I., 1992. *Disasters and the small dwelling*. Oxford: Pergamon Press.
5 Barakat, S., 2003. Housing reconstruction after conflict and disaster. *Humanitarian Practice Network paper no. 43*. London: Overseas Development Institute.
6 Casutt, D., 2007. *Change and continuity after disasters: the interplay between vulnerability, options and choices at community level and the influence of external actors on the reconstruction and rehabilitation process*. Thesis (Master's). University of Zurich.
7 Clinton, W.J., 2006. *Key propositions for building back better: a report by the UN Secretary General's Special Envoy for Tsunami Recovery*. New York: United Nations.
8 Davis, I., 1978. *Shelter after disaster*. Oxford: Oxford Polytechnic Press.
9 Duyne Barenstein, J., 2006. Challenges and risks in post-tsunami housing reconstruction in Tamil Nadu. *Humanitarian Exchange*, 33 (March), 38–9.
10 Duyne Barenstein, J., 2006. Housing reconstruction approaches in post-earthquake Gujarat: a comparative analysis. *Humanitarian Practice Network paper no. 54*. London: Overseas Development Institute.
11 Duyne Barenstein, J., and Pittet, D., 2006. *Towards sustainable post-disaster housing reconstruction: an empirical assessment of a housing reconstruction project in two tsunami-hit villages in coastal Tamil Nadu*. Lugano: World Habitat Research Unit.
12 Duyne Barenstein, J., and Pittet, D., 2007. Post-disaster housing reconstruction: current trends and sustainable alternatives for tsunami-affected communities in coastal Tamil Nadu. *Point Sud*, 8, 5–8.
13 Government of India, Ministry of Home Affairs, 2004. Disaster management in India: a status report. New Delhi: Government of India, Ministry of Home Affairs, National Disaster Management Division.
14 Government of Maharashtra, 2005. *Maharashtra emergency earthquake rehabilitation programme (MEERP)* [online]. Available at http://mdmu.maharashtra.gov.in/pages/meerp/profile.htm [Accessed 15 January 2009].
15 Government of Tamil Nadu/Government of Pondicherry, 2005. *India emergency tsunami reconstruction project* [pdf]. Available at http://www.tn.gov.in/tsunami/Tsunami_ESMF.pdf [Accessed 15 January 2009].
16 Gujarat State Disaster Management Authority, 2005. *Grit and grace: the story of reconstruction*. Gandhinagar: Gujarat State Disaster Management Authority Press.
17 Inglin, S., 2008. *The impacts of compensation payments after tsunami on artisan fishery: a case study from a south Indian fisher village*. University of Zurich

(unpublished manuscript).

18 Jigyasu, R., 2000. From 'natural' to 'cultural' disaster: consequences of post-earthquake rehabilitation process on cultural heritage in Marathwada region, India. *In International conference on seismic performance of traditional buildings* [online], 16–18 November, Istanbul. Available at http://www.icomos.org/iiwc/seismic/Jigyasu.pdf [Accessed 15 January 2009].

19 Jigyasu, R., 2002. *Reducing disaster vulnerability through local knowledge and capacity: the case of earthquake prone rural communities in India and Nepal.* Thesis (Dr. Eng). Trondheim: Norwegian University of Science and Technology.

20 Joshi, V., and Duyne Barenstein, J., 2005. *The role of humanitarian aid in the restoration of livelihoods in post-earthquake Gujarat: analysis and interpretation of a questionnaire-based citizens' survey*. Chennai: Ecosmart (unpublished manuscript).

21 Naimi-Gasser, J., 2008. The impact of tree loss upon social life: a call for cultural considerations in post-disaster housing reconstruction projects. Thesis (M.A.). University of Zurich.

22 Office for the Coordination of Humanitarian Affairs, 2008. *Transitional settlements and reconstruction after natural disasters* [pdf]. Geneva: United Nations. Available at http://www.sheltercentre.org/library/Transitional+settlement+and+reconstruction+after+natural+disasters [Accessed 15 January 2009].

23 Parasuraman, S., 1995. The impact of the 1993 Latur-Osmanabad earthquake on lives, livelihoods and propoerty. *Disasters: The Journal of Disaster Studies, Policy and Management*, 19 (2), 152–69.

24 Salazar, A., 1999. Disasters, The World Bank and participation: relocation housing after the 1993 Earthquake in Maharashtra, India. *Third World Planning Review*, 21 (1), 83–105.

25 Salazar, A., 2002. *Normal life after disaster? 8 years of housing lessons, from Marathwada to Gujarat: a response to K.S. Vatsa* [online]. Available at http://www.radixonline.org/gujarat6.htm [Accessed 15 January 2009].

26 Salazar, A., 2002. The crisis of modernity of housing disasters in the developing countries: participatory housing and technology after the Marathwada (1993) earthquake. *In International conference on post-disaster reconstruction: improving post-disaster reconstruction in developing countries* [pdf], 23–5 April, Montreal. Montreal: i-Rec. Available at http://www.grif.umontreal.ca/pages/papersmenu.html [Accessed 15 January 2009].

27 Scawthorn, C., 2007. Handbook on housing reconstruction following disasters: dialogue on housing – pre and post disaster [presentation]. *Stockholm forum for disaster reduction and recovery* [pdf], 23 October, Stockholm. Available at http://siteresources.worldbank.org/EXTDISMGMT/Resources/SCAWTHORNOCT23.pdf [Accessed 15 January 2009].

28 Sphere, 2004. Minimum standards in shelter, settlement and non-food items, Chapter 4. *Sphere humanitarian charter and minimum standards in disaster response handbook* [pdf]. Geneva: Sphere Project. Available at http://www.sphereproject.org/component/option,com_docman/task,cat_view/gid,17/Itemid,203/lang,english/ [Accessed 15 January 2009].

29 Tenconi, D., 2007. *L'impatto del terremoto sulla cultura abitativa e sull'organizzazione sociale dell'ambiente costruito in un villaggio del Kutch (India) (The impact of the earthquake on the social organization and housing culture in a village in Kutch, India)*. Thesis (Master's). University of Zurich.

30 Trachsel, S., 2008. *Die Wiederherstellung, der Wiederaufbau und Konflikte an der vom Tsunami 2004 betroffenen Küste Tamil Nadus.* (*Recovery, reconstruction and conflicts in 2004 tsunami-affected coastal Tamil Nadu, India*). Thesis (Master's). University of Zurich.

31 Trachsel, S., 2008. Post-tsunami reconstruction in a South Indian fishing village: the impact on elderly people's social security. Unpublished paper. University of Zurich.

32 United Nations Disaster Relief Organization – UNDRO, 1982. *Shelter after disaster: guidelines for assistance*. New York: UNDRO.

33 UN-Habitat, 2007. *Building back better in Pakistan* [pdf]. Nairobi: UN-Habitat. Available at http://www.unhabitat.org/downloads/docs/4627_75789_GC%20 21%20Financing%20Field%20Report%20Pakistan.pdf [Accessed 15 January 2009].

34 United Nations Development Program – UNDP, 2001. *From relief to recovery: the Gujarat experience*. Delhi: UNDP.

35 Vatsa, K. 2002. *Rhetoric and reality of post-disaster rehabilitation after the Latur earthquake of 1993: a rejoinder*. Available at http://www.radixonline.org/gujarat5.htm [Accessed 2 April 2009].

36 Vincentnathan, S.G., 1996. Caste, politics, violence and the panchayats in a South Indian Community. *Studies in Society and History*, 38 (3), 484–509.

37 World Bank and Asian Development Bank, 2001. *Gujarat earthquake recovery program: assessment report* [pdf]. New Delhi: World Bank. Available at http://siteresources.worldbank.org/INDIAEXTN/Resources/Reports-Publications/gujarat-earthquake/full_report.pdf [Accessed 15 January 2009].

9 The politics of participation: involving communities in post-disaster reconstruction

1 Anderson, M., and Woodrow, P., 1989. *Rising from the ashes: development strategies in times of disaster*. Boulder, CO: Lynne Rienner.

2 Arnstein, S.R., 1969. A ladder of citizen participation. *Journal of the American Institute of Planners*, 35 (4), 216–24.

3 Bankoff, G., Freks, G. and Hilhorst, D., eds., 2004. *Mapping vulnerability: disasters, development and people*. London: Earthscan.

4 Bourdieu, P., 1977. *Outline of a theory of practice*. Cambridge: Cambridge University Press.

5 Bourdieu, P., 1986. The forms of capital. *In* J. Richardson, ed. *Handbook of theory and research for the sociology of education*. New York: Greenwood Press, 241–58.

6 Bradshaw, S., 2001. Reconstruction roles and relations: women's participation in reconstruction in post-Mitch Nicaragua. *Gender and Development*, 9 (3), 79–87.

7 Chambers, R., 1987. *Rural development: putting the last first*. London: Longman.

8 Chambers, R., 1997. *Whose reality counts? Putting the first last*. London: Intermediate Technology Publications.

9 Chamlee-Wright, E., 2006. After the storm: social capital regrouping in the wake of hurricane Katrina. *Mercatus Center working paper series*, August. Arlington, VA: Mercatus Center at George Mason University.

10 Chamlee-Wright, E., 2007. The long road back. Signal noise in the post-Katrina context. *The Independent Review*, 12 (2), 235–59.

11 Choguill, M.B.G., 1996. A ladder of community participation for underdeveloped countries. *Habitat International*, 20 (3), 431–44.

12 Chossudovsky, M., 1996. *The globalization of poverty: impacts of IMF and World Bank reforms*. Atlantic Highlands, NJ: Zed Books.

13 Cleaver, F., 2001. Institutions, agency and the limitations of participatory approaches to development. *In* B. Cooke and U. Kothari, eds. *Participation: the new tyranny?* London: Zed Books, 36–56.

14 Coleman, J., 1990. *Foundation of social theory*. Cambridge, MA: Harvard University Press.
15 Cooke, B., and Kothari, U., eds., 2001. *Participation: the new tyranny?* London: Zed Books.
16 Cornwall, A., 1998. Gender, participation and the politics of difference. *In* I. Guijt and M. Shah, eds. *The myth of community: gender issues in participatory development*. London: Intermediate Technology, 46–57.
17 Cornwall, A., 2003. Whose voices? Whose choices? Reflections on gender and participatory development. *World Development*, 31 (8), 1325–42.
18 Cuny, F.C., 1983. *Disasters and development*. New York: Oxford University Press.
19 Cupples, J., 2007. Gender and hurricane Mitch: reconstructing subjectivities after disaster. *Disasters: The Journal of Disaster Studies, Policy and Management*, 31 (2), 155–75.
20 Davidson, C.H., *et al.*, 2007. Truths and myths about community participation in post-disaster housing projects. *Habitat International*, 31 (1), 100–15.
21 Davis, I., 1978. *Shelter after disaster*. Oxford: Oxford Polytechnic Press.
22 Duyne Barenstein, J., 2006. Housing reconstruction in post-earthquake Gujarat. A comparative analysis. *Humanitarian Practice Network paper no. 54*. London: Overseas Development Institute.
23 Enarson, E., 1998. Through women's eyes: a gendered research agenda for disaster social science. *Disasters: The Journal of Disaster Studies, Policy and Management*, 22 (2), 157–73.
24 Escobar, A., 1995. *Encountering development: the making and unmaking of the third world*. Princeton, NJ: Princeton University Press.
25 Etzioni, A., 1996. Positive aspects of community and the dangers of fragmentation. *Development and Change*, 27 (2), 301–14.
26 Ferguson, J., 1994. *The anti-politics machine: "development", depoliticization and bureaucratic power in Lesotho*. Minneapolis: University of Minnesota Press.
27 Foucault, M., 1977. *Discipline and punish: the birth of the prison*. Harmondsworth: Penguin.
28 Foucault, M., 1979. *History of sexuality: an introduction*. Harmondsworth: Penguin.
29 Freire, P., 1973. *Education for critical consciousness*. New York: Seabury Press.
30 Giddens, A., 1984. *The constitution of society: outline of the theory of structuration*. Cambridge: Polity Press.
31 Gossiaux, J.F., 2004. Communauté (Community). In *Dictionnaire de l'ethnologie et de l'anthropologie*. Paris: Presses Universitaires de France, 165–6.
32 Guijt, I., and Shah, M.K., eds., 1998. *The myth of community: gender issues in participatory development*. London: Intermediate Technology.
33 Hewitt, K., 1997. *Regions of risk: a geographical introduction to disasters*. London: Longman.
34 Hickey, S., and Mohan, G., eds., 2004. *Participation: from tyranny to transformation*. London: Zed Books.
35 Huizer, G., 1972. *El potencial revolucionario del campesino en America Latina, (The revolutionary potential of peasants in Latin America)*. Lexington, MA: Heath-Lexington Books.
36 Hyndman, J., 1998. Managing difference: gender and culture in humanitarian emergencies. *Gender, Place and Culture*, 5 (3), 241–60.
37 Jigyasu, R., 2001. From Marathwada to Gujarat – emerging challenges in post-earthquake rehabilitation for sustainable eco-development in South Asia. *In International conference on post-disaster reconstruction: improving post-disaster*

reconstruction in developing countries [pdf], 23–5 April, Montreal. Montreal: i-Rec. Available at http://www.grif.umontreal.ca/pages/papersmenu.html [Accessed 5 December 2008].

38 Kay, A., 2005. Social capital, the social economy and community development. *Community and Development Journal*, 41 (2), 160–73.

39 Long, C., 2001. *Participation of the poor in development initiatives*. London: Earthscan.

40 Long, N. and Long, A., eds., 1992. *Battlefields of knowledge: the interlocking of theory and practice in social research and development*. London: Routledge.

41 Mohan, G., 2001. Beyond participation: strategies for deeper empowerment. *In* B. Cooke and U. Kothari, eds. *Participation: the new tyranny?* London: Zed Books, 153–67.

42 Mosse, D., 2001. People's knowledge, participation and patronage: operations and representations in rural development. *In* B. Cooke and U. Kothari, eds. *Participation: the new tyranny?* London: Zed Books, 16–35.

43 Nelson, N., and Wright, S., eds., 1995. *Power and participatory development: theory and practice*. London: Intermediate Technology.

44 Oliver-Smith, A., 1990. Post-disaster housing reconstruction and social inequality: a challenge to policy and practice. *Disasters: The Journal of Disaster Studies, Policy and Management*, 14 (1), 7–19.

45 Pelling, M., 2007. Learning from others: the scope and challenges for participatory disaster assessment. *Disasters: The Journal of Disaster Studies, Policy and Management*, 31 (4), 73–85.

46 Ponthieux, S., 2006. *Le capital social* (Social capital). Paris: La Découverte.

47 Putman, R., 1993. The prosperous community: social capital and public life. *The American Prospect*, 4 (13), 35–42.

48 Rahnema, M., 1997. Participation. *In* W. Sachs, ed. *The development dictionary*. London: Zed Books.

49 Rossi, I., 1993. *Community reconstruction after an earthquake: dialectical sociology in action*. Westport, CT: Praeger.

50 Schilderman, T., 2004. Adapting traditional shelter for disaster mitigation and reconstruction: experiences with community-based approaches. *Building Research and Information*, 32 (5), 414–26.

51 Sliwinski, A., 2007. Désastre humanitaire dans la vallée des hamacs: les logiques de la reconstruction au Salvador (Humanitarian disaster in the valley of the hammocks: the logics of reconstruction in El Salvador). *Anthropologie et Sociétés*, 31 (2), 113–31.

52 Spaling, H., and Vroom, B., 2007. Environmental assessment after the 2004 tsunami: a case study, lessons and prospects. *Impact Assessment and Project Appraisal*, 25 (1), 45–52.

53 Stiglitz, J., 2002. *Globalization and its discontents*. New York: Norton.

54 Tönnies, F., 1887. *Community and society*. Translated by C.P. Loomis, 1957. East Lansing: Michigan State University Press.

55 Williams, R., 1976. *Keywords: a vocabulary of culture and society*. New York: Oxford University Press.

56 Wisner, B., *et al.*, 2004. *At risk: natural hazards, people's vulnerability and disasters*. 2nd ed. London: Routledge.

10 User requirements and responsible reconstruction

1 Balta, E., 1998. *Earthquake and social change: the case of Dinar*. Thesis (Master's). Ankara: Middle East Technical University.

2 Bayraktar, N. and Aksu, A., 1995. Kültür farklılığının konut tasarımında veri olarak değerlendirilmesinin gerekliliği (Necessity of evaluation of cultural

differences as the data for house design). In *VII international building and life congress: culture and space*, 25–30 April, Bursa. Bursa Branch of the Chamber of Architects, 235–46.
3 Demiröz, G., 1996. *A research on long-term effects of state resettlement projects in vernacular settings in rural areas: the case of Yüzüncü Yıl, Mudurnu*. Thesis (Master's). Ankara: Middle East Technical University.
4 Dikmen, N., 2005. *A provision model and design guidelines for permanent post-disaster housing in rural areas of Turkey based on an analysis of reconstruction projects in Çankırı*. Thesis (PhD). Ankara: Middle East Technical University.
5 Hofstede, G., 1980. *Culture's consequences: international differences in work-related values*. Newbury Park, CA: Sage.
6 Oliver, P., and Aysan, Y., 1987. *Housing and culture after earthquakes: a guide for future policy making on housing in seismic areas*. Oxford: Oxford Polytechnic Press. Quote from page 10.
7 Rapoport, A., 1969. *House form and culture*. Englewood Cliffs, NJ: Prentice-Hall.
8 Rapoport, A., 1982. *The meaning of the built environment: a nonverbal communication approach*. Beverly Hills: Sage.

11 Space and place after natural disasters and forced displacement

1 Bachelard, G., 1964. *The poetics of space*. New York: Orion Press.
2 Benjamin, D.N., 1995. *The home: words, interpretation, meanings and environments*. Aldershot, UK: Avebury.
3 Boano, C., 2007. *Dynamics of linking reconstruction and development in housing and settlements for forced migrants in post disaster situations*. Thesis (PhD). Oxford: Oxford Brookes University.
4 Brookings-Bern, 2008. *Protecting internally displaced persons: a manual for law and policy makers* [pdf]. Washington: The Brookings Institution. Available at http://www.brookings.edu/~/media/Files/rc/papers/2008/1016_internal_displacement/10_internal_displacement_manual.pdf [Accessed 14 January 2009].
5 Buchanan-Smith, M., and Christopolos, I., 2003. Natural disasters in complex political emergencies. *In DFID seminar hosted by the British Red Cross Society*, 6 November 2003. London: British Red Cross Society.
6 Canter, D.V., 1977.*The psychology of place*. London: Architectural Press.
7 Cardona, O.D., 2003. The need for rethinking the concepts of vulnerability and risks from a holistic perspective: a necessary review and criticism for effective risk management. *In* G. Bankoff, G. Frerks and D. Hilhorst, eds. *Mapping vulnerability: disasters, development and people*. London: Earthscan, 37–51.
8 Connolly, W.E., 1991. Democracy and territories. *Millennium Journal of International Studies*, 20 (3), 163–84.
9 Corsellis, T., and Vitale, A., 2005. *Transitional settlement: displaced populations*. Oxford: Oxfam.
10 Davis, I., 1978. *Shelter after disaster*. Oxford: Oxford Polytechnic Press.
11 Dayaratne, R., 2000. *Attachment to place and the urban rural dichotomy in Sri Lanka in Architexts*. Colombo: Vishvalekha.
12 de Certeau, M., 1984. *The practice of everyday life*. Berkeley: University of California Press.
13 Dovey, K., 1985. Home and homelessness. *In* I. Altman and C. M. Werner, eds. *Home environments*. New York: Plenum Press, 33–64.
14 Duyne Barenstein, J., and Pittet, D., 2007. Post-disaster housing reconstruction: current trends and sustainable alternatives for tsunami-affected communities in coastal Tamil Nadu. *Point Sud*, 8, 5–8.

15 El-Masri, S., and Kellett, P., 2001. Postwar reconstruction: participatory approach to rebuilding the damaged villages of Lebanon: a case study of Al-Burjam. *Habitat International*, 25 (4), 535–57.

16 Etlin, R.A., 1997. Space, stone, and spirit: the meaning of place. *In* S. Golding, ed. *The eight technologies of otherness*. London: Routledge, 306–19.

17 Gupta, A., and Ferguson, J., 1997. Beyond "culture": space, identity and the politics of difference. *In* A. Gupta and J. Ferguson, eds. *Culture, power, place: explorations in critical anthropology*. Durham, NC: Duke University Press, 33–52.

18 Hansen, A., and Oliver-Smith, A., 1982. *Involuntary migration and resettlement: the problems and responses of dislocated peoples*. Boulder: Westview Press.

19 Harmer, A., and Macrae, J., 2004. *Beyond the continuum: the changing role of aid policy in protracted crises. Humanitarian Practice Group report no. 18*. London: Overseas Development Institute.

20 Heidegger, M., 1971. *Poetry, language and thought*. New York: Harper Row.

21 Hunnarshala, 2008. *Community driven housing* [online]. Available at http://hunnar.org/cdh.htm [Accessed 31 July 2008].

22 Hurwits, A., Studdard, K. and Williams, R., 2005. *Housing, land property and conflict management: identifying policy options for rule of law programming* [pdf]. New York: International Peace Academy. Available at http://www.state.gov/documents/organization/98035.pdf [15 January 2008].

23 Hyndman, J., 2004. *House matters: displacement and sanctuary in a transnational context. In Norwegian University of Science and Technology research network conference on internal displacement; house: loss, refuge and belonging*, 16–18 September, Trondheim. Unpublished paper.

24 Jalali, R., 2002. Civil society and state: Turkey after the earthquake. *Disasters: The Journal of Disaster Studies, Policy and Management*, 26 (2), 128.

25 Kälin, W., 2008. *A human rights perspective for major natural disasters* [online]. Washington: The Brookings Institute. Available at http://www.brookings.edu/speeches/2008/0114_disasters_kalin.aspx [Accessed 14 January 2009].

26 Kellett, P., and Moore, J., 2003. Routes to home: homelessness and home-making in contrasting societies. *Habitat International*, 27 (1), 123–41.

27 Kemeny, J., 1992. *Housing and social structure: towards a sociology of residence. School for Advanced Urban Studies working paper, no. 12*. University of Bristol.

28 Lambert, B., and Pougin de la Maisonneuve, C., 2007. *UNHCR's response to the tsunami emergency in Indonesia and Sri Lanka, December 2004 – November 2006: an independent evaluation* (PDES/2007/01). Geneva: United Nations High Commissioner for Refugees.

29 Macrae, J., 1999. *Aiding peace ... and war: UNHCR, returnee reintegration, and the relief development debate*. Geneva: United Nations High Commissioner for Refugees.

30 Markus, T.A., 1993. *Buildings and power: freedom and control in the origin of modern building types*. London: Routledge.

31 Oliver-Smith, A., 1999. What is a disaster? Anthropological perspectives on a persistent question. *In* A. Oliver-Smith and S.M. Hoffman, eds. *The angry earth: disaster in anthropological perspective*. London: Routledge, 18–35.

32 Overseas Development Institute, 2005. *The currency of humanitarian reform. Humanitarian Practice Group briefing note* [pdf], November. London: Overseas Development Institute. Available at http://www.odi.org.uk/hpg/papers/Humanitarian_reform.pdf [Accessed 15 January 2009].

33 Porteous, D., and Smith, S., 2001. *Domicide: the global destruction of home*. Montreal: McGill-Queen's University Press.

34 Quarantelli, E.L., 1995. Patterns of shelter and housing in US disasters. *Disaster Prevention and Management*, 4 (3), 43–53.

35 Rakoff, R., 1977. Ideologies in everyday life: the meaning of the house. *Politics and Society*, 7, 85–104.
36 Rapoport, A., 1995. A critical look at the concept "home." *In* D.N.A Benjamin and D. Stea, eds. *The home: words, interpretations, meanings, and environments*. Aldershot: Avebury, 25–52.
37 Roy, A., 2006. Praxis in the time of empire. *Planning Theory*, 5 (1), 7–29. Quote from page 21.
38 Rypkema, D., 1996. The dependency of place. *Places*, 10 (2), 58–63. Quote from page 58.
39 Saegert, S., 1985. The role of housing and the experience of dwelling. *In* I. Altman and C. Werner, eds. *Home environments. Human behaviour and environments: advances in theory and research, volume 8*. New York: Plenum Press, 287–309.
40 Skotte, H., 2004. Tents in concrete? Housing the internally displaced. In *House: loss, refuge and belonging conference report* [pdf], 16–18 September, Trondheim. Oxford: Forced Migration Review, 3. Available at http://www.fmreview.org/FMRpdfs/Supplements/House.pdf [15 January 2008].
41 Sphere, 2004. *Sphere humanitarian charter and minimum standards in disaster response handbook* [pdf]. Geneva: Sphere Project. Available at http://www.sphereproject.org/component/option,com_docman/task,cat_view/gid,17/Itemid,203/lang,english/ [Accessed 15 January 2009].
42 Stoddard, A., *et al.*, 2007. *Cluster approach evaluation*. London: Overseas Development Institute.
43 Telford, J., and Cosgrave, J., 2007. The international humanitarian system and the 2004 Indian Ocean earthquake and tsunami. *Disasters: The Journal of Disaster Studies, Policy and Management*, 31 (1), 1–28.
44 Tuan, Y.F., 1971. Geography, phenomenology and the study of the human nature. *Canadian Geographer*, 15 (3), 188–92.
45 Tuan, Y.F., 2004. Home. *In* S. Harrison, D. Pile and N. Thrift, eds. *Patterned ground: the entanglements of nature and culture*. London: Reaktion Books, 164–5.
46 Turner, J.F.C., 1972. *Freedom to build: dweller control of the housing process*. New York: Macmillan.
47 United Nations High Commissioner for Refugees – UNHCR, 2005. *Practical guide for the systematic use of standards and indicators in UNHCR Operations*. Geneva: UNHCR.
48 United Nations High Commissioner for Refugees – UNHCR, 2006. *IDP camp coordination and camp management. A framework for UNHCR offices*. Geneva: UNHCR.
49 United Nations Office for the Coordination of Humanitarian Affairs, 2008. *Transitional settlements and reconstruction after natural disasters* [pdf]. Geneva: United Nations. Available at http://www.sheltercentre.org/library/Transitional+settlement+and+reconstruction+after+natural+disasters [Accessed 15 January 2009].
50 USAID Interaction, 2006. Gaining a sense of the sector. *In Participatory workshop on shelter and settlements activities* [pdf], 22 September, Washington. Washington: USAID Interaction, 3. Available at http://www.sheltercentre.org/sites/default/files/USAID_GainingaSenseOfSector.pdf [15 January 2009].
51 Zetter, R.W., 1995. Shelter provision and settlement policies for refugees: a state of the art review. *Studies on emergencies and disaster relief, no. 2* [pdf]. Uppsala: Nordiska Afrikainstitutet. Available at http://www.brookes.ac.uk/schools/planning/dfm/pdf/zetter-shelter.pdf [15 March 2007].
52 Zetter, R.W., 2005. Land, housing and the reconstruction of the built environment. *In* S. Barakat, ed. *After the conflict: reconstruction and development in the aftermath of war*. London: I.B. Taurus.

53 Zetter, R., and Boano, C., 2007. *Gendering space for forcibly displaced women and children: concepts, policies and guidelines. Working paper commissioned by Inter-University Committee on International Migration for United Nations Population Fund*. New York: United Nations Population Fund.
54 Zetter R.W., Hamdi, N. and Ferretti, S., 2001. *From roofs to reintegration – a study to enhance the competencies in housing and resettlement programmes for returnees*. Berne: Swiss Agency for Development and Co-operation.

12 The importance of institutional and community resilience in post-disaster reconstruction

1 Agarwal, B., 1990. Social security and the family in rural India: coping with seasonality and calamity. *Journal of Peasant Studies*, 17 (3), 341–412.
2 Asgary, A., and Willis, K.G., 1997. Households' behaviour in response to earthquake risk: an assessment of alternative theories. *Disasters: The Journal of Disaster Studies, Policy and Management*, 21 (4), 354–65.
3 Bosher, L.S., 2007. *Social and institutional elements of disaster vulnerability: the case of South India*. Bethesda, MD: Academica Press.
4 Bosher, L.S., ed., 2008. *Hazards and the built environment: attaining built-in resilience*. London: Taylor & Francis.
5 Bosher, L.S., Penning-Rowsell, E. and Tapsell, S., 2007. Resource accessibility and vulnerability in Andhra Pradesh: caste and non-caste influences. *Development & Change*, 38 (4), 615–40.
6 Boyce, J.K., 2000. Let them eat risk? Wealth, rights and disaster vulnerability. *Disasters: The Journal of Disaster Studies, Policy and Management*, 24 (3), 254–61.
7 Burton, I., Kates, R.W. and White, G., 1993. *The environment as hazard*. 2nd ed. London: Guilford Press.
8 Dainty, A.R.J., and Bosher, L.S., 2008. Afterword: integrating resilience into construction practice. *In* L.S. Bosher, ed. *Hazards and the built environment: attaining built-in resilience*. London: Taylor & Francis, 357–72.
9 Dynes, R., and Quarantelli, E.L., 1977. *Organisational communications and decision-making in crises, series 17* [report]. Columbus: Ohio State University, Disaster Research Centre.
10 Green, R., 2008. Informal settlements and natural hazard vulnerability in rapid growth cities. *In* L.S. Bosher, ed. *Hazards and the built environment: attaining built-in resilience*. London: Taylor & Francis, 218–37.
11 Jigyasu, R., 2002. From Marathwada to Gujarat – emerging challenges in post earthquake rehabilitation for sustainable eco-development in South Asia. *In International conference on post-disaster reconstruction: improving post-disaster reconstruction in developing countries* [pdf], 23–5 April, Montreal. Montreal: i-Rec. Available at http://www.grif.umontreal.ca/pages/papersmenu.html [Accessed 15 January 2009].
12 Jigyasu, R., 2004. Sustainable post-disaster reconstruction through integrated risk management. Learning from post-disaster reconstruction for pre-disaster planning. In *2nd international conference on post-disaster reconstruction: planning for reconstruction*, 22–3 April, Coventry. Coventry University.
13 Jigyasu, R., 2008. Structural adaptation in South Asia: learning lessons from tradition. *In* L.S. Bosher, ed. *Hazards and the built environment: attaining built-in resilience*. London: Taylor & Francis, 74–95.
14 Kaushik, S.K., and Islam, S., 1995. Suitability of sea water for mixing structural concrete exposed to a marine environment. *Cement and Concrete Composites*, 17 (3), 177–85.
15 Lizarralde, G., and Davidson, C. H., 2007. Learning from the poor. *In*

D. Alexander, C.H. Davidson, A. Fox, C. Johnson and G. Lizarralde: eds. *Post-disaster reconstruction: meeting stakeholder interests,* Florence: Firenze University Press, 393–403.

16 Maskrey, A., 1989. *Disaster mitigation: a community based approach*. Oxford: Oxfam.

17 Menoni, S., 2001. Chains of damages and failures in a metropolitan environment: some observations on the Kobe earthquake in 1995. *Journal of Hazardous Materials*, 86 (1–3), 101–19.

18 Neville, A.M., 1995. *Properties of concrete. 4th and final ed.* London: Longman.

19 Parasuramam, S., and Unnikrishnan, P.V., eds., 2000. *India disasters report: towards a policy initiative*. New Delhi: Oxford University Press.

20 Petal, M., *et al.*, 2008. Community-based construction for disaster risk reduction *In* L.S. Bosher, ed. *Hazards and the built environment: attaining built-in resilience*. London: Taylor & Francis, 191–217.

21 Rashid, S.F., 2000. The urban poor in Dhaka City: their struggles and coping strategies during the floods of 1998. *Disasters: The Journal of Disaster Studies, Policy and Management*, 24 (3), 240–53.

22 Reddy, A.V.S., Sharma, V.K. and Chittoor, M., 2000. *Cyclones in Andhra Pradesh: a multidisciplinary study to profile cyclone response in coastal Andhra Pradesh, India*. Hyderabad: Bookline.

23 Twigg, J., 2004. *Disaster risk reduction: mitigation and preparedness in development and emergency programming*. London: Overseas Development Institute.

24 United Nations International Strategy for Disaster Reduction – UN/ISDR, 2004. *Living with risk: a global review of disaster reduction initiatives*. Geneva: UN/ISDR.

25 White, G.F., 1964. *Choice of adjustments to floods. Research paper no. 93*. Chicago: University of Chicago, Department of Geography.

26 Wisner, B., *et al.*, 2004. *At risk: natural hazards, people's vulnerability and disasters*. 2nd ed. London: Routledge.

13 From complexity to strategic planning for sustainable reconstruction

1 Davidson, C.H., 1988. Building team. *In* J.A. Wilkes and R.T. Packard, eds. *Encyclopedia of architecture: design, engineering & construction,* vol. 1. New York: John Wiley & Sons, 509–15.

2 Hall, A.D., 1962. *A methodology for systems engineering*. Princeton, NJ: Van Nostrand.

3 Johnson, C., Lizarralde, G. and Davidson, C.H., 2005. Reconstruction in developing countries – a case for meta-procurement. *In International symposium of CIB Working Commission W92, procurement systems: the impact of cultural differences and systems on construction performance, 8–10 February, Las Vegas*. Tempe, AZ: Arizona State University PBSRG, 87–97.

4 Project Management Institute Standards Committee – PMI, 1996. *A guide to the project management body of knowledge ("pmbok guide")*. Upper Darby, PA: PMI.

5 Roesch da Silva, R., 1980. *La participation de l'usager dans le processus de construction (Participation of the user in the construction process)*. Thesis (PhD). University of Montréal.

6 Winerman, L., 2009. Crisis communication. *Nature*, 457, 376–8.

Editors and contributors

Editors

Gonzalo Lizarralde is a founding member of i-Rec (Information and Research for Reconstruction) and Director of the IF Research Group (grif) at the Université de Montréal (grif is a leader group in the study of processes associated with the development of construction projects). He is Professor of Architecture at Université de Montréal, and has taught at the University of Cape Town, McGill University, and the Pontificia Universidad Javeriana. He holds a PhD from the Université de Montréal and a post-doctorate from the University of Cape Town.

Cassidy Johnson is Lecturer at the Development Planning Unit, University College London, and a founding member of i-Rec. She has a background in urban development and is interested in Interdisciplinary studies concerning cities, vulnerability and disasters. Turkey is the regional focus of her work. She holds a PhD from Université de Montréal, has taught at McGill University and Concordia University and has been a post-doctoral fellow at the Earth Institute at Columbia University.

Colin Davidson is Emeritus Professor of Architecture, Université de Montréal, where, since 1968, he taught and carried out research related to technology transfer, innovation and communication, and organization of the building team. He is a founding member of i-Rec and a member of the International Council for Research and Innovation in Building and Construction (CIB). He holds a Masters degree in architecture from MIT.

Contributors

James Amdal, an architect/urban planner by background, has been actively involved in neighborhood activism in two of New Orleans' most vibrant neighborhoods for over 25 years: the historic Warehouse District and Algiers Point. He currently serves as Director of the University of New Orleans' (UNO) Transportation Center, an applied research unit within the College of Liberal Arts. He also serves as Chairman of the city's CBD

Historic Districts Landmark Commission. In these capacities, Mr Amdal has been directly involved in all phases of post-Katrina planning in New Orleans, with a special emphasis on District 5, a collection of seven distinct neighborhoods near UNO's Lakefront Campus.

Camillo Boano is an architect and currently Lecturer and Director of the MSc Building and Urban Design program of the Development Planning Unit, University College London. He is also Senior Researcher at the World Habitat Research Unit at the Institute for Applied Sustainability of the Built Environment, University of Applied Science of Southern Switzerland in Lugano. His work and research interests are particularly focused on urban development, post-disaster shelter and housing, reconstruction and recovery, architecture and planning in contested spaces, and the transition between emergency and development.

Lee Bosher is Research Fellow in the Department of Civil and Building Engineering at Loughborough University, England. In 2004 he completed his doctorate on the social and institutional aspects of resilience in South India; since then, he has specialized in research related to integrating disaster risk reduction into the design, construction and management of the built environment. His books include *Social and Institutional Elements of Disaster Vulnerability in South India* (Academica Press, 2007) and *Hazards and the Built Environment: attaining built-in resilience* (Taylor & Francis, 2008).

Graeme Bristol, a Canadian architect, has been teaching at King Mongkut's University of Technology Thonburi in Thailand since 1998. He is also the founder and Executive Director of the Centre for Architecture and Human Rights, a Canadian foundation advancing a rights-based approach to development in the practice of architecture, engineering and planning. He holds a Masters degree in architecture from the University of British Columbia and a Masters in human rights law from Queen's University Belfast.

Nese Dikmen has been Assistant Professor of Architecture at Suleyman Demirel University since 2006. Her principal areas of research lie in the fields of reconstruction after disasters, traditional and contemporary construction techniques, and thermal performance of buildings. She is a member of i-Rec and the Turkish Constructional Steelwork Association. She holds a Masters degree in art from Hacettepe University and a PhD in building science in architecture from Middle East Technical University (METU).

Jennifer Duyne Barenstein has a PhD in social anthropology. She is the Head of the World Habitat Research Unit at the Institute for Applied Sustainability of the Built Environment, University of Applied Science of Southern Switzerland. She has over 20 years of professional and research experience in South Asia and has led several interdisciplinary research projects and evaluations on housing and post-disaster recovery and reconstruction in India, Indonesia, Sri Lanka, Bangladesh, Nicaragua, Argentina and the Philippines.

Rohit Jigyasu is a conservation architect and risk-management consultant from India, and he is presently working as Invited Professor at Ritsumeikan University, Kyoto. After undertaking his post-graduate degree in architectural conservation, he obtained a doctoral degree in engineering from the Norwegian University of Science and Technology, Trondheim.

Isabelle Maret is Associate Professor of Urban Planning at the Université de Montréal, where she teaches courses and conducts research on issues related to resiliency and sustainability. She was previously an adjunct professor at the University of New Orleans, where she actively took part in the recovery process post-Katrina. She is still involved with research on resilience and challenges to rebuild viable communities, especially in New Orleans. She is a member of i-Rec and holds a PhD from the Sorbonne University, Paris IV.

Alicia Sliwinski is Assistant Professor in Global Studies at Wilfrid Laurier University in Waterloo, Ontario, Canada. She has a PhD in social anthropology from the Université de Montréal, specializing in the local dynamics of humanitarian aid and post-disaster reconstruction in El Salvador. She has worked as a consultant in international project and program evaluation, and she is a member of i-Rec.

Roger Zetter is Professor of Refugee Studies and has been the Director of the Refugee Studies Centre at the University of Oxford since 2006. He has nearly 30 years of research, publication, teaching and consultancy experience in forced migration, refugee and humanitarian issues. His work focuses on institutional and policy dimensions and on the impacts of humanitarian assistance on refugees and asylum seekers. His research has addressed all stages of the "refugee cycle", from exile to reception and settlement policies, the experience of protracted exile and integration, repatriation and post-conflict reconstruction. Research on shelter and settlement for the forcibly displaced is a dominant theme of his work.

Index

Entries in **bold** denote references to figures and tables.